Mental Health Promotion

Mental Health Promotion

A Lifespan Approach

Edited by Mima Cattan and Sylvia Tilford

 Open University Press

Open University Press
McGraw-Hill Education
McGraw-Hill House
Shoppenhangers Road
Maidenhead
Berkshire
England
SL6 2QL

email: enquiries@openup.co.uk
world wide web: www.openup.co.uk

and Two Penn Plaza, New York, NY 10121-2289, USA

First published 2006

Copyright © Mima Cattan and Sylvia Tilford 2006

A catalogue record of this book is available from the British Library

ISBN-10: 0335 21966 7 (pb)   0335 21967 5 (hb)
ISBN-13: 978 0335 21966 7 (pb)   978 0335 21967 4 (hb)

Library of Congress Cataloging-in-Publication Data
CIP data has been applied for

Typeset by RefineCatch Limited, Bungay, Suffolk
Printed in Poland by OZ Graf S.A.
www.polskabook.pl

The *McGraw·Hill* Companies

Contents

List of figures, tables and boxes

Figures

Tables

Boxes

List of contributors

Mima Cattan is Senior Lecturer in Public Health/Health Promotion at Leeds Metropolitan University. She spent several years as a specialist and senior manager in health promotion where she was involved in a range of local and national health promotion initiatives in relation to mental health promotion and older people. She has a PhD from the University of Newcastle for research into effective health promotion interventions targeting social isolation and loneliness among older people. She currently teaches on postgraduate modules such as professional practice, health promotion and older people, and mental health promotion. Her research interests include accessibility of the social and physical environment and mental health and older people's contributions to transport planning.

Sylvia Tilford is Visiting Professor in Health Promotion at Leeds Metropolitan University. Before working for over 20 years at Leeds Met in postgraduate training for health promotion she worked in school and adult education. She has a special interest in international developments in health promotion. She was also the Director of the Centre for Health Promotion Research at Leeds Met. Her interest in mental health promotion has been longstanding and related activities have included teaching, the review and dissemination of the evidence base for mental promotion and involvement in community health promotion projects. She is a co-author with Keith Tones of a widely used academic textbook, *Health Promotion, Effectiveness, Efficiency and Equity*.

Glenn MacDonald has worked in industry and has taught in secondary schools for several years prior to working as a health promotion specialist. He is currently the Course Director for the undergraduate and postgraduate studies in health development at the University of Central England in Birmingham. He also directs Health Development Projects at UCE which undertakes a range of health development work including research, mental health promotion, consultancy, and the national Health Development Conference. He is the Society of Health Education and Promotion Specialists lead on Education and Training, and mental health promotion. He has presented papers on mental health promotion and other aspects of health development theory and practice to national and European conferences. He is currently completing research into the organizational experiences of health promotion specialists.

Associate Professor **Louise Rowling** has established a national and international reputation for her work on health promoting schools, drug abuse prevention, loss and grief and mental health promotion. She was a chief investigator for the development phase of MindMatters, the National Mental Health Promotion in Schools Project, funded by the Australian government. Louise's publications include *Mental Health Promotion and Young People: Concepts and Practice* (2002) and *Grief and School Communities: Effective*

Support Strategies (2003). She recently contributed to the WHO publication, *Promotion of Mental Health: Concepts, Evidence and Practice* (2005). Louise has been a consultant to the World Health Organisation, working in Asia and the South Pacific and has contributed to the development of materials for the WHO Global School Health Initiative. She is President of INTERCAMHS (International Alliance for Child and Adolescent Mental Health and Schools).

Foreword

There is no doubt about it, my graduate students at the University of Bergen are the greatest source of my inspiration – more so than even the most famous and productive contributors to the health promotion literature. My ideas about various aspects of health promotion are in constant flux precisely because daily discussions with graduate students and collaborative writing with them forces me to keep tilling the ground. The intensity with which my students influence my understanding of health promotion has increased in recent years, as we have placed problem-based learning at the core of our instructional methods at the Research Centre for Health Promotion in Bergen. As a tutor to groups of emerging professionals, struggling with real world health promotion problems, there is plenty of time to listen and reflect, interjecting every now and again a few words of encouragement and advice, while making frequent mental notes of the type, 'I've got to dig into *that* subject just to keep up!'

So, stimulated as I am by my own students, I felt real delight to read in the Preface to this book that Mima Cattan and Sylvia Tilford were stimulated to write it by their interactions with their students. Even better, their discussions with their students were a significant factor in determining the anatomy and physiology of the book – and the result is simply excellent.

It is fashionable nowadays for Forewords to have little to do with the books they introduce, but that fashion will not be followed here. It has always been fashionable for Forewords to claim that the books they front are really needed, and that fashion *will* be adhered to here – not because I wish to be genial, but because it is the plain truth.

In the 1990s quite a few books having to do with mental health promotion were published, and I have what I consider to be some of the best of them on my office shelves. Yet there is easily room for Mima's and Sylvia's new book, because there is no other like it in my collection, and it fills an empty niche that really needs filling. Blane's (1999) review of scientific developments that highlight the need for a lifespan perspective includes these points:

- health in adulthood is affected by health earlier in life;
- childhood social circumstances influence health status through the remainder of life;
- intra-uterine and infant living conditions can programme adult health; and
- these biological and social processes interact in complex ways that can only be appreciated by taking a lifespan perspective.

These understandings have bolstered interest in the field of public health in a life course approach that acknowledges the importance of early life for adult health, that recognizes the importance of programming of health during critical periods of early life, and that emphasizes the risk as accumulating through life (Kuh and Ben-Shlomo

1997). This volume contributes uniquely to the existing knowledge base on health through the lifespan because it addresses mental health, rather than the chronic diseases that epidemiology has tended to focus on, and because it succeeds in the difficult task of weaving together scientific developments from the lifespan perspective with key ideas about mental health, and key ideas about health promotion.

In an edited book, the burden of ensuring quality is shared by the editor(s) and usually quite a few chapter authors. The production of this book is the result of a collaboration involving just four people – Mima, Sylvia, Glenn MacDonald, who is presently at the University of Central Birmingham, and Louise Rowling, an Australian who adds a refreshing international dimension that should enhance the book's appeal beyond the borders of the United Kingdom. In fact, the great majority of the book was written by Mima and Sylvia, who between them have an extraordinary range of experience in mental health promotion practice, teaching and research. It gives substantial comfort, knowing that when so much responsibility is concentrated in so few hands, those hands are strong and capable!

While there are some who quibble about whether 'mental' health promotion should have an identity distinct from health promotion generally, it seems mental health promotion is here to stay, and I for one am happy about that. In too many quarters, the term 'mental health promotion' actually refers to mental illness prevention, and it is past time that we win the term over to 'our' side. This book makes a sound case for mental health promotion across the span of life, and it is practical enough to be both a text and a handbook . . . enjoy!

Maurice B. Mittelmark
University of Bergen
President of the International Union for Health Promotion and Education

References

Blane, D. (1999) The life course, the social gradient, and health, in M. Marmot and R. G. Wilkinson (eds) *Social Determinants of Health*. Oxford: Oxford University Press.

Kuh, D. and Ben-Shlomo, Y. (1997) Introduction: a life course approach to the aetiology of adult chronic disease, in D. Kuh and Y. Ben-Shlomo, (1997) *A Life Course Approach to Chronic Disease Epidemiology*. Oxford: Oxford University Press.

Preface

The idea for *Mental Health Promotion: A Lifespan Approach* came about as a result of a lively discussion with a group of students studying mental health promotion as part of their Masters in public health and health promotion course. In several sessions we had explored the philosophy and theory of mental health and mental health promotion, differing perspectives on mental health and mental health promotion, the evidence base and mental health promotion policy into practice, when one of the students exclaimed: 'Yes, but what I really want to know is how do I relate all this to my own practice. In other words, how can I become a good mental health promoter?' The result was a session where we considered the population groups the students in their professional capacity worked with in relation to what had been covered in the previous sessions. The chart we drew on the white board was entitled 'Life stages and mental health promotion practice', and was adapted from a set of tables on risk and protective factors from the 'old' National electronic Library for Health website (National electronic Library for Health 2003). It became clear that to be able to promote mental health and well-being effectively students needed something they could relate to in their working lives. As most of them worked with specific population groups rather than generically or in settings the lifespan approach appealed to them because they could apply it directly to their practice. Since that session we have refined our mental health promotion module to fit more directly with this approach, which has been a great success with the students. It has occasionally been suggested to us that a 'settings approach' might be more appropriate for addressing mental health promotion. However, we have found that although settings can be useful for providing a 'stage' for activities and interventions the lifespan approach (despite some overlap) provides a cross-cutting framework enabling students to consider the relationship between the wider determinants of mental health and different age groups. This also helps students to identify meaningful priorities when developing mental health promotion activities. As our students come from a very wide range of disciplines and backgrounds it would seem that a lifespan approach isn't just useful for those 'doing mental health promotion', but also for those who want to have a better understanding of how their work fits in with mental health promotion.

Mima Cattan and Sylvia Tilford

Reference

National electronic Library for Health (2003) Mental health promotion: risk and protective factors, *Mental Health*. London: NHS National electronic Library for Health. Available at http://www.nelmh.org (accessed 27 October 2005).

Acknowledgements

First our thanks go to the students at Leeds Metropolitan University whose insight and critical comments led to the idea for this book. Our thanks also go to our colleagues in the Department of Public Health/Health Promotion for their encouragement, support and helpful ideas. In particular we would like to thank Joy Walker and James Woodall for their contributions to Chapters 4 and 6, and Gary Raine for invaluable information support.

Our thanks go to the many projects around the world who responded favourably to requests for information and input, and to Alyson Learmonth for last minute comments on the main chapters.

Finally we would like to thank our partners and families who have supported us throughout the whole writing process, and in particular Richard for helping out with the final proofreading.

List of abbreviations

ACE	Adverse childhood experience
AMHS	Adult Mental Health Services
BGOP	Better Government for Older People
CAMHS	Children and Adolescent Mental Health Services
CBR	Community-based rehabilitation
DfDS	Department for Education and Skills
GBV	Gender based violence
GRR	Generalized resistive resources
HAZ	Health Action Zone
HEA	Health Education Authority
HPS	Health Promoting School
HRBQ	Health Related Behaviour Questionnaire
MOOTS	Moving Out Of The Shadows
NHMRC	National Health and Medical Research Council
NHS	National Health Service
NHSS	National Healthy School Standard
NGO	Non-government organization
NICE	National Institute for Health and Clinical Excellence
NSF	National Service Framework
Ofsted	Office for Standards in Education (England)
PRECEDE-PROCEED	Framework for systematic development and evaluation of health promotion programmes
PSE	Personal and social education
PSHE	Personal, social and health education
QCA	Qualifications and Curriculum Authority
RCT	Randomized controlled trial
SSA	Same-sex attracted
SOC	Sense of coherence
UNISEF	United Nations Children's Fund
WHO	World Health Organization

1 Introduction

Mima Cattan

Mental health promotion is a fairly young discipline. When you explore the literature it becomes obvious that there is a great deal of debate and confusion around what constitutes 'mental health', 'mental well-being', 'mental ill health' and 'mental illness' and the differences between 'mental health promotion', and 'mental ill health/illness prevention'. One of the World Health Organization's (WHO) definitions of mental health is: 'a state of well-being in which the individual realises his or her own abilities, can cope with the normal stresses of life, can work productively and fruitfully, and is able to make a contribution to his or her community' (World Health Organization 2001: 1).

The WHO also makes an attempt to distinguish between health promotion and prevention and suggests that:

> Mental health promotion aims to promote positive mental health by increasing psychological well-being, competence and resilience, and by creating supporting living conditions and environments [while] . . . Mental disorder prevention has as its target the reduction of symptoms and ultimately of mental disorders. It uses mental health promotion strategies as one of the means to achieve these goals. Mental health promotion when aiming to enhance positive mental health in the community may also have the secondary outcome of decreasing the incidence of mental disorders.
>
> (World Health Organization 2004a: 17)

In this book we take a broad view of mental health and mental health promotion because in our opinion there are so many grey, overlapping areas that to try and restrict the definitions would ultimately reduce the value of the text. The purpose of the book is to provide a comprehensive text on mental health promotion practice using a lifespan approach. It is intended to demonstrate how health promotion principles and theory link with mental health promotion, and to provide examples of cross-cutting themes across the lifespan. Our starting point are the principles underpinning health promotion which emphasize, 'holistic approaches to health, respect for diverse cultures and beliefs, promoting positive health as well as preventing ill-health, working at structural not just individual levels, using participatory method' (Secker 1998: 57). However, as will be seen, these principles are far from universal in the practice of mental health promotion. In fact, some might argue that mental health promotion is moulded not by health promoters but by a heterogeneous group of health disciplines ranging from psychologists to psychiatrists. The debate about what is 'mental health' and 'mental well-being' and 'mental health promotion' will undoubtedly continue for some time and the purpose of Chapters 2 and 3 is to demonstrate the breadth of some of that debate. The WHO European Ministerial Conference on Mental Health concluded that:

> Mental health and well-being are fundamental to quality of life, enabling people to experience life as meaningful and to be creative and active citizens. Mental health is an essential component of social cohesion, productivity and peace and stability in the living environment, contributing to social capital and economic development in societies. Public mental health and lifestyles conducive to mental well-being are crucial to achieving this aim. Mental health promotion increases the quality of life and mental well-being of the whole population, including people with mental health problems and their carers. The development and implementation of effective plans to promote mental health will enhance mental well-being for all.
> (WHO European Ministerial Conference on Mental Health 2005: 1)

The conference report goes on to offer a framework for action to achieve the above. The framework aims to ensure that mental health promotion is central to public health policy; raise awareness and tackle the stigma of mental health problems; promote activities that are sensitive to vulnerable stages in life; prevent mental health problems and suicide; establish accessible and acceptable mental health information; and ensure that mental health services are accessible, appropriate and competent (WHO European Ministerial Conference on Mental Health 2005). It illustrates the way mental health promotion is for the most part considered to interact with the prevention of mental ill health and the promotion of well-being among those affected by mental health problems.

This notion sits uncomfortably with some mental health promoters who claim that it medicalizes mental health. Some community mental health workers would argue that mental health promotion is about promoting the well-being of the community and individuals within that community rather than the prevention of mental ill health. Others again, particularly in the health services, have viewed mental health as the absence of mental illness (see, for example, World Health Organisation 2004a; Rankin 2005). Seedhouse (2002), on the other hand, argues that both the distinction between mental health and mental illness and physical and mental are artificial categories and that therefore 'mental health promotion' does not exist. Instead he suggests the development of 'total health promotion' through the use of rational fields, formed by problem-solving behaviour, to create a critical approach and autonomy. This idea goes beyond the (evidenced) concept that mental and physical health are not separate entities but closely linked through a wide range of inter-related factors (World Health Organisation 2004b).

Other debates in mental health promotion include who or what mental health promotion is aimed at, and the factors that impact on mental health. Much of the time mental health promotion is associated with promoting the mental health of individuals rather than that of communities or societies. Expressions such as 'resilience', 'positive sense of well-being', 'sustaining relationship' and 'capacity to cope' (Health Education Authority 1997; Mentality 2003) illustrate an individualistic approach to mental health promotion. Mentality (2003) goes on to state that mental health promotion is concerned with how individuals, families, organizations and communities think and feel. However, it is clear from their description that it is the mental health needs of the individuals within the organizations and communities that are to be addressed rather than the mental well-being of the communities at large. This view is increasingly being challenged, and while it seems to be accepted that mental health is linked to human development through social and economic determinants it may be that in order to achieve a mentally healthy society the promotion of mental health needs to focus on the wider community or environment. If, as has been suggested, there is a strong association between health, mental health and social capital, then mental health promotion could be used to further social capital (World Health Organisation 2004b). Social capital has been said to describe social relationships within societies or communities, and consists of community networks, civic engagement, sense of belonging, norms of cooperation and trust (De Silva et al. 2005). Perhaps there is an association between the French word 'milieu' – which over time, in several languages, has come to mean the whole social, cultural, economic and natural environment and all interactions that occur within these settings – and social capital. It has been said that social capital has the potential to explain the interaction between the environment and social factors. Maybe 'milieu' is the arena where a holistic approach to mental health promotion takes place, thereby enhancing and maintaining social capital.

When considering the factors that impact on mental health it would seem that most current documents agree that there are a large number of personal, physical, behavioural, social, economic, cultural and environmental determinants which contribute to mental health and mental well-being (see, for example, Korkeila et al. 2003; Scottish Executive 2003; Friedli et al. 2004; World Health Organisation 2004b; Commission of the European Communities 2005; WHO European Ministerial Conference on Mental Health 2005), although how these are prioritized may differ. Interestingly, for example, the European Union focuses on micro level determinants by proposing to promote mental health and address mental ill health through preventive action based on the 'functional model of mental health' (Korkeila et al. 2003; Commission of the European Communities 2005). The functional model of mental health suggests that society and culture through precipitating factors (e.g. life events), individual resources and social context provide a framework for mental health. The most likely outcome of adopting this model is to develop action that targets individual mental health behaviour, which is exactly what is being proposed in the European Green Paper (Commission of the European Communities 2005). The WHO attempts to base its recommendations for mental health promotion on the wider determinants of mental health, but again most examples of action tend to be in the micro-sphere of mental health promotion. However, there is an acknowledgement that indirect interventions, such as tackling poverty, transport and housing improvements may have an impact on mental well-being (World Health Organisation 2004b). It would seem that one of the main problems here is the lack of 'evidence' of the effectiveness of interventions targeting the wider determinants in improving or maintaining mental health (National electronic Library for Health 2004). This will be seen quite clearly in the ensuing chapters.

So why is mental health promotion becoming increasingly important now? According to Arnett (2002) the influence of globalization on psychological development in the next decades is going to be substantial. He suggests that identity issues, such as the development of bicultural identities, identity confusion, defining and selecting cultures and emerging adulthood are the consequences of rapid transformation in the social environment. Could this be one of the reasons why mental well-being is also affected? Certainly the impact of societal transformation on community and individual mental health is explored in many academic papers and reports. The evidence is discussed in Chapters 4–7.

If we consider the global transformations taking place that go beyond identity, such as demographic changes, environmental disasters, political and cultural changes, wars and rapid communication, then perhaps we are beginning to see some of the influences on mental health and well-being. This may be the very reason why mental health promotion on a macro-level now and in the future is likely to have a pivotal role. This does not, however, exclude mental health promotion at an individual level. The WHO makes the point that public health policies should encompass multiple prevention interventions to be able to address multiple causal trajectories for populations at risk (World Health Organisation 2004a). And, although we may agree in principle with the notion that mental health promotion needs to 'take a step outside the box' and consider the wider global determinants of mental health, in reality most mental health promoters will either be working in the prevention sphere or in settings where the focus is on the promotion of mental health and well-being of local communities and individuals within those communities.

In reality the distinction between mental health and mental ill health is often blurred. If mental health promotion is about promoting the mental health of mentally well individuals or environments we could almost argue that in the purest form mental health promotion is impossible because a totally mentally healthy individual or 'milieu' does not exist. Is it possible to categorize mental health from, for example, 0–10? Seedhouse (2002) of course argues that it is not, even without including any mental illness classifications. A European health monitoring programme on the other hand claims that it is possible and suggests the establishment of a set of mental health indicators to monitor mental health in Europe (Korkeila et al. 2003). The purpose of such monitoring would be to evaluate the impact of good practice and mental health policies. Another question we might wish to reflect on is, if we accept the impact of the wider social determinants on mental health is it possible or even desirable to equate different mental health promotion interventions with one another? In other words, is mental health in different geographical locations experienced in the same way, do men and women, different ethnic groups or different socio-economic groups experience mental well-being similarly?

When asked, many people will say that one of the main roles of mental health promotion is to combat stigma. But, it is the stigma of mental illness, not the stigma of mental health that is being referred to. The argument often used is that the stigma of mental illness needs to be tackled in order to achieve a mentally well community or society. Does this mean that mental health promotion will tackle the stigma of mental illness but not engage in the prevention of mental ill health? And, consequently, does it follow that mental health (or mental wellness) co-exists with mental illness?

Secker (1998: 64) suggests that the development of a holistic mental health promotion agenda based on health promotion principles might include the following:

- Drawing on health promotion theory to reconceptualize mental health and illness;
- A commitment to exploring and valuing lay understandings of mental health;
- A proactive approach to defining the boundary between prevention and promotion based on needs assessment and evaluation research;
- Alliances with anti-poverty and other organizations aiming to address social and economic inequalities;
- The validation of participatory methods through evaluation research;
- The development of research strategies which are themselves consistent with health promotion principles.

These points are addressed in this book, either through debate and discussion or through examples and evidence. The book is structured in such a way that the first two chapters introduce the reader to the debates around the meanings and perspectives of mental health and mental well-being and the current status of mental health promotion. The reader is also given a brief introduction to the principles and theoretical underpinning of mental health promotion and the focus of national and international policies providing guidance on the practice of mental health promotion. These chapters are intended to provide the grounding for the core of the book in that much of what is debated here is applied in the next chapters.

The following four chapters address mental health promotion using a lifespan approach. We have deliberately used the expression 'lifespan' rather than 'life course' or 'life stage' to indicate the differences between age groups and to illustrate some of the corresponding effective practice for each age group. The expressions 'life course' and 'life stage' are used by other disciplines with different meanings, such as psychological and biological life stages, and could therefore be misleading. The age groups we have chosen could be perceived as arbitrary. However, if we accept that a person's chronological age is not necessarily the same as their functional or health age, we also accept that if we attempt somehow to categorize according to chronological age there will always be differences and overlaps in terms of functional or health age. We could almost devote an entire chapter to the debate of terms such as childhood, adolescence, middle-age, older and so on. Therefore, although we have chosen chronological age groups to set the chapters, we have also described what we see as the main life events in those age groups, accepting that 'entering adulthood' may not necessarily be the same chronological age everywhere. Where ambiguity has occurred we, as editors, have taken a decision where the topic should be discussed based on 'best fit'.

The idea behind the four lifespan chapters is that by having a common thread running through the chapters the reader should be able to access relevant information readily about each age group and also be able to compare similar information across the age groups. Common themes include the determinants of mental health, evidence-based practice and 'good practice', significant policy and the application of health promotion principles and theory. Although these are distinct sections occasionally the evidence is drawn on in other parts of the chapter to illustrate the links between the determinants and current research and practice. Good practice in this context refers to (mostly local) mental health promotion activity, which is often widely accepted and considered to be effective. Such activity has usually either not been evaluated or has been evaluated locally without the rigour of a research study. Our main concern is that the examples of practice reflect the needs of the communities they are intended for, but also that they are do-able for those at the forefront of mental health promotion. In writing this book we recognize that many of the themes covered in these four chapters are cross-cutting rather than specific to one or other age group. This is addressed in two ways: first, the chapters highlight the 'uniquenes' of the theme to each age group, and, second, some themes are dealt with in-depth in one chapter because of the particular significance to that age group even though they may be relevant in all ages. Examples of this include employment and mental health which is dealt with in Chapter 6 and social isolation and loneliness covered in Chapter 7.

The concluding chapter discusses the role and importance of mental health promotion and reflects on the key themes and issues that have been highlighted throughout the book. It also considers neglected areas and how these might be addressed. Finally, the chapter discusses the future of mental health promotion practice in relation to political will and resource implications.

A final important point to make here is that the book is not intended as a comprehensive encyclopaedia of mental health and mental health promotion. Instead we see it as text which might challenge the reader's perspectives on mental health promotion a little, and hopefully also provide the reader with some ideas for acceptable and realistic practice. We have not attempted to provide a full systematic review of research evidence and good practice. Rather, the evidence and examples of practice that are given should provide the reader with a good overview of current applicable knowledge. There are four contributors in this book and consequently four personal perspectives of mental health and mental health promotion. This is not necessarily a bad thing because it highlights the diversity of opinions and approaches in the field. It also gives the reader a sense of the dilemmas in mental health promotion. A recent editorial in the *BMJ* headed, 'Get happy – it's good for you' (Delamothe 2005: 1489–90) suggests that the way to achieve well-being is to have a loving relationship, lots of friends, a fulfilling job and a meaningful and spiritual existence through community involvement. Although we agree in principle, it is also our view that good mental health demands more than simply personal responsibility. The core philosophy of this book emphasizes the wider principles of mental health promotion and provides responding evidence-based and realistic solutions.

References

Arnett, J. J. (2002) The psychology of globalisation, *American Psychologist*, 57(10): 774–83.

Commission of the European Communities (2005) *Improving the Mental Health of the Population: Towards a Strategy on Mental Health for the European Union*. Brussels: European Union.

De Silva, M. J., McKenzie, K., Harpman, T. and Huttly, S. R. A. (2005) Social capital and mental illness: a systematic review, *Journal of Epidemiology and Community Health*, 59: 619–27.

Delamothe, T. (2005) Get happy – its good for you, *British Medical Journal*, 331: 1489–90.

Friedli, L., Maxwell, M., McCollam, A. and Woodhouse, A. (2004) *Evidence into Practice: Evaluating Mental Health Improvement Interventions*. Edinburgh: Scottish Development Centre for Mental Health.

Health Education Authority (1997) *Promoting Mental Health: Older People*, World Mental Health Day Fact Sheet. London: Health Education Authority.

Korkeila, J., Lehtinen, V., Bijl, R. et al. (2003) Establishing a set of mental health indicators for Europe, *Scandinavian Journal of Public Health*, 31: 451–9.

Mentality (2003) *Mental Health Promotion: Current Debates*. Available at: http://www.mentality.org.uk/services/promotion (accessed 8 January 2006).

National electronic Library for Health (2004) Mental health promotion: know-how that works, *Specialist Library, Mental Health*. Available at: http://rms.nelh.nhs.uk/mental-Health/default (accessed 8 January 2006).

Rankin, J. (2005) *Mental Health in the Mainstream*. London: Institute for Public Policy Research.

Scottish Executive (2003) *National Programme for Improving Mental Health and Well-Being*. Edinburgh: Scottish Executive.

Secker, J. (1998) Current conceptualizations of mental health and mental health promotion, *Health Education Research*, 13(1): 57–66.

Seedhouse, D. (2002) *Total Health Promotion: Mental Health, Rational Fields and the Quest for Autonomy*. Chichester: John Wiley & Sons.

WHO European Ministerial Conference on Mental Health (2005) *Mental Health Action Plan for Europe: Facing the Challenges, Building Solutions*. Helsinki: World Health Organisation.

World Health Organisation (2001) *Strengthening Mental Health Promotion*. Helsinki: World Health Organisation. Available at: http://www,who.int/inf-fs/en/fact220.html (accessed 15 February 2002).

World Health Organisation (2004a) *Prevention of Mental Disorders*. Geneva: WHO.

World Health Organisation (2004b) *Promoting Mental Health: Concepts – Emerging Evidence*. Geneva: WHO in collaboration with the Victorian Health Promotion Foundation (VicHealth) and the University of Melbourne.

2   What is mental health?

Glenn MacDonald

Editors' foreword

The question, 'What is mental health?' has been debated across disciplines, among politicians and by those who have experienced 'mental ill health'. In order to understand mental health promotion, in what way it is effective and how we might apply it in our practice we need to understand first the different perspectives of mental health and mental well-being. This chapter considers the range of approaches to mental health, the distinctions and similarities between mental health, mental well-being and mental illness and the ongoing philosophical debate regarding mental health. The author does not attempt to provide a definitive answer to, 'What is mental health?' but offers a challenging and perhaps slightly controversial perspective on the debates. The chapter starts with a discussion about terminology and goes on to consider this in a cultural context. Theoretical concepts are explored next and the chapter concludes with a discussion about the measurement of mental health. The chapter provides a challenging starting point for Chapter 3 on mental health promotion.

Introduction

There is no succinct and universally agreed answer to this question. Some people feel that there should be a clear and unequivocal answer and have developed strategies for improving mental health based on this assumption. Others argue against what they see as a simplistic and **reductionist**[1] view and claim that mental health is a complex and relative issue that cannot be easily defined or treated in the same objective fashion as, say, physical ailments and disorders.

The aim of this chapter is to help develop an understanding of mental health and to sort through some of the claims and arguments that have been made. In doing so, we need to remember that arguments to do with mental health and illness – what they are, how they are improved and how they are damaged – are not trivial, academic or abstract, but central to people's everyday lives.

An important starting point is to acknowledge the strength and depth of emotion involved. Many writers report the all-pervading effects on an individual's personal and social life when mental health falls short of what is needed to cope (for example,

Lazarus 1966; Rowe 1983). On the other hand, Hay argues, 'When we create peace and harmony and balance in our minds, we will find it in our lives' (Hay 1988: 7). And Field writes about being enchanted by life, open and trusting, at the centre of your own universe. You feel powerful and creative and you are full of self-esteem (Field 1993).

Dealing with mental health problems has never been without criticism and controversy. Many aspects of the medical treatment of mental illness are claimed to be dehumanizing and exploitative (Ingleby 1981). Basaglia (1981) and Laing (1964) have criticized the role of the medical professions in the 'treatment' of mental health problems. Albee argues that 'chemical or organic treatment is a reactionary form of symptomatic relief that is part of a long history of oppression and failure' (Albee 1982: 1043). Many psychiatrists hold to a mechanistic or organic view of mental health problem as something to be tackled at an individual level, assuming there to be something wrong with the way the 'patient'[2] is functioning physiologically. On the other hand, Szasz (1979) has argued, 'the criteria for mental illness are most usually some deviation from social, ethical or legal norms and not physical or bodily characteristics' (in Graham 1986: 45). And as Schofield (1964) put it, 'The psychiatrist has expanded the domain of mental illness to include all degrees and kinds of psychological distress, failing to appreciate that the human suffers pain not because he is sick but because he is human' (in Graham 1986: 46).

These criticisms of the medical approach underline the contentious nature of mental health and mental illness. This is not surprising given that in the health promotion world, the nature of 'health' is never unquestionable (Seedhouse 1997, 2001).

In the UK, the question, 'What is mental health?' has been addressed in recent years by regional groups, national conferences and at local level following the impetus given by the inclusion of mental illness as a key area in *The Health of the Nation* (DoH 1993). This trend has continued with the inclusion of mental health as one of the four main target areas in the *Saving Lives: Our Healthier Nation* White Paper (DoH 1999a) and the *Mental Health National Service Framework* (DoH 1999b). Within psychology, however, there is a longer tradition of dealing with this question (Jahoda 1958; Secker 1998).

Mental 'health', mental 'well-being' and mental 'illness'

Many people are used to hearing 'mental health' as a euphemism for 'mental illness'. A real problem in talking about mental health is that very often we are led into a way of thinking based on ideas and assumptions about mental illness – issues like depression, suicide, paranoia, schizophrenia come to the fore.

On the other hand, it can be argued that mental health has very little if anything to do with mental illness. But the problem is that for so long the 'mental health as mental illness' euphemism has been a stable part of our ordinary language and the illusion sticks. So it becomes very hard to think of mental health as anything other than something affected by the values, myths and fears that often surrounds mental illness.

In this chapter it will be argued that it is possible and desirable to agree to a characterization of mental health without resorting to 'mental illness' discourses. But it may not be helpful to fudge the issue by introducing new terms like 'mental well-being' or 'emotional intelligence', as these may only tell part of the story. And in any case, many people feel quite angry about the hijacking of the term 'mental health' by what they see as the power of the mental illness field. I want to reclaim a more positive, humanistic and celebratory meaning of the term 'mental health'.

However, this cannot be achieved unless our thinking about mental illness is very clear, and how thinking about mental *health* can be different. One very common attempt to make this distinction is to imagine a continuum with mental health at the one end and mental illness at the other (Trent 1993):

mental health ⸻⸻⸻⸻⸻⸻⸻⸻⸻ mental illness

Or to claim that mental health is simply the absence of mental illness (Cox 1992):

mental health = ~~mental illness~~

Both these represent what is known as the pathogenic view of mental health. For many health professionals and people with mental health problems, this is the reality of mental health – the idea that we are healthy until something happens or something goes wrong and we become 'mentally ill'. Some people see mental illness as something to be frightened of, to be embarrassed about, and to fear. Some who have mental health problems will go to some length to deny or avoid being labelled as 'mentally ill' because of this fear, because of the stigma and **victim blaming**,[3] because of what it might lead to in terms of their job, their relationships and their own sense of worth. Others are accepting of the label and are even glad to have it – they feel they are being taken seriously, they feel their problems have been identified and acknowledged. Both of these are understandable and valid views and it is not appropriate to be judgemental about people who embrace the term or those who deny it applies to them.

However, it is important to consider some of the problems that arise with the concept of mental illness, especially in relation to an understanding of mental health. One problem with the pathogenic view is that the starting point for recognition and intervention is the opinion of those who have the knowledge and influence to decide what is mental health and who is mentally ill. The argument against this view can be summarized by a long-standing health promotion principle of needing to 'start where people are at' – people who may not share this 'medicalization' of their problems. As Ingleby (1981) observes, the norms of mental 'health' and 'illness' are essentially matters of cultural judgement, although **positivism** misrepresents them as matters of empirical fact.

Another point is that life can be profoundly shaken by traumatic events and unresolved chronic problems, and these can assault our very foundation and raise broad questions about one's life such as: 'Does my suffering have a purpose and meaning?' or 'Am I responsible for my suffering?' (Van Egeren 2000). So maybe we need to do more for people than fix their mental illness.

Other arguments are that the pathogenic model frequently leads to the disempowering of the 'patient', and that it creates a dependency for those who are categorized as ill for treatment provided by those doing the categorizing. Also, the main focus of any prevention work is the identification or elimination of a specific pathogen and so resources are concentrated or diverted onto technologies to deal with the pathogen rather than the host or the context in which the host lives her or his life.

Another important problem with the pathogenic view is that the focus is on 'what makes people ill', not 'what makes people healthy', and involves a very narrow and mechanistic model of being human. Antonovsky argues strongly against this: 'It is impermissible to identify or equate a rich, complex human being with a particular pathology, disability or characteristic, or a particular set of risk factors' (Antonovsky 1987: 14).

Perhaps the strongest argument against the pathogenic model is its assumption that a focus on curing or preventing disease in individuals is the most effective way of improving the health of populations. This has been challenged because it avoids or even diverts attention from systemic determinants of health (environmental, social, economic). It does nothing for people 'waiting to be ill' – the idea (returned to later) that given the environmental, economic and social conditions some people live their lives within, it is not a question of, 'Will they get ill?' but, 'When?' It can also be argued that the pathogenic model assumes there will always be an adequate supply of carers to meet the demands of those who need the care. Albee (1992: 6) argues: 'one to one intervention is hopeless . . . it's humane, it's kind but it's hopeless . . . because of the unbridgeable gap between the large numbers in need and the small numbers of helpers'.

So these problems with the pathogenic view make it untenable to define 'mental health' as the absence of 'mental illness'. Maybe the field of 'mental illness' has enough unresolved problems to make it an unacceptable starting point for a useful account of mental health.

Mental health: individuals, culture and society

The search for an answer to, 'What is mental health?' frequently involves well meaning people articulating a meaning for mental health by attempting a definition. Some examples of definitions[4] are:

1   Mental health consists of the ability to live happily, productively, without being a nuisance (Preston 1943).
2   Mental health is the capability of personal growth and development (Chwedoro-wicz 1992).
3   Health of the psyche is a matter of maturity (Winnicott 1988).
4   Mental health means *harmony* between values, interests and attitudes with the scope of action of the individuals and consequently, realistic life planning and purposeful implementation of life concepts (Neumann et al. 1992).
5   Mental health is the capacity to live life to the full in ways that enable us to realize our own natural *potentialities* (Guntrip 1961).
6   Mental health is the emotional resilience which enables us to enjoy life and to survive pain, disappointment and sadness. It is a positive sense of well-being and an underlying belief in our own, and others', dignity and worth (HEA 1996).

While some of these seem to make initial sense, there are several problems with definitions – not least the fact that at least 20 competing definitions have been published – how does anyone decide between them? How does anyone decide about *which* needs, skills, feelings and beliefs are involved in mental health, and hence which ones need promoting? And what is the rationale for this choice? Who of any of us has the right to decide this on behalf of other people? Whatever answers are given to our questions here, the point to remember is that these definitions are arbitrary and relative to the values and assumptions of those doing the defining. And these answers are given on behalf of people whose mental health we are concerned about, using language, norms and assumptions that may not be shared by those people. Secker (1998) argues that this goes against what is one of the basic principles of health promotion, namely a respect for diverse cultures and beliefs. This raises an important point about the ethics of trying to do mental health promotion *to* people, which is returned to in Chapter 3. It also raises the issue of cultural variation in how 'mental health' is understood and experienced, something which is returned to later in the chapter. Secker also argues that these attempts to define mental health are essentially a reductionist venture that contradicts the holistic principles of health promotion.

Another problem with many of the definitions of mental health is that they see mental health as static and stable. This does not accord with how we live our lives: although about balance, mental health also encompasses experiences at the extremes, e.g. being happy and sad, hopeful and despairing; although about stability, mental health is also about the variability which is seen by many (see, for example, Potter and Wetherell 1987; Stainton-Rogers 1991) as being an essential part of social living, e.g. the ability and the right to alter, to change, to 'be in two minds'.

As well as the paternalistic values likely to be wrapped up in attempts to define mental health, a rather less obvious but perhaps equally serious issue concerns the individualization that is also frequently involved (Secker 1998). If we are to judge from the definitions available in the literature, it would seem that mental health consists mainly of skills, attributes or behaviours such as:

- 'the ability to live productively, without being a nuisance;
- the capacity to live life to the full;
- the ability to work, love and cooperate with others;
- adjusting to the world;
- being effective, efficient, and maintaining an even temper and so on.

or capacities, emotions or senses such as:

- being happy;
- being content;
- capable of personal growth and development;
- having emotional resilience to enjoy life and to survive pain;
- having spiritually;
- having a sense of trust, challenge, competency, accomplishment, humour; and so on.

(MacDonald and O'Hara 1998)

What is striking about this analysis is how the emphasis in the definitions has been placed on mental health as a combination of the emotional life of an individual, and his or her actions in the world. The focus is very much on the individual. Nowhere is there any reference to actually being *in* relationships (only being able to have them); or of *having* our own worth validated (only doing it for ourselves); or being *allowed* to grow personally (only being capable of personal growth); or being *treated* as emotionally intelligent (only having an alert emotional intelligence).

In short, there is no acknowledgement or recognition of the *social conditions and processes* that contribute to an individual's mental health, and no acknowledgement of an individual's need for these things. To ignore these needs is to replace a focus on individual pathology with a new focus on individual psychology. The above definitions seem fixated with the features and qualities of individuals rather than the features and qualities of the environments in which we live our lives.

It is worth pointing out that the predominant thinking about 'mental illness' also shares this over-concentration on the individual. UK mainstream mental health services have become much more interested – until fairly recently – in these individual malfunctions, and in creating treatments that allegedly correct them. Recent developments from this norm have focused on the idea of recovery. However, here too it isn't always clear if supporters of recovery are holding tight to a pathogenic theory of mental illness that people are recovering *from*, or whether they have a clear idea what it is that people are trying to recover *to*.

Rather than thinking of mental illness as a clear-cut, objective set of individual factors or conditions, it could be argued that it is more accurate to see it as a set of *descriptions* that have been built up over time through a process known as reification. This is 'the process of taking a complex and amorphous mixture of observed events, experiences, accounts and ideas, conceptually turning them (or having them turned) into a "thing" and then giving that "thing" a name . . . constraining people to see the world in a particular way' (Stainton-Rogers 1991: 9). An important point about this (following Taussig 1980; Young 1980) is that processes like reification do not happen randomly or in a neutral fashion. They are not merely practical solutions to practical problems (such as finding a convenient name for a new phenomenon). While they may seem commonsensical, what they are in fact doing is 'constructing and then promoting a particular version of reality . . . not just "naming names" but, more powerfully (and indeed, in some cases more insidiously and subversively), constraining people to see the world in a particular way' (Stainton-Rogers 1991: 19). It could be argued that reification and defining can be seen as very similar processes albeit conducted at different speeds with different levels of consciousness or intent.

If we accept the view that 'mental illness' is more of an arbitrarily reified concept and less of an organic, objective reality, we begin to see that at least some 'mental illness' is normal human reaction to living in damaging environments, in conditions of stress and exploitation, with minimal coping mechanisms and resources, **self-esteem** or social support. But the damage caused is not the fault of the people living in those circumstances, nor an abnormality, but a normal, understandable response. Wilkinson (1996) talks about a sense of deprivation, anger, bitterness, learned helplessness or aggression that he argues are totally understandable responses to various social, economic and material difficulties that people have to live their lives within. People who have problems dealing with their mental world are probably best understood as victims of circumstance rather than adding to their problems by blaming them for their inabilities to cope. And if society were organized differently, then it might be possible for people to enjoy better mental health than many do at the moment.

Around the world, societies clearly *are* different. And in consequence the overall level of mental health differs from one society to another (Wilkinson 1996, 2005), but also the meaning of 'mental health' alters.

The fact that mental health and mental illness have been characterized by various Western authors in essentially individualistic ways says more about *their* cultural values, norms and academic orientation than it does about the reality of people's mental experiences.[5] In other cultures this emphasis on individualism cannot be assumed to be the norm. In Japanese culture for example, the idea of 'self' is experienced as 'one's share of the shared life space' – a much more interdependent notion of 'self' (Markus and Kitayama 1991).

Another example of this cultural variation is that there are times when 'resilience' is *not* appropriate – times when it is all right *not* to cope. And these times and circumstances are different from culture to culture (the British 'stiff upper lip' is not universal). In other cultures, the point at which resilience and coping become inappropriate will vary. Another variation is whether things like 'resilience' – or even mental health in general – is seen and experienced as a personal, social, religious or spiritual issue.

Ideas about mental health and mental illness are, according to Haque (2005: 184) 'addressed minimally in Eastern cultures'. He observes that there continue to be apprehensions, myths and taboos about mental illness in the East, and in this respect, there are similarities with how it is viewed in the West. That said there are interesting and important Eastern perspectives that need to be addressed – both in this chapter and by mental health and mental health promotion services.

To a large extent, this variation of ideas and experience of mental health and mental illness derives from the various religions around the world. The general belief within Islam is that mental disorders are an outcome of abandoning or neglecting of Islamic values. Similarly, within Christianity, true mental health is not possible without the right relationship with God. In Islam, the idea of balance is important – the balance between the body's need for physical pleasure and spiritual adherence. The belief is that movement away from God causes imbalance resulting in mental malady, whereas purification of thought and deed leads a person closer to God and keeps them mentally healthy. In the Qur'an, the state of mental health or psychological well-being is referred to as *inshirah al sadr* or *taqwa*, and other references are made to psychological imbalance (*dhaiq al sadr*); psychological stress (*dhaiq nafsi*); a stressed life (*hayatan dhaniqah*) (Haque 2005).

Chinese culture identifies health with good emotional state. The circulation of ch'i influences the body's basic function and is in turn affected by the emotions. Anger makes the ch'i rise; joy relaxes it; sorrow dissipates it; fear makes it go down; cold contracts it; heat makes it leak out; fright makes its motions chaotic; exhaustion consumes it; worry congeals it. Balance is again a key idea. In Chinese culture, the individual is responsible for the society rather than the other way around. Society cannot be blamed for one's emotions and their influence on one's ch'i.

In Buddhist philosophy, life is full of sufferings (*dukkha*) for those who crave for this world, but can be ended by a ceasing of desire, which leads to a state of ultimate happiness (*nirvana*). Poor mental health is seen as resulting from negative behaviours done in the past. Many studies show the benefits of Buddhist meditation on mental health. Qualities such as right understanding, right thought, right action, right livelihood and right mindfulness are seen as necessary for good mental health. Meditation also is important.

In Hinduism, health constitutes an appropriate balance among three entities – mind (*sattva*), soul (*atma*) and body (*sharira*). There is no distinction made between physical and mental health. Disease results from an unhealthy mind and unhealthy body even though the soul may be pure. Balance in the body is determined by every word, thought, action, experience, of the person. Diet is important, as is one's relationship with the gods, teachers and the Brahmins.

Cultural belief as well as or combined with religious belief are sometimes significant. In Malaysia, for example, feelings of confusion are thought of and believed to be due to a loss of '*semangat*' or soul substance. Experiences of nervousness, hallucination and delusion are experienced as '*angin*' or the wind present in the stomach. Another physical expression of what in the West we would label as a mental health problem relates to ideas about possession by spirits. For these physical experiences, people may turn to guidance from traditional healers. For example, in Malaya '*Santau*', or black magic, is applied by using traditional ingredients mixed in food or drinks (Haque 2005: 185).

This variety of cultural meaning shows there can be no 'culture free' definition of mental health. Rather than the invariant, objective state envisaged by the science and medicine of the West, we need to acknowledge that the meaning and experience of 'mental health' varies from culture to culture. To attempt to reach a universal, 'objective' definition is an alienating process which of itself demotes the mental health of those whose lives and values will inevitably be excluded or marginalized by the definition, and the act of defining (see also Fernando 1995).

So far it has been argued that mental health needs to be thought of a lot less individualistically and a lot more socially and culturally than is often the case. Similarly, it needs to be thought of a lot less 'objectively' and more relative to the culture, language and experiences of people's lives. Social and cultural norms affect it, social values dictate how it is responded to, social actions illustrate its richness and diversity, social interaction creates and recreates its meaning.

Even though human needs are sometimes alluded to, the predominant overall focus of contemporary literature in the West is on individualistic, psychological constructs, not on the social conditions, structures, contexts and processes in which individuals' experiences are grounded. It can be argued that the consequence of this is to miss the point, to provide patriarchal, normative starting points and to fail to understand or address the very things that will actually make the difference.

Given these arguments, it would seem that we should not be expending all our efforts trying to treat people 'diagnosed' with a (fairly arbitrary) category of mental 'illness', or trying to promote a version of 'mental health' derived from a fairly arbitrary definition. Instead, we should be investing in the people themselves (their behaviours, resources, thoughts, feelings, actions and aspirations) as well as the wide range of social, environmental and cultural factors conditions in which these behaviours, feelings and actions are embedded; are staged against; are influenced by; make sense within; and derive their significance from. This type of approach has been called ecological – that is 'seeing people as developing persons living in a context within an immediate and wider environment' (Dodd and Loeb 1994).

The need for an ecological approach

An abundance of literature points to the shortcomings of attempting to improve the health of populations by interventions aimed at individuals (McKeown 1979). There are, for example, the very real psychological dynamics that often play against the usual behaviour change approaches to promoting health (RUHBC 1989; Conner and Norman 1996). As Albee observes, 'no mass disorder afflicting human kind has ever been eliminated or controlled by attempts at treating the affected individual, or by training large numbers of individual practitioners' (1992: 11). This is because, as Blane et al. (1966: preface) put it, 'There is a growing recognition that the most powerful determinants of health in contemporary populations are to be found in social, economic and cultural circumstances'. And 'health remains highly sensitive to socio-economic circumstances even in the most affluent societies'. This evidence includes *Inequalities in Health* (Townsend and Davidson 1980); *The Health Divide* (Whitehead 1987); the two 'Whitehall' studies (Marmot et al. 1978, 1991; Marmot and Bobak 2000); and the work of Wilkinson (1996, 2005).

Within this less individualistic, more social, ecological account of the determinants of health, it is clear that it is the inequalities brought about through social exclusion, stressful environments, environmental deprivation, and the persistent downgrading of emotional life that count. Another point which has already been made is again relevant here: 'this [individualistic] approach is very limited because it does nothing about those forces in society that cause our problems in the first place and that will continue to provide a fresh supply of at-risk people, forever' (Syme 1996: 26). We know enough about the impact of structural factors on health to be able to predict that for many people, it is only a matter of time.

These points about ecological determinants of health are of particular importance given UK government rhetoric about reducing health inequalities. The growing tide of evidence confirms that health inequalities are not resultant from individual behaviours, but from social and economic contexts (Syme 1996; Wilkinson 2005). Hence, to reduce inequalities in mental health it is necessary to address the structural inequalities that, to a very large extent, determine which of us will be healthy or not.

So far this chapter has dealt with a range of issues and arguments about mental health and its promotion. What we need to do now is examine a number of contemporary theories and models of mental health to see which if any provide a practical way forward in the debate about the promotion of mental health while avoiding the irresolvable difficulties of pathologizing, reification, individualizing, victim-blaming and labelling which we have discussed so far.

Theories of mental health

Resilience theories

There are a number of references to resilience in mental health promotion writing. For example, Joubert and Raeburn (1998) place considerable emphasis on 'resilience' which they see as 'a dynamic and human concept' (p.16) and central to their model of mental health.

In the UK the then Health Education Authority's (HEA) treatment of mental health also had a heavy emphasis on resilience: 'Mental health . . . is the emotional *resilience* which enables us to enjoy life and to survive pain, disappointment and sadness. It is a positive sense of well-being and an underlying belief in our own, and others' dignity and worth' (HEA 1996: 2).

One of the problems with this is that although Joubert and Raeburn emphasize 'supportive environments' (1998: 16) which are needed to enhance and develop individual resilience, they also leave unmentioned the social and ecological factors for which such resilience is often needed. This omission was also made by the HEA and Orley and Birrell Weisen (1998). Although some of life's disappointments and sadness, such as bereavement and loss, are going to happen to everyone, many of life's 'ups and downs' are not inevitable but rather they are socially created, and things could be constructed differently. Many of the 'downs' are the result of social injustices, inequalities and health-demoting policies that need to be challenged and improved – not just accepted – if we are to improve mental health.

Another related point about resilience is that there are some people in the world who have a great deal more resilience than most of us will ever have or need. They would simply not survive without it. For them, it is not a 'requisite capacity' or 'latent resourcefulness' in need of awakening (Joubert and Raeburn 1998: 19). Instead it is something they would rather not have to use quite so routinely. The appropriate argument may be less about 'awakening' and more about social justice. So although Joubert and Raeburn are right to place their faith in 'the human spirit' and the potential this has for things to be done, there is a problem with such a single emphasis. They ignore the **meso** and **macro**-ecological systems and structures which are there in society, which cannot be neutral in their propensity for promoting or demoting health, and which in many cases need addressing.

Antonovsky's sense of coherence theory

As we have seen, the pathogenic view sees health as being the absence of disease and sees treatment, such as pharmaceutical drugs, as an **allopathic system** of opposite forces to correct the sickness. This is reductionist and mechanistic, reducing the problem down to pathogens or risk factors.

A theory that turns the argument around is called salutogenesis. This suggests that we need to look at those who stay well despite being high on risk factors. What is different about them? How do they cope? What helps the person to cope? Why do some people cope better than others do? Salutogenesis sees health as a continuum – 'We are all terminal cases. And we are all, so long as there is a breath of life in us, in some measure healthy' (Antonovsky 1987: 3). Salutogenesis sees treatment as enhancing the coping mechanisms not just to one specific illness but in general, helping people to move towards the healthy end of the health–illness continuum.

A salutogenic theory of health starts from the assumption that the human and living systems are subject to unavoidable entropic processes (the damage and deterioration caused by life and aging), and unavoidable death. In reading the work of Antonovsky (1987: 90), you will find a metaphor of health based on the idea of a river.

> Contemporary Western medicine is likened to a well organized heroic, technologically sophisticated effort to pull drowning people out of a raging river. Devotedly engaged in this task, often quite well rewarded, the establishment members never raise their eyes or minds to inquire upstream, around the bend in the river, about who or what is pushing all these people in.

But Antonovsky questions the accuracy of this metaphor and redefines the river as the 'stream of life'. He argues that 'none walk the shore safely, so the nature of one's river and the things that shape one's ability to swim must all be considered' (1987: 90). Therefore, the object is to study the river and to find out 'what facilitates the capacity to swim well and joyously for some and, for others, makes even staying afloat a constant struggle?' (Antonovsky 1987: 127). Therefore he argues that we are all in the dangerous river of life.

The question that interested Antonovsky was why some of us do so much better in the river of life – why did he or she survive despite being so high on risk factors?

Antonovsky (1987) argued that:

- We need to understand the movement of people towards health.
- This movement to health cannot be explained by simply being low on risk factors.
- It is impermissible to identify or equate a rich, complex human being with a particular pathology, disability or characteristic, or a particular set of risk factors.
- Pathogenic narrowness is simply poor care.

From his research,[6] Antonovsky identified a range of factors that seemed to play a role in helping the people cope and survive. He called these generalized resistive resources (GRRs). These are the properties of a person, (or a collective) which have facilitated successful coping with the inherent stressors of human existence.

What all the GRRs seemed to have in common was that they contributed to or created something he termed a sense of coherence (SOC). He argued that the GRRs he identified in his research all fostered repeated life experiences which helped someone to see the world as *making sense* cognitively, instrumentally or emotionally. Antonovsky began using the term in 1979 but refined it in later years to mean,

> a global orientation that expresses the extent to which one has a pervasive, enduring though dynamic, feeling of confidence that one's internal and external environments are predictable and that there is a high probability that things will work out as well as can reasonably be expected
>
> (1987: xiii)

He argued that this *making sense* was a significant factor in the movement towards health. Someone (or some collective) with a strong SOC will:

- Believe the challenge is understood (*comprehensibility*).
- Believe that the resources to cope are available (*manageability*).
- Wish to and be motivated to cope (*meaningfulness*).

Comprehensibility

A person with a high SOC sees confronting events as making sense in that they will be expected. If events are unexpected they will be ordered or explicable. This is not simply a matter of individual perception or delusion. Some people's lives *are* neither ordered nor explicable due to the social circumstances they live within.

Manageability

A person with a high SOC has the view that 'there was a high probability that things will work out as well as can be reasonably expected' (Antonovsky 1987: 17). People with low SOC see themselves as the ones things always happen to. This outlook is defined by Antonovsky as being linked to the extent to which someone perceives that the resources at their disposal are adequate to meet the demands posed by the life events that are bombarding them. Again this is not mere perception. People's lives simply may not contain adequate resources given the scale of what has to be managed.

Meaningfulness

People with a strong SOC speak of areas of their life that are important to them, that they very much cared about and that made sense to them. People with a weak SOC 'gave little indication that anything in life seemed to matter particularly to them' (Antonovsky 1987: 18). Again, this can clearly have a social origin – people can be forced through a life of serial meaninglessness by the societal conditions in which they live.

This ability to believe that the best possible outcome will occur helps one through bad periods of life. Seeing these difficult events as 'challenges' more than as crushing blows may challenge one's SOC but it will not undermine it completely. Of course there can be mistakes and failures, but the person with a strong SOC learns from these and is not doomed to repeating them. Again, this is not just a matter of individual resources. As well as individual factors, our ability to stay afloat and thrive in the river of life depends on its turbulence, its hidden rocks and the support we get from those around us.

Social capital

Cowley and Billings (1999) have argued that a salutogenic perspective links to qualities such as social capital, capacity building and citizen engagement. These qualities and the salutogenic point of view both seek to maximize the health and quality of life of individuals, families and communities.

Putnam has written most widely on social capital and defines it as the: 'features of social organisation such as networks, norms and social trust that facilitate coordination and collaboration for mutual benefit' (Putnam 1993: 65). It can be thought of as:

- 'A measure of the capacity of the social linkages and their resilience or fragility'
- 'As something iterative and experientially developed'
- 'As requiring levels of trust and competence in social interaction'

(Cox 1997)

An important feature of social capital is that it is a property of groups rather than of individuals (McKenzie et al. 2002). Social capital therefore is a mechanism that links individuals with institutions and organizations through certain types of social and civic networks. It is not just the existence of these networks that count, but their quality and ability to be outward looking (Gillies 2001). People's active participation in these networks builds the social trust which in turn underpins cohesiveness and collaboration. These are seen as two important resources for health and health creation (Brehm and Rahn 1997). Social capital therefore is an idea that emphasizes cooperation, participation and **social inclusion**. However, it ought to be pointed out that the presence of social capital is not always seen to be entirely positive (Cullen and Whiteford 2001). McKenzie et al. (2002) note that societies with high social capital are sometimes intolerant of 'deviant' behaviour and demand obedience to norms.

Whitehead and Finn (2001) note that social capital means different things to different people (as with all constructs in social life). There seems to be a lack of agreement on how the concept should be operationalized in research (McKenzie et al. 2002). Also, Shrader and Anirduh (1999) found that what counts as 'social capital' for men may not count as such for women, as there are differences in the way that men and women utilize social resources. In addition, access and utilization of social capital tends to differ among urban and rural settings (Grant 2000).

Henderson and Harvey (2003) noted that a relationship between social capital and mental health has intrinsic appeal, but they conclude that 'stronger evidence, rather than well-intended enthusiasm, is needed' (Henderson and Harvey 2003: 505). McKenzie et al. (2002) argue that any effects of social capital are likely to be complex, and that the few studies that have been carried out are prone to methodological limitations. The wide ranging review by Whitley and McKenzie (2005) concludes there is a lack of strong evidence supporting the hypothesis that social capital protects mental health. However, Sartorious (2003: 101) has claimed that 'an increase of social capital supports mental health and that the promotion of mental health and its improvement (as well as the successful treatment of mental disorders) contributes to the growth of social capital'.

Seedhouse's Foundation Theory

Seedhouse (1997, 1998) seems to be right about a good many things to do with mental health promotion: right about the shortcomings of replacing 'mental health' with equally unclear terms like 'well-being'; right to flag up that health promotion has limits; right that mental health promotion should not be a separate health promotion activity; and right to acknowledge that practice is necessarily based more on values and 'untestable beliefs' than on evidence (Seedhouse 1998: 8).

His basic idea is that health requires various foundations which include:

1   The basic needs of food, drink, shelter, warmth and purpose in life.
2   Access to the widest possible information about all factors which have an influence
    on a person's life.
3   The skill and confidence to assimilate this information.
4   The recognition that an individual is never totally isolated from other people and
    the external world.

There are however two possible concerns with the Seedhouse approach.[7] First,
there is a point which has already been made by a number of writers on the subject
from Trent (1993) to Tudor (1996) to the HEA (1997): that his focus is too individualistic and the emphasis is on what we need to do for or to the *individual* to promote
mental health. Even in his fourth 'foundation', I don't think he goes far enough to
bring the social into the analysis.

A second, though related, point can be identified when we look at his claim that we
must understand, 'the purpose of health work to be the identification, and if possible
removal of obstacles to worthwhile (or "enhancing") human potentials' (Seedhouse
1998: 8). The problem here is that what counts as 'worthwhile' and 'enhancing' (or
other terms he uses such as 'enabling', *'appropriate* foundations', *'basic* means', *'chosen*
goals', 'optimum' and 'realistic' [my italics]) is open to question yet not clarified. So
I think he ought to acknowledge more forcefully than he does that these things are
socially constructed and culturally determined. He misses out on the opportunity
to underline that it is precisely these *social constructions and cultural determinations* of
mental health that we would do well to focus upon in our efforts to promote mental
health.

MacDonald and O'Hara's Ten Element Map

The starting point for the MacDonald and O'Hara (1998) analysis is an analysis
provided by Albee and Ryan Finn (1993). Although based on research about factors
known to reduce or increase mental illness, they claim that this empirical evidence base
is also an appropriate starting point to consider what might reduce or increase mental
health. Albee and Ryan Finn (1993) summarize their analysis of the research evidence
and provide a 'formula' for the prevention of mental 'illness' as follows:

$$\text{Mental illness} = \frac{\text{Organic factors} + \text{Stress} + \text{Exploitation}}{\text{Coping skills} + \text{Self-esteem} + \text{Social support}}$$

According to this formula, mental 'illness' can be prevented by decreasing the factors or
elements on the top of the equation such as organic factors or exploitation, and by
increasing the factors or elements on the bottom such as self-esteem and social support.

Other theories of mental health have been put forward following this tactic of
identifying elements or factors within mental health. Trent (1993) lists five *senses* of
mental health, namely the senses of trust, challenge, competency, accomplishment
and humour. Similarly, the NHS Health Advisory Service (quoted by the HEA in its
Quality Framework project, 1997) lists four *abilities*. Neither of these includes wider
structural elements. Also, Tudor (1996) lists eight *'elements* of mental health', namely:

coping; tension and stress management; self-concept and identity; self-esteem; self-development; autonomy; change; and social support and movement. However, for things like 'self-development' or 'autonomy' there is always another side to the story, namely the conditions and processes that promote or demote these sorts of individual developments. So these theories fall down because they omit either social influences, demoting influences or both.

Building on the Albee and Ryan Finn (1993) analysis, MacDonald and O'Hara (1998) identify ten elements of mental health, its promotion and its demotion. According to the map, mental health can be promoted by increasing or enhancing the elements above the dotted line, and by decreasing or diminishing the elements below it (see Figure 2.1).

The mapping provides a deconstruction of the abstract term 'mental health' into elements that have a greater lay understanding. The elements themselves can of course be open to interpretation but MacDonald and O'Hara (1998) provide accounts of what meaning they see as attaching to the elements, and also an account of where this meaning comes from. The basic idea is that a qualitative examination of ordinary language (Wittgenstein 1958) will show up features or markers as to how people live their lives and the shared, social meanings that are attached to their actions and discourse.

Within the mapping, MacDonald and O'Hara (1998) identify three ways in which elements or levels should not be looked at in isolation, but in interaction and in interrelatedness with each other. The first of these comes from an acknowledged overlap

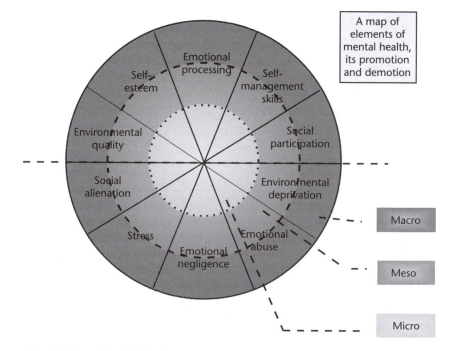

Figure 2.1   MacDonald and O'Hara's (1998) ten element map

between each element. Because of this, they claim there is a need for mental health promotion to act on these interactions between the elements. For example, as well as being a direct attack on self-esteem, emotional abuse will relate to environmental deprivation, emotional negligence, stress or **social exclusion**. Similarly, good self-esteem makes emotional processing much easier to develop, and in its turn, better emotional processing will lead to more effective self-management skills and in turn, more socially participative and supportive behaviour. Hosman and Vetman (1990) lend support for the need to acknowledge and respond to this interaction. They claim that a multi-component approach would increase the effectiveness of mental health promotion programmes.

The second interaction is that experiences in one element can have an effect on mental health much later on in life. Because of this there is a need for mental health promotion to aim for cumulative interaction. In terms of salutogenic theory, Antonovsky (1987) claims that sense of coherence has established and stabilized by the end of their young adulthood, and Bosma and Hosman (1994) may lend support to this notion. Their research suggested that in general, programmes working with young people were more effective than programmes working with adults.

The third aspect of interdependence in the ten element map is the claim that all of the ten elements can occur or relate to three levels: the **micro-**, meso-, and macro-level. The argument is that mental health promotion needs to work at all these levels, building on the interaction between the levels, not just at the micro-, individualistic level. For example, at the individual (micro-) level, social support would include those skills which enable individuals to develop their support systems. At the organizational and institutional (meso-) level, it would mean facilitating support systems and networks by providing opportunities and resources for their formation, development and maintenance. The example of the family as a support system provides us with an example of *incongruity* between the various structures and systems. For as the twentieth century family evolves, and roles within families – particularly those of women – change, problems often arise. These are caused because 'changes at the social (macro-) level of the system lag behind changes at the family level, and, therefore, fail to validate and support the changes (Carter and McGoldrick 1989). Examples of this incongruity include poor policy on childcare provision for women who wish/need to work; inadequate legislation on paternity leave for men wishing or needing to develop a less 'traditional' male role; and so on.

A good example illustrating all three of these interdependencies is work to promote the mental health of young people. First, the cumulative interaction is that work on self-management skills within a school's personal and social education (PSE) curriculum is likely to be more effective if it is done earlier on to help build a sense of coherence during the most opportune time. In terms of interaction between the elements of mental health, PSE work is again likely to be more effective if it involves the development of better emotional processing and self-esteem as well as self-management skills. Clearly this complementarity is going to be jeopardized if incongruity exists, such as good PSE work being undermined by bullying behaviour by staff, parents or other children. And, in addition, the work is likely to be more effective if it addresses interaction between the levels of mental health by including other interpersonal issues in the life of the school and its community (e.g. how teachers, parents and children communicate with each other; approaches to reward and punishment; etc.) rather than just concentrating on micro-level work with individuals.

MacDonald and O'Hara (1998) claim that these three interactions have clear implications for the way that mental health promotion needs to be planned, delivered and evaluated: good mental health promotion will *acknowledge and build* on such interaction, and will integrate various policy developments and interventions into a strategically determined whole. Poor mental health promotion will ignore it.

Weighing up the theories and models

The discussions in the chapter so far have identified some of the strengths and weaknesses of theories and models of mental health. All of these have avoided the reductionism incurred by pathologizing mental health. All bar one have taken on board some aspect of ecological thinking. Not all acknowledge the cultural variability of meanings of terms like 'mental illness' and 'mental health' or show awareness of the reification at work in cultures to socially construct and reconstruct meaning of these terms. Some are theoretical models and others are based on some level of empirical data. These factors are summarized in Table 2.1. There may well be other criteria which could be used to compare these theories and models. In the end, the one you feel happy with will depend on your own circumstances and ontology (see Labonte and Robertson 1996).

I have argued against the **positivist belief** that there is one single 'truth' about mental health. So no one theory or model can claim to be 'true'. Instead I have argued the **social constructionist** case that there are many 'truths' about mental health, and so all of these theories are valid attempts to make sense of mental health. However, taking this relativist position does not mean that all of the theories are *equally* valid – they have strengths and weaknesses mapped out by the criteria given in the table, and perhaps by others such as helping to develop your thinking, or not.

Measuring mental health

The final part of this chapter considers what can or should be done to measure mental health. Clearly, from the arguments already made, those who think mental health is the absence of mental illness will make a different measurement from those who take a salutogenic view. Those who see it in individualistic terms will measure it differently than those who look at mental health in population terms.

Stewart-Brown (2002) argues that many current population surveys tend to measure the prevalence rates of mental illness rather than of mental health. Instruments such as the General Health Questionnaire (Goldberg and Hillier 1979) that do measure positive aspects of mental health tend to skew the results so that most of the population reports near perfect mental health and thus offers little room for improvements.

Stewart-Brown (2002) surveyed six instruments against 17 different aspects of mental health: both positive and negative. Illustrating the earlier point, one of these instruments (the Psychological Well-being scale; see Ryff and Keyes (1995)) concentrates on those elements of mental health identified through a literature review as being considered important by psychotherapists. Another instrument (the General Health

Table 2.1 Comparison of theories relating to mental health promotion

	Albee and Ryan Finn	Resilience theories	Antonovsky's sense of coherence theory	Seedhouse's foundation theory	Trent, HEA, Tudor, etc.	MacDonald and O'Hara
Mental illness or mental health?	Mental illness	Mental health	Mental health	Mental health	Mental health	Mental health
Individualistic or ecological?	Both	Individual	Both	Both	Individual	Both
Comprehensive enough to capture complexity of mental health?	Nearly	No	Possibly	Possibly	No	Yes
Acknowledges the interaction between different elements of mental health?	Possibly	No	Yes	Possibly	No	Yes
Acknowledges the influence of social factors on mental health?	Yes	No	Yes	Yes	No	Yes
Acknowledges both promoting and demoting factors?	Yes	No	Yes	No	No	Yes
Acknowledges the social construction and variability of 'mental illness' and 'mental health'?	No	No	Yes	No	No	Yes
Any empirical support?	Yes	??	Yes	No	No	Yes
Useful as a planning tool?	Yes	No	Possibly	Possibly	Possibly	Yes

Questionnaire; see Goldberg and Hillier (1979)) includes elements such as happiness, optimism and resilience, but excludes what Stewart-Brown (2002: 6) identifies as, 'widely regarded components of positive mental health' such as assertiveness, auton- omy and agency. The instrument that comes out as being the most comprehensive is the Affectometer 2 scale (Kammann and Flett 1983). This instrument uses two sets of questions with Likert-type responses: one about yourself (for example, 'My life is on the right track'; 'I wish I could change some part of my life'), and one about how you feel (for example, 'I feel: satisfied; impatient; confident; loving; helpless'). However, this instrument has no element regarding 'autonomy' which some may regard as too important to omit.

There is a need to see how well the Affectometer scale (developed in New Zealand) transfers to the UK, and how sensitive it is in detecting changes in population mental health. There is also an international need. A report in 2005 from the WHO observed that 'internationally agreed measures of the mental health of populations are often inadequate or unavailable and lack relevance to policy' (WHO 2005: 1). Measuring the mental health (not just the absence of disease) of whole populations would enable truer international comparisons to be made. Stewart-Brown (2002) also argues that population measures of positive mental health are needed because:

- Mental health does not fit into traditional epidemiological distributions, which means that there is no obvious cut off point within a population that could be used as a targeting device.
- Any empirical evidence for the effectiveness of mental health promotion work is only going to be generated if there are ways of measuring the mental health status of populations, and if these can be fairly compared pre and post intervention.

Conclusions

The aim of this chapter has been to help develop an understanding of mental health while acknowledging that there are no succinct or uncontentious answers. But this does not imply that a totally eclectic position is appropriate or tenable. There are several reasons for this.

First, it has been argued that mental health has very little, if anything, to do with mental illness. Reasons include the problems of power, knowledge and influence to decide what is mental health; the concern that treating mental illness forgets the assault on our whole being that this has; the unacceptability of disempowering of the 'patient'; the inappropriate focus on 'what makes people ill' rather than on 'what makes people healthy'; the mistaken belief that preventing disease in individuals is the most effective way of improving the health of populations.

Second, a range of problems with arbitrary definitions of mental health were identified: how does anyone decide between them; again, the problem of power, knowledge, influence and language; the reductionist approach built into the act of defining, which ignores health promotion's commitment to holistic approaches, and which seems to forget the complex messiness within which people actually live their lives.

Third, the individualization that is frequently involved in definitions of mental health and mental illness has been argued against. There is seldom a proper acknowledgement of the *social conditions and processes* that contribute to an individuals' mental health. Rather than the universal, individualized, objective state envisaged by the science and medicine of the West, we need to acknowledge that the meaning and experience of 'mental health' varies from culture to culture.

So the argument put forward is that mental health needs to be thought of a lot less individualistically and a lot more socially and culturally than is often the case. Similarly, it needs to be thought of a lot less 'objectively' and more as being relative to the culture, language and experiences of people's lives. Not to do this will be to miss the point about mental health, to provide patriarchal, normative starting points and to fail to understand or address the very things that will actually make the difference.

All this points to a need for an ecological approach. An abundance of literature points to the shortcomings of attempting to improve the health of populations by interventions aimed at individuals, an approach which does nothing about those forces in society that cause our problems in the first place and that will continue to provide a fresh supply of at-risk people, forever. And to seriously tackle inequalities in mental health it is necessary to address the structural inequalities that, to a very large extent, determine which of us will be healthy or not.

A number of theories of mental health have been discussed in the chapter. The notion of resilience is one common theory of mental health that seems to forget that many of life's 'ups and downs' are not inevitable but socially created. The Salutogenic theory responds to a need to understand the movement of people towards health. I think that salutogenic theory is an extremely powerful way of re-thinking our theories and practices of mental health promotion because it avoids many of the irresolvable difficulties of pathologizing, reification, individualizing, victim-blaming and labelling.

Another theory which emphasizes the social and structural nature of mental health is social capital. Some have claimed that an increase of social capital supports mental health although others claim there is a lack of strong evidence. Perhaps the problem here is that social capital theory again tries to reduce the issue to just one factor.

Some theories identify more than one factor – lists of elements or categories of mental health. In many of these, the focus is again too individualistic. The ten element map of mental health promotion emphasizes the conditions and processes that promote or demote individual developments. These elements and levels should not be looked at in isolation, but in ways that acknowledge their interaction.

From this discussion of theories of mental health, a number of criteria were identified to compare their strengths and weaknesses. The salutogenic theory of Antonovsky and MacDonald and O'Hara's (1998) ten element map are the only ones that I think are comprehensive enough to capture complexity of mental health; to acknowledge the interaction between different elements and levels of mental health promotion; to sufficiently acknowledge the influence of social factors on mental health including demoting factors; and to have any usefulness as a tool for auditing mental health promotion activities or planning them.

Finally the issue of measuring mental health has been discussed. Clearly, how we measure mental health will depend on what meaning we place upon it, or what theory of mental health we apply. It was argued that many current population surveys tend to measure the prevalence rates of mental illness, not mental health. However, we need to find ways of measuring the mental health (not the absence of disease) of whole populations to enable truer international comparisons to be made. And we need such a measure to tell us whether at the population level our mental health promotion is doing any good at all.

Box 2.1   Questions to reflect on regarding the concepts of mental health

- Consider what the different definitions of mental health have in common and what their differences are.
- How might different concepts of mental health influence your practice?
- In what way does culture affect the meaning and interpretation of mental health?
- Consider some of the dilemmas that might arise in mental health promotion as a result of potential tensions between an individualistic and an ecological approach.
- Does the current theory base draw on practice or does practice draw on theory?

Notes

1   This refers to a theory that any complex system can be fully understood in terms of its simple, component parts.

2   Terms that I have put in quote marks – like 'patient', 'illness', etc. – signify that I think there is something not quite right about accepting these terms at face value. I am trying to indicate that we need to be wary of how these terms are being used and the meanings they carry.

3   Crawford (1977) introduces the term to describe the emergence of an ideology which seeks to justify retrenchment from rights and entitlements (to health care and to health protection) and to divert attention from the 'social causation of disease in the commercial and industrial sectors' (Crawford 1977: 663).

4   These are admittedly a small and Western selection of definitions. However, perhaps the act of seeking knowledge by defining things is a particularly Western approach. Ways of thinking about mental health derived from non-Western cultures are dealt with later in the chapter.

5   This is an argument based on a word view called social constructivism. For a good introduction, see Burr 1995.

6   Antonovsky undertook unstructured interviews with 51 people described as having undergone severe trauma : 18: severe disability; 11: the loss of a loved one; 10: difficult economic conditions; 8: concentration camp; 4: immigration from the USSR.

7   See MacDonald, G. (2000) for a fuller analysis of Seedhouse's contribution.

References

Albee, G.W. (1982) Preventing psychopathology and promoting human potential, *American Psychologist*, 37(9): 1043–50.

Albee, G.W. (1992) Keynote speech, in D.R. Trent and C. Reed (eds) *Promotion of Mental Health*, vol.2. Aldershot: Avebury.

Albee, G.W. and Ryan Finn, K.D. (1993) An overview of primary prevention, *Journal of Counselling and Development*, 72(2): 115–23.

Antonovsky, A. (1987) *Unravelling the Mystery of Health*. San Franscisco: Jossey-Boss.

Antonovsky, A. (1996) The Salutogenic model as a theory to guide health promotion, *Health Promotion International*, 11(1): 11–18.

Basaglia, F. (1981) *Breaking the Circuit of Control*, in D. Ingelby (ed.) *Critical Psychiatry*. London: Penguin.

Blane, D., Brunner, E. and Wilkinson, R. (eds) (1966) *Health and Social Organization: Towards a Health Policy for the Twenty-First Century*. London: Routledge.

Bosma, M. and Hosman, C. (1994) *Preventie op waarde geschat*. Nijmegen: Beta boeken.

Brehm, J. and Rahn, W. (1997) Individual level evidence for the causes and consequences of social capital, *American Journal of Political Science*, 41: 999–1023.

Burr, V. (1995) *An Introduction to Social Constructionism*. London: Routledge.

Carter, B. and McGoldrick, M. (1989) *The Changing Family Life Cycle: A Framework for Family Therapy*. Boston: Allyn and Bacon.

Chwedorowicz, M. (1992) Psychic hygiene in mental health promotion, in D.R. Trent (ed.) *Promotion of Mental Health*, vol. 1. Aldershot: Avebury.

Conner, M. and Norman, P. (1996) *Predicting Health Behaviour: Research and Practice with Social Cognition Models*. Buckingham: Open University Press.

Cowley, S. and Billings, J. R. (1999) Resources revisited: salutogenesis from a lay perspective, *Journal of Advanced Nursing*, 29: 994–1004.

Cox, J. (1992) Guest speaker presentation, in D. Trent and C. Reed (eds) *Promoting Mental Health*, vol. 2. Aldershot: Avebury.

Cox, E. (1997) Building social capital, *Health Promotion Matters*, 4: 204.

Crawford, R. (1977) You are dangerous to your health: the ideology and politics of victim blaming, *International Journal of Health Services*, 7(4): 663–80.

Cullen, M. and Whiteford, H. (2001) *The Interrelations of Social Capital with Health and Mental Health*, June. Available at http://www.mentalhealth.gov.au (accessed 21 January 2006).

Dodd, C. and Loeb, D. (1994) Mental health: a way of working, in D.R. Trent and C. Reed (eds) *Promotion of Mental Health*, vol. 4. Aldershot: Ashgate.

DoH (Department of Health) (1991) *The Health of the Nation*. London: HMSO.

DoH (Department of Health) (1993) *Health of the Nation Key Area Handbook on Mental Illness*. London: HMSO.

DoH (Department of Health) (1999) *Saving Lives: Our Healthier Nation*, Green Paper. London: The Stationery Office.

DoH (Department of Health) (1999a) *Saving Lives: Our Healthier Nation*. London: The Stationery Office.

DoH (Department of Health) (1999b) *Mental Health National Service Framework*. London: The Stationery Office.

Fernando, S. (ed.) (1995) *Mental Health in a Multi-ethnic Society: A Multi-Disciplinary Handbook*. London: Routledge.

Field, L. (1993) *Creating Self Esteem*. Shaftesbury: Element Books.

Gillies, P. (2001) Social capital and its contribution to public health, in D. Harrison and E. Ziglio (eds) *Accademia Nazionale di Medicina*, – Italy. Available at www.accmed.net (Supplement No. 4, forum trends in experimental and clinical medicine).

Goldberg, D.P. and Hillier, V.E. (1979) A scaled version of the General Health Questionnaire, *Psychological Medicine*, 9: 189–272.

Graham, H. (1986) *The Human Face of Psychology*. Buckingham: Open University Press.

Grant, E. (2000) Meeting on social capital and health. Workshop report, Washington, DC, 19 May, in M. Cullen and H. Whiteford (eds) (2001) *The Interrelations of Social Capital with Health and Mental Health*. Available at http://www.mentalhealth.gov.au (accessed 21 January 2006).

Guntrip, H. (1961) *Personality Structure and Human Interaction the Developing Synthesis of Psychodynamic Theory*. London: Hogarth.

Haque, A. (2005) Mental health concepts and program development in Malaysia, *Journal of Mental Health*, 14(2): 183–95.

Hay, L. (1988) *You Can Heal Your Life*. London: Eden Grove.

HEA (Health Education Authority) (1996) *Health Promotion and Health Gain in a Primary Care Led NHS*. London: HEA.

HEA (Health Education Authority) (1997) *Quality Framework for Mental Health Promotion*. London: HEA.

Henderson, S. and Harvey, W. (2003) Social capital and mental health, *The Lancet*, 362(9383): 505.

Hosman, C. and Vetman, N. (1990) *Prevention in Mental Health: A Review of the Effectiveness of Health Education and Health Promotion*. Utrecht: Dutch Centre for Health Promotion.

Ingleby, D. (ed.) (1981) *Critical Psychiatry*. London: Penguin.

Jahoda, M. (1958) *Current Concepts of Mental Health*. New York: Basic Books.

Joubert, N. and Raeburn, J. (1998) Mental health promotion: people, power and passion, *International Journal of Mental Health*, Inaugural Issue.

Kammann, R. and Flett, R. (1983) Affectometer 2: a scale to measure current levels of general happiness, *Australian Journal of Psychology*, 35: 256–65.

Labonte, R. and Robertson, A. (1996) Delivering the goods, showing our stuff: the case for a constructivist paradigm for health promotion research and practice, *Health Education Quarterly*, 23(4): 431–47.

Laing, R.D. (1964) *Sanity, Madness and the Family*. London: Penguin.

Lazarus, R.S. (1966) *Psychological Stress and the Coping Process*. New York: McMillan.

MacDonald, G. (2000) Problems, possibilities, people power and passion; what mental health promotion is and what it is not: a response to the Inaugural Issue, *International Journal of Mental Health Promotion*. Brighton: Pavillion.

MacDonald, G. and O'Hara, K. (1998) *Ten Elements of Mental Health: Its Promotion and Demotion. Implications for Practice*. London: Society of Health Education and Promotion Specialists.

McKenzie, K., Whitley, R. and Weich, S. (2002) Social capital and mental health, *The Royal College of Psychiatrists*, 181: 280–3.

McKeown, T. (1979) *The Role of Medicine: Dream, Mirage or Nemesis?* Oxford: Blackwell.

Markus, H. and Kitayama, S. (1991) Culture and the self: implications for cognitions, emotion and motivation, *Psychological Review*, 98: 224–54.

Marmot, M.G. and Bobak, M. (2000) International comparators and poverty and health in Europe, *British Medical Journal*, 321: 124–8.

Marmot, M.G., Rose, G., Shipley, M. and Hamilton, P.J.S. (1978) Employment grade and coronary heart disease in British civil servants, *Journal of Epidemiology and Community Health*, 3: 244–9.

Marmot, M.G., Smith, G.D., Stansfield, S. et al. (1991) Health inequalities among British civil servants: the Whitehall II study, *Lancet* 337: 1387–93.

Neumann, J., Schroeder, H. and Voss, P. (1992) *Mental Health Within the Health Promotion Concept*. Copenhagen: WHO.

Orley, J. and Birrell Weisen, R. (1998) *Mental Health Promotion: What it is and What it is Not. International Journal of Mental Health*, Inaugural Issue: 40–4.

Potter, J. and Wetherell, M. (1987) *Discourse and Social Psychology*. London: Sage.

Preston, G.H. (1943) *The Substance of Mental Health*. New York: Farrar & Rinehart.

Putnam, R.D. (1993) The prosperous community: social capital and public life, *American Prospect*, 13: 35–42.

RUHBC (Research Unit in Health and Behavioural Change), University of Edinburgh (1989) Health-related behavioural change, *Changing the Public Health*. Edinburgh: John Wiley & Sons.

Rowe, D. (1983) *Depression: The Way Out of Your Prison*. London: Routledge & Kegan Paul.

Ryff, C.D. and Keyes, L.M. (1995) The structure of psychological well-being revisited, *Journal of Personality and Social Psychology*, 69(4): 719–27.

Sartorius, N. (2003) Social capital and mental health, *Current Opinion in Psychiatry*, 16 (Supplement 2): S101–S105.

Schofield, W. (1964) *Psychotherapy: The Purchase of Friendship*. Englewood Cliffs, NJ: Prentice Hall.

Secker, J. (1998) Current conceptualizations of mental health and mental health promotion, *Health Education Research*, 13(1): 57–66.

Seedhouse, D. (1997) *Health Promotion: Philosophy, Prejudice and Practice*. Chichester: Wiley.

Seedhouse, D. (1998) Mental health promotion: problems and possibilities. *International Journal of Mental Health Promotion*, Inaugural issue: 4–9.

Seedhouse, D. (2001) *Health: The Foundations of Achievement*, 2nd edn. Chichester: Wiley.

Shrader, E. and Anirduh, K. (1999) *Social Capital Assessment Tool*, prepared for the Conference on Social Capital and Poverty Reduction. The World Bank, Washington, D.C., 22–4 June 1999.

Stainton-Rogers, W. (1991) *Explaining Health and Illness: An Exploration of Diversity*. London: Routledge.

Stewart-Brown, S. (2002) Measuring the parts most measures do not reach: a necessity for evaluation in mental health promotion, *Journal of Mental Health Promotion*, 1(2): 4–8.

Syme, L. (1996) To prevent disease: the need for a new approach, in D. Blane, E. Brunner and R. Wilkinson (eds) (1996) *Health and Social Organisation*. London: Routledge.

Szasz, T.S. (1979) *The Myth of Psychotherapy: Mental Healing as Religion, Rhetoric and Repression*. Oxford: Oxford University Press.

Taussig, M. (1980) Reification and the consciousness of the patient, *Social Science and Medicine*, 14b: 3–13.

Townsend, P. and Davidson, N. (1980) *Inequalities in Health*. London: Penguin.

Trent, D. (1993) The concept of mental health, *Promoting Mental Health: Everyone's Business*. Surrey: NW Surrey Health Authority.

Tudor, K. (1996) *Mental Health Promotion*. London: Routledge.

Van Egeren, L. (2000) Stress and coping and behavioral organization, *Psychosomatic Medicine*, 62: 451–60.

Whitehead, M. (1987) *The Health Divide: Inequalities in Health in the 1980s*. London: Health Education Council.

Whitehead, M. and Finn, D. (2001) Social capital and health: tip-toeing through the minefield of evidence, *The Lancet*, 358.9277: 165.

Whitley, R. and McKenzie, K. (2005) There is a lack of strong evidence supporting the hypothesis that social capital protects mental health, *Harvard Review of Psychiatry*, 13(2): 71–84.

WHO European Ministerial Conference on Mental Health (2005) *Mental Health Action Plan for Europe. Facing the Challenges, Building Solutions*. EUR/04/5047810/7. Helsinki: WHO.

Wilkinson, R. (1996) *Unhealthy Societies: Afflictions of Inequality*. London: Routledge.

Wilkinson, R. (2005) *The Impact of Inequality: How to Make Sick Societies Healthier*. London: The New Press.

Winnicott, D.W. (1988) *Babies and Their Mothers*. London: Free Association Press.

Wittgenstein, L. (1958) *Philosophical Investigations*. Cambridge: Blackwell.

Young, A. (1980) The discourse on stress and the reproduction of conventional knowledge, *Social Science and Medicine*, 14b: 133–46.

3   Mental health promotion

Sylvia Tilford

Editors' foreword

Chapter 2 provided a detailed analysis of the concept of mental health and introduced models that can be drawn on in mental health promotion. This chapter extends the discussion of mental health promotion and raises issues that will be developed further in later chapters. The chapter begins with an outline of the foundations and principles of health promotion prior to consideration of the nature of mental health promotion and its relationship with general health promotion. Selected debates about mental health promotion will then be discussed. The importance of public policy to support health is integral to mental health promotion and relevant policies will be considered. The final section of the chapter discusses the theory base of mental health promotion and appraises the application of theory in a lifespan approach to mental health promotion.

Foundations and principles of health promotion

A report on the health of the Canadian population (Lalonde 1974) and the Alma Ata Conference (WHO 1978) are widely cited as key contributions in setting the early agenda for health promotion. Certainly it is from this time that the term 'health promotion', although not a new term, began to be widely used. The foundations of health promotion were complex and differed between countries and regions of the world but three are widely noted. The first was a change in perceptions of the key determinants of health. In Europe, and in other parts of the world, there was consider-able optimism in the mid-twentieth century about the contribution that modern medicine could make to health and a widespread tendency to equate health with avail-ability and access to health care. As a result other contributions to health were under-recognized. Gradually, however, this situation began to change. Lalonde refocused attention on the multiple determinants of health categorizing them into four interact-ing groups: health behaviours, social factors, biological determinants and health care. In the UK a seminal book by McKeown (1979) entitled, *The Role of Medicine*, examined the decline of infectious diseases in those countries which had moved through the **epidemiological transition** from infectious diseases to chronic diseases as the major causes of illness and death. He documented the relative contributions of different influences to the changes since the nineteenth century. He demonstrated that improvements in water and sanitation, and later in nutrition, were significantly more important than health care interventions in the decline of infectious diseases. McKeown's work, and that of others at the time (McKinlay and McKinlay 1977) helped to remind people of the importance of basic aspects of public health in developing the health of populations. The shift to chronic diseases in higher income countries also highlighted the fact that people's lifestyles were important in the causal pathways of such diseases which were mostly incurable. Prevention, therefore, assumed major importance. In the UK a number of documents (DHSS 1976, 1977) promoted the idea that prevention was everybody's business and focused heavily on individual responsibility for health and the need to make changes in health related behaviours. While the role of social determinants of health was acknowledged in these documents relatively little attention was given to them leading to allegations of 'victim blaming'. At this time there were also developments of what was called 'The New Public Health' moving public health beyond public health medicine to action on the wider social and environmental determinants of population health.

Health education was a second important foundation. While education for health is an integral part of lay cultures health education, as a formalized activity, expanded during the twentieth century. Typically this was as a component of other professional roles but also, in a few countries such as the UK, as a specialist role. It has been customary to make specific allegations about 'traditional' health education, describing it as narrowly focused either on behaviour change or on simple educational goals such as information provision (Rodmell and Watt 1986). From the 1970s there was awareness of these concerns and health education activities broadened. Educational activities for individuals extended to develop empowerment and informed decision-making. Education about the social determinants of health and radical actions to improve it also increased (Freudenberg 1981).

The third foundation was a growing awareness of the wide differences between the health of industrialized and developing countries. In 1977 the World Health Assembly considered these differences and initiated the slogan of Health For All by the Year 2000 and a series of targets were set (WHO 1998a) with targets focused not only on health care services but also on the determinants of public health. Although most low income countries had traditional systems of health care they lacked access to modern medicine. There was a widespread tendency to undervalue the contributions of the former, and overvalue those of the latter, to health care. The provision of primary care through 'barefoot doctors' in China and similar initiatives in other countries had been noted. In 1978 the Alma Ata Conference presented a new philosophy of primary health care. This addressed the provision of first line preventive and treatment services in low income countries within a context of actions directed towards key determinants of health such as water, sanitation and nutrition. Effective primary health care was to have health education as a core activity and be built on community participation. Many countries went on to develop programmes of primary health care as laid out in Alma Ata but it became clear that the focus was often more strongly on the basic health services rather than the development of full primary care (Mull 1990). Although health in developing countries was the main focus of Alma Ata it was intended that its concept of primary care should be relevant to all countries (Kaprio 1979). Those, however, with established primary care medical services paid little attention to the idea (Green 1987).

The rapid development of health promotion thinking and practice began in the early 1980s. A key early influence was a discussion paper in 1984 often referred to as the Copenhagen document (WHO 1984). This presented a socio-ecological model of health and considered the principles of health promotion, areas of action and priorities for the development of policies. Health was seen as a resource for everyday life, with an emphasis on social and personal resources, as well as physical capacities, and viewed positively rather than as the absence of disease. Health promotion was described as: 'the process of enabling people to increase control over, and to improve their health', a statement which was widely adopted. The document outlined five key principles of health promotion:

- It should involve the population as a whole rather than focusing on people at risk for specific diseases.
- It should be directed towards action on the determinants or causes of health and required, therefore, cooperation of sectors beyond health services.
- It should combine diverse, but complementary, methods including communication, education, legislation, fiscal measures, organizational change and community development.
- It should aim at effective and concrete public participation.
- Health promotion was not a medical service but health professionals had an important role in nurturing and enabling it and had a special contribution in education and health advocacy.

Thinking about health promotion was refined further through a series of conferences and associated documents (WHO 1986, 1988, 1991, 1997, 2000, 2003). Possibly because it came early in the development process the Ottawa Charter (WHO 1986) has been the document most widely quoted. It endorsed the above definition for health promotion and set out the prerequisites for health as: peace; shelter; education; food; income; a stable ecosystem; sustainable resources; and social justice. In order to secure health improvements three prerequisites were needed:

- advocacy for health representing the interests of disadvantaged groups and lobbying to influence policy;
- enablement: achieving **equity** in health through reducing differences in health and ensuring equal opportunities and resources to enable all to achieve health potential;
- mediation: social groups, professionals and health personnel had a major responsibility to mediate between differing interests in society for the pursuit of health.

The key action elements of health promotion listed in the Ottawa Charter and consistently used thereafter to categorize practice were:

- Building healthy public policy

- Creating supportive services
- Strengthening community action
- Re-orienting health services
- Developing personal skills

The Ottawa Charter also referred to the importance of the contexts in which health was developed and said that 'health is created and lived by people within the settings of their everyday life: where they learn, work, play and love'. This recognition of context laid the foundations of what came to be called the 'settings approach' to health promotion. Health promotion required that all elements of settings such as schools, workplaces, prisons and hospitals should promote health and the settings should not simply be seen as locations for health education activities. The main themes of the subsequent WHO documents are as shown in Box 3.1.

Box 3.1   WHO health promotion documents

Adelaide 1988

This examined healthy public policy in greater detail. Healthy public policy was characterized by an explicit concern for health and equity in all areas of policy and by accountability for health impact. The main aim of health public policy was to create a supportive environment to enable people to lead healthy lives. Four main areas for health public policy were identified:

- supporting the health of women;
- food and nutrition;
- tobacco and alcohol;
- creating supportive environments.

Sundsvall 1991

Sundsvall was described as the first global conference on health promotion. It examined the creation of supportive environments for health emphasizing two key principles:

- equity as a key priority; and
- the recognition that public action for supportive environments must recognize the interdependence of all living beings.

Four key public health action strategies to secure supportive environments were set out:

- Strengthening advocacy through community action, particularly through groups organized by women.
- Enabling communities and individuals to take control over their health and environment through education and **empowerment**.

- Building alliances for health and supportive environments in order to strengthen the cooperation between health and environmental campaigns and strategies.
- Mediating between conflicting interests in society in order to ensure equitable access to supportive environments for health.

Jakarta 1997

This conference reflected on what had been learned to date about effective health promotion, re-examined the determinants of health and identified directions and strategies for the twenty-first century. It concluded that there was evidence that:

- comprehensive approaches to health development are the most effective;
- specific settings offered practical opportunities for the implementation of comprehensive strategies;
- participation was essential to sustain efforts;
- health learning fostered participation.

It was the first of the international meetings to involve the private sector and to emphasize a need for cooperation between public and private sectors and the creation of new partnerships for health.

Mexico 2000

This meeting focused on bridging the equity gap and emphasized again that: the promotion of health and social development is a central duty and responsibility of governments that all sectors of society share, and 'health promotion must be a fundamental component of public policies and programmes in all countries in the pursuit of equity and health for all'. This would require new funding mechanisms. The organizational base of the infrastrucure should be settings for health. The necessity of health for social and economic development was emphasized and the need for a global health promotion alliance to speed progress with the World Health Organization taking the lead.

Bangkok 2003

The Bangkok Charter identified actions, commitments and pledges required to address the development of health in a globalized world through health promotion and highlighted:

- progress towards a healthier world required strong political action, broad participation and sustained advocacy; and
- the repertoire of proven effective strategies in health promotion which needed to be fully utilized.

A series of *actions* were stated:

- Advocacy for health based on human rights and solidarity.
- Investment in sustainable policies actions and infrastructures to address determinants of health.

- Capacity building for policy development, leadership, health promotion practice, knowledge transfer, and research and **health literacy**.
- Regulation and legislation to ensure high level of protection from harm and enable equal opportunity for health and well-being of all people.
- Partnerships and alliances involving public, private, international organizations, non-government organization (NGOs) and civil society to create sustainable action.

Key commitments were to make the promotion of health:

- central to the global development agenda;
- a core responsibility for all governments;
- a key focus of communities and civil society; and
- a requirement for good corporate practice.

A number of values can be traced through the WHO documents and these are now widely associated with health promotion thinking and practice (Tilford et al. 2003). Main values are:

- equity and the reduction of health inequalities
- empowerment
- participation
- evidence-based practice
- ecological model of health
- health as a human right
- partnership working
- justice.

Over the years many definitions of health promotion have been offered. For example:

> Health promotion is an approach to improving public health that requires broad participation. It may be understood as actions and advocacy to address the full range of potentially modifiable determinants of health, including actions that allow people to adopt and maintain healthy lives and those that create living conditions and environments that support health.
>
> (WHO 1998, in Herrman et al. 2004: 9)

Tones (Tones and Tilford 2001) used a useful formula for health promotion which strips it down to essentials:

health promotion = health education × healthy public policy

This formula serves to remind of the centrality of health education within health promotion where education may be directed towards policy makers or towards individuals and communities.

The 51st World Health Assembly (WHO 1998a) produced its first resolution on health promotion and listed a number of priorities, the first four of which had emerged at the 1997 Jakarta Conference:

* promote social responsibility for health;
* consolidate and expand partnerships for health;
* increase community capacity and empower the individual;
* secure an infrastructure for health promotion;
* strengthen consideration of health requirements and promotion in all policies; and
* adopt an evidence-based approach to health promotion policy and practice using quantitative and qualitative methodologies.

Interestingly the important emphasis of health promotion on the reduction of health inequalities was not explicitly brought out in this list of priorities.

Having set out in some detail the development of health promotion and its constituent principles, with particular reference to the WHO literature, it is important to emphasize that the term is not always conceived in the way outlined so far. For example, in some contexts of health care practice while the use of health promotion as a term has largely replaced health education the activities have continued to focus predominantly on education directed towards individuals with little, if any, recognition of social contextual influences on health and the importance of complementing education with healthy public policy.

Differences in interpretation of the nature of health promotion and its activities have been formalized into a number of 'approaches' or 'models' specifying alternative goals and the processes for achieving them, and underpinned, to some extent, by distinctive sets of values. These approaches were initially developed within health education then taken over within health promotion. Typologies of approaches, differing in sophistication, have been developed. Some simply map the content of practice while others present alternative ideological positions. Naidoo and Wills (2000) list preventive, medical, empowerment and social change approaches. Tones' categorization has changed in a number of ways over the years and most recently he has distinguished preventive, educational and empowerment models (Tones and Tilford 2001; Tones and Green 2004). Approaches are fully described and reviewed in general health promotion texts (Naidoo and Wills 2000; Ewles and Simnett 2001; Tones and Tilford 2001; Tones and Green 2004).

A specific model of health promotion practice that is widely used was developed by Beattie (1979, 1991). It presents a 2 × 2 relationship of processes and levels of action distinguishing between 'top–down' and 'bottom–up' in identifying a range of mental health promotion activities which can be related to different value positions as illustrated in Figure 3.1.

Running through the different typologies are distinctions between levels of action – micro-, meso- or macro-level and the purposes of action at the respective levels. For example, there is a clear distinction at the micro-level between the widely used preventive medical and empowerment models. Work informed by the former is designed to provide information and build knowledge, form and change attitudes, and to develop new or change existing behaviours linked, on the basis of evidence, to health

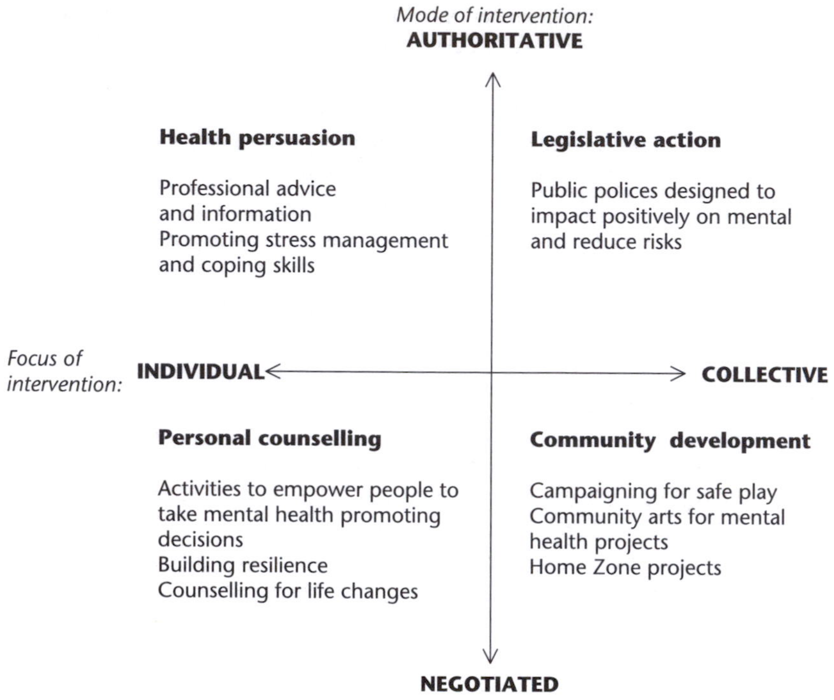

Mode of intervention:
AUTHORITATIVE

Health persuasion

Professional advice
and information
Promoting stress management
and coping skills

Legislative action

Public polices designed to
impact positively on mental
and reduce risks

Focus of   **INDIVIDUAL**← ——————————————→ **COLLECTIVE**
intervention:

Personal counselling

Activities to empower people to
take mental health promoting
decisions
Building resilience
Counselling for life changes

Community development

Campaigning for safe play
Community arts for mental
health projects
Home Zone projects

NEGOTIATED

Figure 3.1   Beattie's model of health promotion applied to mental health

outcomes. This approach is essentially top–down and professionally led and the methods used will include persuasion and others known to achieve attitude and behaviour change. The values underpinning an empowerment approach and the methods used are different. The ultimate goal is to empower individuals, or communities to take health related decisions by developing **critical literacy, self-efficacy**, self-esteem, coping skills, etc. and building activities on the basis of participatory needs assessment. It is this latter approach which fits health promotion as presented in the series of WHO documents. In reality, although individuals may hold a commitment to a specific model it is not always appropriate or possible to work solely within the one model. For example, where individuals cannot, for whatever reasons, take responsibility for their own decisions, or where the health of the public takes precedence over individual rights to choose, a preventive model of practice may be justified. Selection of a model may also be influenced by:

- The characteristics of groups with whom work is being undertaken. In working with young children the question is posed of whether there are age restrictions in using an empowerment model.
- The expressed wishes of individuals or groups to work in accordance with the approaches and goals associated with a specific model.
- The requirement imposed on some health promotion workers to account for the success of practice in terms of outcomes associated with a specific model. For

example, **community development** projects funded by health authorities can be asked to justify themselves in terms of health outcomes associated with the preventive model rather that in terms of outcomes associated with the empowerment model which underpins community development.

When mental health promotion programmes are reviewed in subsequent chapters observations will be made, where the information is available, on the approach to practice adopted.

At this point comment needs to be made on the relationship between health promotion and public health. In comparison with health education which predominantly focused on individual or community level action health promotion has more in common with public health which focuses on the health of populations and the determinants of health. For some writers the differences between the two are limited, or even non existent, and public health and health promotion are as a result used as interchangeable terms. In other cases health promotion is distinguished as the term for the processes used in securing public health. In some countries a very clear distinction is maintained between public health and health promotion. The former is associated with the activities of public health medicine with a major emphasis on prevention and the control of disease and health promotion operates independently. In the UK there is now the concept of the wider public health workforce to which a number of professional groups contribute at various levels. Within this structure some wish to support retention of the term health promotion to signal the particular perspective offered by specialist practice (Society of Health Education and Promotion Specialists (SHEPS) 1998). Most recently this was summarized as consisting of:

- Building the capacity of the wider public health workforce
- Supporting people to develop health literacy and personal health skills
- Involving local people
- Empowering organizations and groups
- Ensuring different settings are used to maximize potential
- Building partnerships and alliances
- Applying theoretical models and principles of health promotion practice
- Translating policy and strategy into effective action.

(DoH/Welsh Assembly 2005)

It is not possible to make a clear distinction between the two activities of health promotion and public health which would be universally acknowledged. Clearly they share many features such as the importance of reducing inequalities in health and a population level focus but may place differing emphases, both within and across countries on the constituent activities.

The nature of mental health promotion and the association with health promotion

The simplest description of mental health promotion would be to describe it as health promotion focused on mental rather than physical health. Adapting the WHO definition used earlier mental health promotion would then be defined as 'the process of enabling people to take control over and to increase their mental health'.

An alternative succinct statement is, 'action to maximize mental health and well-being among populations and individuals' (Commonwealth Department of Health and Aged Care 2000, in Scanlon 2002: 58).

Two definitions bring out its complementary activities operating at differing levels:

> Mental health promotion is an umbrella term that covers a variety of strategies, all aimed at having a positive effect on mental health. The encouragement of individual resources and skills and improvements in the socio-economic environment are among them.
>
> (WHO 2001: 1)
>
> Mental health promotion is the process of enhancing the capacity of individuals and communities to take control over their lives and improve their mental health. It uses strategies that foster supportive environments and individual resilience, while showing respect for equity, social justice, interconnections and personal dignity.
>
> (Canadian Public Health Association 1996)

It is appropriate to question whether separate definitions of mental health promotion are necessary. Since health promotion adopts an holistic definition of health logically its actions are directed towards mental as well as physical health and mental health promotion is an integral part of general health promotion. At the same time if mental health is subsumed in general definitions of health promotion there is some risk that it can be overlooked in the priority often accorded to physical health. There is evidence that this has been the case. Few of the early general WHO health promotion documents, for example, gave special attention to mental health. What is also important to recognize is that mental health promotion has developed, to a certain extent, independent of general health promotion and generated its own thinking and practice. Mental health (illness) professionals have contributed to this development as have psychologists and educationists. Of the many people currently involved in mental health promotion some may be strongly influenced by the thinking in general health promotion while others may be more influenced by the separate mental health promotion tradition.

The relationship between mental health promotion and health promotion has been discussed. For Raeburn (2001), mental health promotion can most fruitfully be seen as a combination of established health promotion values and principles (as embodied especially in the Ottawa Charter) and of the unique features of the domain of mental health, especially those aspects which emphasize living skills, personal control and well-being. Spirituality, he said, our deepest or most essential dimension is especially important for mental health promotion – although he observes that this did not rate a mention in the Ottawa Charter. In the adoption of a wider sociopolitical view of the context for mental health promotion he makes no distinction between health promotion and mental health promotion. It is only at the individual health level where Raeburn suggests that the two differ in their focus of interest – mental health promotion on experienced well-being and coping with life and health promotion interested in physical health and the lifestyle behaviours associated with it.

Moving beyond definitions there have been various attempts to provide models of mental health promotion practice. Chapter 2 used Albee and Ryan Finn's (1993) formula for mental illness – we can turn this around to describe mental health promotion as increasing the factors above the line and reducing those below:

$$\frac{\text{Coping skills} + \text{Self-esteem} + \text{Social support}}{\text{Organic factors} + \text{stress} + \text{exploitation}}$$

As previously noted these particular factors were drawn from a review of literature and identified as key factors. Social support is defined by Albee and Ryan Finn as support at the individual level so we gain no strong impression from the top line of the influence of factors at the macro or even, perhaps, at the meso level which promote mental health.

Macdonald and O'Hara (1998) drew on this model in developing the Ten Element Map, discussed in detail in Chapter 2, dividing factors into those which, if increased, enhance mental health and those which need to be diminished. The model takes into account the differing levels at which mental health is promoted; micro, meso and macro level. Macdonald and O'Hara recognize that the individual elements of the model can be queried although they do make clear their definitions and the source of the meanings given. Barry (2001), on the other hand, has extended Mrazek and Haggerty's (1994) half circle risk reduction model which sets prevention within a spectrum of mental treatment and rehabilitation and produced a whole circle where mental health promotion activities of competence, resilience, supportive environment and empowerment constitute the bottom circle. A succinct categorization of mental health promotion which makes explicit its levels of action is that offered by Mentality (2005). See Box 3.2. A mental health programme, even if its activities focus predominantly on one of these levels, should recognize the others and the interactions between and influences on action at a specific level, as Macdonald emphasized in the previous chapter. Programmes which integrate levels of action, the healthy settings initiatives being a good example, are the kinds of programmes that will be looked for in consideration of evidence in the lifespan chapters.

Box 3.2   How does mental health promotion work?

- *Strengthening individuals*: increasing emotional resilience through interventions designed to promote self-esteem, life and coping skills, such as communicating, negotiating, relationship and parenting skills.
- *Strengthening communities*: this involves increasing social inclusion and participation, improving neighbourhood environments, developing health and social services which support mental health, anti-bullying strategies in schools, workplace health, community safety, childcare and self-help networks.
- *Reducing structural barriers to health*: through initiatives to reduce discrimination and inequalities and to promote access to education, meaningful employment, housing services and support for those who are vulnerable.

Mental health promotion debates

In literature and practice there are issues which are debated. These concern the goals of mental health promotion activity, the levels and focus of actions and how success is to be assessed. We will comment briefly on these issues.

Prevention versus promotion and which is the more effective

Three positions can be identified:

1   mental health promotion focuses solely on the promotion of positive mental health;
2   mental health promotion focuses on the prevention of ill health – at primary (the prevention of new incidence), secondary (early identification of signs of ill health) and tertiary (prevention of relapse and return to health when illness is established); and
3   mental health promotion combines promotion and prevention.

Support for these positions may be based on ideology, beliefs about evidence of effectiveness or context of practice. Those involved in health promotion informed by the values and principles described above are those most likely to advocate a solely promotion approach with this approach seen as relevant to people who are well and equally to people experiencing mental health difficulties. In contrast, a focus on prevention, informed by a medical model, is typified by much of what is labeled as mental health promotion within health care settings. In the promotion approach success is evaluated in positive mental health terms with no reference to mental ill health outcomes. When working in accordance with the prevention model success is measured by primary, secondary or tertiary outcomes. In sum, the promotion approach is successful in so far as it increases positive mental health – the preventive approach in so far as it prevents mental ill health. A number of writers have argued in support of maintaining the conceptual difference between promotion and prevention (Tudor 1996; Raeburn and Rootman 1998). This is possible if a two continuum model of mental health and illness is used (Downie et al. 1990; Tudor 1996). It is more difficult if mental health and illness are placed on a single continuum:

Maximal mental illness	Minimal mental illness
Optimal mental health	Minimal mental health
Mental health	Mental ill health

In practice, however, many who support a promotion approach in principle and prioritize positive health outcomes also recognize, implicitly or explicitly, the fact that in so doing mental illness will also be prevented. Others supporting a prevention approach cite positive health outcomes from their programmes as will be seen in later chapters.

There are a number of influential contributors to mental health promotion who support the third position of combining positive mental health and the prevention of ill health as a basis for activities. Weare (2004), for example, in discussing mental health promotion in schools, while endorsing a positive mental health promotion perspective recognizes the magnitude of the task in achieving mental health and stresses that the full continuum of mental health promotion, early intervention and treatment should be represented. Barry (2001) also proposed an integrative approach which 'locates a central role for strategies promoting mental within the broader spectrum of intervention activities', as described above. The combination of promotion and prevention within a single programme can, of course, be challenged on ideological grounds.

If either of the first two approaches is adopted where mental ill health and mental health exist on separate continuums the success of each is measured within its own terms. Where the combined approach of promotion and prevention is supported it becomes relevant to ask if a promotion approach, in addition to promoting positive mental health is also effective in relation to the prevention of ill health even if this is not its stated purpose. Those concerned to reduce mental ill health may legitimately ask whether resources given to promoting positive health might also make a contribution to their task. If we take the population as a whole, the majority, at any one time, are mentally healthy and it is therefore logical to identify and promote those actions that the evidence suggests sustain and improve this positive situation. The conclusions of many who have reviewed mental health promotion programmes is that there is a growing body of evidence that actions at the individual and group level demonstrate effectiveness in relation to indicators of positive mental health. Barry (2001: 30), in fact concluded that 'competence enhancing programmes carried out in collaboration with families, schools and wider communities have the potential to impact on multiple positive outcomes across social and personal health domains'. As will be seen in the following chapters the evidence base for interventions informed by a preventive approach is often more extensive and easier to obtain than it is for positive mental health promotion. On the basis of a review of preventive and promotive interventions with adolescents meeting stringent criteria for evaluation Patton et al. (2002) concluded that many relevant strategies of mental health promotion have, to date, received little systematic study in instances where improvements in mental health might reasonably have been considered. They considered that while there is evidence that the promotion of protective factors for mental health in the social environment and at individual level is feasible too few indices of positive mental health have included promotion. While a clear ideological distinction can be made between promotion and prevention and some people would wish to adhere to one or the other position combining the two does tend to reflect the reality of much practice. Both researchers and practitioners seem to be quite comfortable combining outcome indicators which appear to reflect both positions. Barry (2001), for example, observed that most competence enhancement programmes which had been reviewed had the dual effect of reducing problems and increasing competences. We will return to this question in the final chapter. Adjudicating between the two positions is not easy even if it is considered relevant to try and do so.

Promoting public health: a population approach versus targeting vulnerable groups

This debate is linked to the previous one. The major writings on health promotion all emphasize the importance of a population approach rather than focusing on individuals or groups defined as vulnerable. At the population level activities can be focused on the promotion of positive mental health, the prevention of ill health or both of these. Raphael combines both in defining a population level approach as attending 'to the mental health status and needs of the whole population, with the view to promoting mental health and preventing the development and onset of, and reducing morbidity associated with mental health problems and disorders across the whole population' (Raphael 2000, in Scanlon 2002: 57). The populations may be all those in specific geographical contexts or subsections such as children, older people and so on.

Two arguments for a focus on vulnerable groups can be made. Where there is a preference for positive mental health promotion across populations it can be recognized that resources delivered in this way can be insufficient to support groups who are facing major challenges to their mental health. Inequalities in health are, therefore, unlikely to be reduced. While a major focus of activity should remain on promoting positive health across the population the vulnerable status of some groups would be recognized and, to achieve equity, additional resources made available. The Sure Start programme discussed in Chapter 4 is a good example of such an approach. Alternatively, and rather more commonly, the priority is to focus simply on vulnerable groups defined as 'at risk' for some aspect of mental ill health and develop appropriate interventions identified as likely to achieve prevention. Informed by a preventive medical model of health it would be argued that such an approach is most likely to help individuals maintain, or return to health. While there is evidence that actions defined as preventive – whether primary, secondary or tertiary – and undertaken with vulnerable groups can be effective the impact of such activities on population level mental health statistics is relatively small.

We can draw a parallel with McKeown's work noted earlier where social and environmental changes at the population level made a more significant impact on decline of infectious illnesses than individually focused preventive measures with defined target groups. In a similar way, we would argue, therefore, that action on such social factors as economic and educational ones has the potential to make greater impact overall on mental health than preventive activities with at risk groups. This is not to be taken as an argument to desist from preventive activities with vulnerable groups but as an indication that in terms of mental health statistics they are likely to make a smaller contribution than population level measures.

To some extent this debate is about the health of individuals versus the health of the collective. The former may be maximized by individually targeted activities but focus on the latter, while having a lesser impact on individuals, generates a greater benefit on population wide statistics. The context of practice will, to a great extent, influence the decisions on level of action. A community health worker working with new mothers in situations of disadvantage will focus primarily on the development of their health and that of their children. However, at the same time, they may campaign as part of a professional group for population level supports for parenting which would reduce, in time, the overall levels of disadvantaged parents and the need, therefore, for individually focused work.

Health of the individual versus the community

Whether the main emphasis of mental health promotion should be on the health of the individual or that of the community can be debated. Within the WHO documents outlined earlier there is strong support for community level approaches and for measuring the success of actions in terms of community rather than individual level indicators. Working at the community level, using participatory approaches is designed to enhance empowerment of the community and the individuals who are part of it. Working with communities, it would be argued, creates greater potential for health creation than working simply with individuals. Where work meets the criteria for being described as community development its activities are geared not only to the immediate health of communities but to enabling those communities to take action to get changes of upstream factors which may improve local determinants of mental health and even impact more widely. For example, a community action to secure a local Home Zone (see Chapter 4) might lead to a city wide decision to create such Zones benefiting the whole population.

To focus on community also fits in better with many cultures which have a communitarian rather than a strong individualist focus. Raeburn (2001), for example, with reference to Maori culture makes a strong case for a community-based approach. Maori ideas place family and community and their relationship to resources and the environment as the core of good mental health. Despite the importance that is given to working with communities in health promotion a considerable proportion of the work does not fully involve communities or fit wholly within a philosophy of empowerment. Communities are often used as locations of activities with participation consisting of little more than compliance in programmes designed by others. While work may be carried out with groups outcomes are measured solely with reference to individuals. Communities addressed will often be more disadvantaged or excluded ones.

The current attention to developing social capital relates to the question of individual versus community as focus for action. Social capital is generally analysed at the community rather than the individual level although it has been debated whether it should be considered solely as a property of groups or also of individuals. According to Da Silva et al. (2005) this continues to be an unresolved issue and researchers have measured social capital ecologically and individually.

The decision about focus for action is also partly related to the ideology held of health promotion and the type of practice. Youth workers, play workers, community workers involved in mental health promotion will prefer community level action – nurses, community health workers, patient educators at the individual level whether on a one to one or a group basis.

The evidence base: is it fit for purpose?

In seeking to promote mental health it is important to ensure that actions achieve the outcomes sought and, of particular importance, do not generate negative effects.

Evidence of success is needed from actions at the three levels at which mental health promotion operates: micro, meso and macro level. At the micro- and meso-level what counts as success depends on whether the intended goals relate to positive mental health or to the prevention of ill health. In the case of the former, either mental health as a whole or one or more defined attributes of it can be measured, although the latter approach is vulnerable to criticisms of reductionism (Secker 1998). In both cases valid measures are required and validity and usability across populations considered. At the macro-level the focus will be on providing evidence related to the development and implementation of policies and related initiatives which address the structural determinants of health.

For some years there has been active debate in health promotion about the kinds of evidence of success that is wanted and also about appropriate approaches to evaluation. In clinical areas the evidence on effective practice relates mainly to individual level outcomes and is drawn from systematic reviews and **meta-analyses** of **randomized controlled trials** (RCTs) and other studies high on what is described as a hierarchy of evidence (see Table 3.1). There are also systematic reviews in health promotion which adopt a similar approach to establishing evidence although there are typically fewer topics with sufficient studies to undertake meta evaluations. Studies included in such reviews tend, on the whole, to be relatively simple programmes, often predomin- antly health education and informed by psychological theory, with individual level outcomes. Typically, therefore they include fewer evaluations of complex health promotion interventions and virtually none of policy actions.

Within health promotion many have argued, with differing degrees of intensity, against prioritizing of evidence derived from experimental studies. A frequently quoted statement from the WHO's European Working Group on Health Promotion Evaluation (WHO 1998b: 5) said 'the use of randomized controlled trials to evaluate health promotion initiatives is in most cases, inappropriate, misleading and unnecessarily expensive'. Since many health promotion interventions cannot realistically be evalu- ated by RCTs a partial impression of success is gained if only evidence from such studies is referred to. Others, while sharing reservations about systematic reviews will accept that experimental or other controlled studies can be ethically undertaken

Table 3.1   The hierarchy of research evidence

Level	Source of research evidence
I	At least one properly designed randomized controlled trial (RCT).
II, I	Well designed controlled trials without randomization. Quasi-experimental studies.
II, ii	Well designed (prospective) cohort studies preferably from more than one centre or research group.
II, iii	Well designed case control studies, preferably from more than one centre or research group.
III	Large differences in comparisons between times and/or locations within/without interventions.
IV	Opinions of respected authorities, based on critical experience, descriptive studies, or reports of expert committees.

Source: NHS Centre for Reviews and Disseminations 1996

for some health promotion interventions, particularly of the health education type and that the evidence obtained can be used to support a preventive approach to practice. At the same time such evidence, it would be argued, should be complemented by further evidence from other types of quantitative and also qualitative studies in order to gain a more complete understanding of the success of mental health promotion.

Despite the reservations about evidence from RCTs and similar studies it remains the case in health promotion that this is often the most easily accessed evidence on activities directed towards individuals. We therefore have a partial picture of effectiveness. Secker noted that the current emphasis of the evidence base in mental health promotion can lead to a self fulfilling prophecy. Since interventions which are psychological 'are evaluated using RCTs these interventions will be singled out as effective with the result that more interventions of this type are undertaken and evaluated and so on' (1998: 64). There have been some changes since this point was made although it remains pertinent. There have been a growing number of evaluations of community-based programmes which have taken a broader approach to evidence, using different models of evaluation, such as realistic evaluation (Pawson and Tilley 1997) and action research approaches and combining quantitative and qualitative data.

If changes which have the potential to promote mental health are to be secured at macro-level evidence appropriate to policy makers is required. There is increasing attention being given to the types of research evidence needed for this and how best to bring it to policy makers' attention (Nutbeam 2001; Rychetnik and Wise 2004). Rychetnik and Wise noted the growing evidence base in health promotion but also asked whether the evidence generated is actually relevant and useful in policy contexts. Evidence is also needed by practitioners to inform decisions about health promotions activities. The types of evidence that will suit their particular needs have to be considered alongside encouraging the actual use of evidence. Nutbeam (2001) has identified a number of challenges to be met in ensuring that both policy development and professional practice are informed by available evidence:

- Improving the quality of evidence that informs policy.
- Finding ways of ensuring that evidence forms part of an inherently fluid political decision-making process.
- Developing skills in the critical appraisal of evidence, and achieving the best fit between available evidence, political priorities and practical actions to achieve desired outcomes.

An important shortcoming of the existing evidence base for mental health promotion is that it is drawn predominantly from a limited number of higher income countries. Herrman et al. (2004) point out that evidence for the effectiveness of mental health promotion is least available in areas that have the maximum need, such as low and middle income countries and also conflict areas, where mental health is especially compromised. The need for a wider source of evidence has been recognized in the role attributed to the WHO of 'generating, reviewing, compiling and updating evidence for mental health promotion especially from low and middle income countries' (2004: 11).

In the following chapters the full spectrum of evidence available will be used in recognition of the various styles, purposes and contexts of mental health promotion practice, with critical comment as and when appropriate.

Policy and mental health

Building healthy public policy is, as discussed earlier, integral to health promotion. Links can be established between all major policy areas and mental health although these are of differing strengths and some are more direct than others. A few policy areas may apply more directly to certain periods of the lifespan but most have relevance across the lifespan. A division can be drawn between policies explicitly labelled as mental health policy and policies which have the potential to impact on the determinants of positive mental health and prevention of mental ill health, whether or not these impacts are made explicit. Where mental health policy is concerned comments have been made in a number of countries about the extent to which it has largely been about mental illness, prevention and treatment rather than the promotion of positive mental health. WHO (2001:1) said that 'national mental health policies should not be solely concerned with mental illness but recognize and address the broader issues affecting the mental health of all sectors of society'. WHO is taking a leading role in making statements about mental health policy. World Health Assembly Resolutions have urged Member States to take actions to promote mental health and prevent mental illness. In 2002 the Assembly asked the Director General to provide information and guidance on suitable strategies towards these ends and Resolution (WHA55.10, in Herrman et al. 2004: 11) called for WHO to:

> 'facilitate effective development of policies and programmes to strengthen and protect mental health'. Its most recent contribution has been a Declaration and Action Plan for Mental Health (WHO 2005).

In most countries the traditional focus of specific mental health policy has been on illness and the responses to it. In the UK, for example, Rogers and Pilgrim (1996) noted this illness focus of mental health policy and stated that to date it had not been influenced by the broader traditions of health promotion. By contrast, they saw that USA had taken a broader focus since the 1960s and suggested three reasons for the differences between the two countries over this period: the radical politics of the 1960s; the community care focus of mental health policy makers; and the nature of psychiatry in the USA which included a strand dedicated to social epidemiology. In a number of countries there is evidence that policies are now broadening and examples will be included in the following chapters.

In addition to looking for specific mental health care policy to include not only mental illness but also primary prevention and, ideally, the promotion of positive mental health, what is also needed is a greater emphasis on public health policy and recognition of the links between its various aspects and mental health. The UK provides an illustrative example of the gradual development of public health policy and attention to mental health. The Government's generation of documents on prevention in the 1970s was noted earlier (DHSS 1976, 1977). While making brief mention of the range of determinants of health the documents emphasized strongly the role of individual behaviour and lifestyle. What has been described as the first public health document since the setting up of the NHS in 1948, *The Health of the Nation* appeared in 1992 (DoH 1992). Although the stated strategy was on improving and maintaining health the targets set were ill health outcomes and the socio-economic determinants of health were neglected. Mental health was one of five key health areas specified but the focus was solely on mental illness. This document was seen as too closely linked with the Department of Health and insufficiently shared by other policy areas which also had important contributions to make to public health. As a result the healthy alliances which were called for in the document were slow to develop (Hunter 2003). Notwithstanding its shortcomings the Health of the Nation provided a basis for the developments which followed. With a change of Government in 1997 a Minister for Public Health was appointed and an explicit commitment made to the creation of a more socially equitable and cohesive society. The responsibility for achieving this was clearly stated to cut across policy areas. A Social Exclusion Unit was set up to focus on narrowing the health gap. Several important initiatives were set up in disadvantaged areas, for example Sure Start, a programme for pre-school years which will be discussed in the next chapter and Health Action Zones discussed in Chapter 6. An Independent Inquiry on Inequalities in Health examined health inequalities and identified effective actions (Acheson 1998). Of its 39 recommendations only three were directly related to the NHS reinforcing the fact that addressing inequalities involved actions across departments. A Consultative Document 'Our Healthier Nation' (DoH 1998) emphasized the need to address inequalities and social exclusion through cross government action but was criticized for maintaining a focus on disease outcomes. Mental health was included but the only target was a reduction of the suicide rate. Comments in response to the consultation requested that a target of 'increasing wellbeing' be added and relevant measures identified. Efforts to address inequalities continued with *Tackling Health Inequalities* (DoH 2001a) and *From Vision to Reality* (2001b). An important series of documents entitled National Service Frameworks (NSFs), drawn on in subsequent chapters, developed standards for health for various aspects of health and population groups. One NSF was specifically on mental health and others on children and older age also included much that is relevant to mental health promotion, including reference to its social determinants (DoH 1999b, 2001c, 2004a). Finally, *Choosing Health* (2004b), a public health White Paper, illustrated a shift in the direction of public health policy – towards partnerships with populations in achieving health. The three main principles of its 'New Public Health' approach were informed choice, personalization and working together. The White Paper stated that information and practical support would be provided to get people motivated and to improve emotional well-being. On the basis of earlier consultation with the public various priorities were identified, including that of mental health. The report gave supporting reasons for improving mental health: because it was crucial to physical health and making healthy choices, because stress was the commonest reported cause of sickness absence and because mental ill health can lead to suicide.

An important task is to try and assess the nature and extent of impact of key policy areas on mental health both singly as well as in interaction. Increasingly the health impact of policies is brought out but it can be asked whether the implications for mental health are always recognized as fully as those for physical health. The relations between key policy areas and health will be discussed in the following lifespan chapters but we can offer introductory comments on selected areas. Policy which impacts on economic status is widely seen as a major priority in promoting all aspects of health. At the global level there is growing recognition of the damaging impact of poverty on whole regions of the world and consideration of strategies that may ameliorate the issues. The links between poverty and mental health will be raised frequently in subsequent chapters. Make Poverty History had a high profile in 2005 and campaigning to address world poverty is an ongoing and sustained campaign. Achieving global policies on trade that will impact on the poverty of poorest nations and communities is slow to achieve. Millennium goals were agreed but progress towards these is slow (see Box 3.3).

A second policy area with major significance for mental health is that of education. By this we mean education as a whole rather than specific education for health. While the links between education and mental health have been widely recognized with respect to children the contribution of education to health throughout life has not always received the same attention. For example, the Acheson Report (1998) recommendations on education were confined to pre-school and school aged children. Those involved in the encouragement of lifelong education have, however, recognized its importance. Adult involvement in education has the potential to impact on mental health directly and indirectly through, for example, increasing employability, and enhancing economic status and social inclusion. Currently, in the UK, resources for post-school education are being targeted towards increasing skills for work in young adults which is clearly important. Similar provision for older adults is also needed but is being reduced along with education for personal development not directly related to work and recreation (Tuckett 2006). The significance of education for promoting positive mental health has been acknowledged, as Tuckett points out, in national mental strategy. Initiatives such as a project to issue doctor's prescriptions for education on the same lines as prescriptions for exercise have been developed in recognition of this link (Challis 1996, in Friedli 2001: 27). The current reductions in adult learning provision illustrate a lack of joined up thinking between education, health and economic policy.

A third area of policy with strong influences of mental health is that which relates to work and employment, including policies which increase opportunities for securing employment, which ensure that work takes place in health promoting settings, and which support prompt return to work following involuntary unemployment or illness. Other policy areas with significance for mental health include housing, transport, leisure and recreation, environment, nutrition and neighbourhood renewal. One policy area where there is growing interest in its links with health is that relating to the arts. While people have always reported the positive impacts on mental health of participation in music, dance and other arts activities this has not always been reflected in policy making. In some countries there are now a growing number of evaluations of arts for health projects generating evidence to support relevant policy actions (see the arts for health network: www.nnah.org.uk).

Are policies promoting mental health or preventing ill health?

The emphasis in many countries has traditionally been on policy dealing with established ill health at tertiary and secondary levels with a gradual move towards greater

---

Box 3.3   *The Millennium Development Goals*

1   Eradicate extreme poverty and hunger
2   Achieve universal primary education
3   Promote gender equality and empower women
4   Reduce child mortality
5   Improve maternal health
6   Combat HIV and AIDS, malaria and other diseases
7   Ensure environmental sustainability
8   Develop a global partnership for development

(United Nations 2000)

---

emphasis on primary prevention. Given the magnitude of problems described as mental illness policies clearly have to be in place to respond to established ill health. At the same time fuller attention towards the range of policy areas that, singly or in interaction, can contribute to the development and maintenance of health and, therefore, to primary prevention has begun to develop. As indicated a number of countries are now taking a wider perspective on mental health and considering the impact of policy on positive health, as well as on the prevention of ill health.

Theory in mental health promotion practice

Caplan and Holland (1990: 22) have stated that 'effective practice in mental health promotion depends on good theory'. Awareness of the wide range of theories is needed, they said, together with a critical attitude to them since theories contain contradictions and may lead users into unforeseen and unwanted implications. What is theory and why is its use important? The role of theory is to untangle and simplify the complexities of nature (Green et al. 1994). Theories present in an abstract way the key features of some aspect of the world. They can address either universal, or more localized phenomena, and can relate to micro-, meso- or macro-levels of analysis. The same aspect of the world can be understood differently according to the theory used. O'Brien has used a nice analogy:

> A simple way of understanding theory is to compare it with a kaleidoscope. As the tube is turned different lenses come into play and the combination of colours and shapes shift from one pattern to another. In a similar way we can see social theory as a sort of kaleidoscope – by shifting theoretical perspective the world under investigation changes shape. Different theories bring different aspects of the world into view.
>
> (O'Brien 1993:10)

The nature and purpose of theory differs according to epistemological (theories of knowledge) position with a simple distinction drawn between positivist and interpretivist positions. According to positivist thinking there is an objective world that can be measured, causal relationships identified, and general theories developed which can be tested against reality. No distinctions are drawn between the natural and social sciences. A definition of theory from this perspective is 'a set of interrelated concepts, definitions and propositions that present a systematic view of events and situations by specifying relations among variables in order to explain, and to predict events or situations' (Glanz and Rimer 1995). Theories can be arrived at through deduction from other existing principles as, for example, in mathematics, or built up by induction from empirical investigations. Good theories are testable, generalizable and have power. Within the alternative intellectual positions that can be taken together and labelled as interpretivism social reality is understood as a meaningful construction based on subjective understandings rather than objective measurements. Through gaining access to these understandings theory can be drawn out from research findings. This can consist of theoretical concepts, presented singly or combined into theoretical models. The resulting theories are seen to relate to the situations from which they were derived and while they may be transferable to similar ones are not claimed to be generalizable. The disciplines which underpin health promotion have drawn on theory within both traditions. Theories can be presented in the form of models which offer meaningful ways of presenting the relationships between events and which can be informed by more than one theory. At the same time it should be emphasized that not all models are theory based with some simply providing visual descriptions of particular situations or processes. Deciding definitively whether a model should, or should not be described as theoretical does, to a considerable extent, depend on the conception of theory being held – positivists being more stringent than interpretivists.

What is theory used for in mental health promotion? First, theory can be used in the analysis of situations or problems of interest in order to understand and explain and, where appropriate, to define areas for action. Second, theory is used to guide the nature and process of interventions and their evaluation. Prior to commenting on mental promotion theory some comment can be made the theory of health promotion in general. This theory base has broadened over time. As health promotion began to evolve from health education theory was drawn from several contributory disciplines – predominantly psychology, epidemiology, education and sociology. As health promotion developed it extended its theory base in accordance with its broad range of activities drawing on social policy, political theory, organizational theory, community studies, marketing, economics, etc. Theory was also, to a certain extent, developed within the discipline itself.

It is necessary to ask whether mental health promotion uses the same theory as general health promotion or whether it has a distinctive theoretical basis. To some extent both questions can be answered in the affirmative. Where a conception of mental health promotion is held which fits with the values and principles of health promotion discussed earlier the same broad theory base is clearly relevant. Secker (1998) has observed, however, that general health promotion theory while clearly applicable to developing mental health had not made considerable impact. As noted earlier the fact that mental health promotion developed to some extent independently from general health promotion has led to some differences between its theory base and that of general health promotion. For example, the development of community mental health centres in the USA in the 1960s associated with the field of community psychology stimulated theory development in mental health promotion before the active development of general health promotion. The values of community psychology and its theory and values are similar to the values of health promotion (Orford 1993) and some of the key people involved in the community mental health movement were influential in the development of health promotion.

There are a number of ways of categorizing the theories and models used in mental health promotion. A simple division is between theory which focuses on analysis of problems prior to identifying action and the theory which relates to the implementation and evaluation of actions. Examples of these are shown in Box 3.4. (For references to reading on respective models and theories see Appendix 1.)

Box 3.4   Theories and models in mental health promotion

Theory relating to the analysis of situations and problems

1   *Theoretical concepts*:
   - self-efficacy;
   - self-esteem;
   - discrimination;
   - stigma;
   - empowerment;
   - equity and **inequity**;
   - social capital;
   - resilience;
   - exclusion; etc.
2   *Theories and models*:
   - ecological models of health and mental health;
   - ecological models of human development;
   - psychosocial models of the influences on health decision-making;
   - developmental psychological theories;
   - social theories on childhood, adulthood, older age;
   - models of psychosocial transitions and change;
   - models of the educational process and its consequences, including mental health.

Theory relating to the implementation and evaluation of actions

   - Communication
   - Learning
   - Community development
   - Communication of Innovations
   - Developmental psychology
   - Political theory
   - Organizational theory and the management of change

- Social marketing
- Programme planning
- Evaluation

Another way is to relate theory to levels of influence on mental health as presented in ecological models such as that of Bronfenbrenner (1979), described in Chapter 4, who distinguished intrapersonal; interpersonal; institutional; community factors; and public policy. This model was adapted by Glanz and Rimer (1995) to group theories.

Some of the concepts and theories in Box 3.4 relate particularly to one of these levels, others to two or more levels.

Application of theory in a lifespan approach to mental health promotion

It is not possible to make categorical statements about mental health promotion theory and any distinctiveness it may have from general health promotion. All disciplines continue to develop their theoretical foundations and this is particularly the case with relatively new ones such as mental health promotion. We can tentatively suggest that psychological theory maintains a higher profile in mental health than in general health promotion. In a discipline with philosophical differences around what should take place in its name there will be differing preferences in the selection of theory. For example, those who conceive of mental health promotion as combining policy and educational work informed by an empowerment model will tend to draw on a different combination of theories than those with a narrower focus on health education informed by a preventive medical model. If working in accordance with a lifespan approach theory relevant to the whole of the lifespan as well as to its differing phases will need to be used. In general the particular theory or combination of theories used in mental health promotion practice will depend on the specific issue to be addressed.

The importance of adopting a critical approach to selection and use of theory was noted earlier. Space precludes any detailed consideration of the critique of the theories used in mental health promotion. In a lifespan book reflections on the notion of lifespan development and developmental theories are particularly relevant. One theory, for example, which has been subject to criticism is Piaget's theory of cognitive development. The general progression of thinking which Piaget described leading from ego-centric through to formal operational is generally supported but the rather rigid presentation of the progression through stages has been questioned through later work (Donaldson 1978). Children, it transpires, can think at more sophisticated levels in relation to some areas of their lives than others and in relation to situations which make sense to them and where they are particularly motivated to understand. Given the emphasis that is placed in health promotion on fostering children's active participation in the decisions that affect them it is important to draw on cognitive developmental theory but not to use it so rigidly that children's competencies are strictly age related.

The usefulness of social cognition models of health related decision-making and behaviour change has been regularly reviewed. Some of these models have been modi-fied over time in response to empirical findings and developments in thinking. For example the Health Belief Model (HBM) and the Theory of Planned Behaviour have incorporated the concept of self-efficacy in response to research evidence (Conner and Norman 1995; Bennet and Murphy 1997). Some models are relatively easy to under-stand and this facilitates their rapid adoption. The Health Belief Model (HBM) and Transtheoretical Stages of Change (Prochaska et al. 1997) are particularly good examples but the ease of adoption may not always lead to appropriate use. In the case of the HBM it has become clear that the model, while providing a useful theoretical framework which has underpinned many studies, has its shortcomings. It is economic in including a relatively small number of factors, but the downside is that it is most useful in relation to less complex behaviours which are actually governed by the par-ticular beliefs contained within the model (Sheeran and Abraham 1995). The evidence in support of the Transtheoretical Stages of Change Model does not appear in the light of some research to be particularly strong and a number of critiques have been offered (Whitelaw et al. 2000; Adams and White 2005).

Some of the critiques of theoretical models can be misplaced. Many models seek for economy by incorporating only sufficient factors to meet their purposes such as to explain and predict. That they could include further factors to explain more fully or predict more accurately will often be acknowledged but a balance is needed between elaboration of a model and its capacity to fulfil a stated purposes. Green et al. (1994) provided a useful contribution on this matter. They commented on the position that theories or models are unusable or unsatisfactory because they are less than com-prehensive in accounting for all the variable operating in a situation, or do not relate explicitly to the precise problem and circumstances in which practitioners find them-selves. This, they said, misses the point of theory. The first demands models or theories of such complexity that they would seldom be read, much less used. The second demands a cook book. Theory must strive for a level of abstraction that generalizes beyond the specific case and a level of simplification that achieves efficiency of explanation without distortion.

Taking up the question of what theory actually is used widely in health promotion, in contrast with what could be used, there does not appear to be a comprehensive survey of this for mental health promotion. Some systematic reviews of mental health promotion interventions have documented the theory base of included studies and these have tended to be theories derived from psychology, as noted earlier. What such reviewers also note is a lack of reported theory, a comment regularly made in reviews of other health promotion areas. In some cases the theoretical underpinnings can be deduced through a careful reading of papers but in others it is not apparent that con-siderations of theory had a part in decision-making. For example Wight et al. (1998) observed with reference to sexual health programmes that few were theoretically based and those that were relied almost exclusively on social cognitive theory. Trifiletti et al. (2004) reviewed the theories used in research geared to injury prevention. They speci-fied a list of behavioural and social science theories, not intending to map fully health promotion theory, but found few applications of main theories to their topic of inter-est. Theory was most often used, they concluded, to guide programme design and implementation and the development of evaluation measures. The most citations were found for the Health Belief Model, Theory of Reasoned Action/Theory of Planned Behaviour, Social Learning Theory and the PRECEED–PROCEED model. Other theories reported in only one or two articles included precaution adoption process model; protection motivation theory; community organization; communication of innovations; and social marketing.

It would be surprising if these findings did not equally apply to mental health promotion. Commenting on theory as reported in journals is not a full picture of theory used in practice but the full range is more difficult to comment on, in the absence of research on this matter. We can gain some insight on theory used in practice from examining what is taught in the context of professional training although this may not be reflected in practice. Given that those who see themselves as involved in some way in mental health promotion go through different types of training ranging from specialist health promotion and public health training through to teaching, community, social work, nurse education and so on, there will be differences in theory that is introduced. To date there has been relatively little research that has reported fully on health promotion practitioners' use of theory, either in analysing situations or in planning and implementing interventions. One example of such research in Australia (Jones and Donovan 2004) reported a gap between the theory of which practitioners were aware and that which they used in practice.

It should also be stressed that theory, while important, is only one factor which governs the development and implementation of mental health promotion programmes. In a study of decisions relating to smoking prevention programmes with young people theory sat alongside use of the evidence base, response to situational pressures, attempts to be innovative and commitment to maintaining, for a number of reasons, existing practice (Tilford et al. 1998). In the subsequent chapters the nature of theories which have informed practice at particular lifespan periods will be noted in describing specific studies, and a full table of studies described plus their associated theory can be found in Appendix 2. The final chapter will include further reflection on mental health promotion theory in the light of the discussion across all chapters.

Conclusions

This chapter has sought to provide a general background overview of the nature and development of health promotion and its relationship to mental health promotion. While there are ideas which have attained some dominance it should have become clear that there are complexities. These have consequences for what is deemed to be important to pursue in seeking to enhance mental health. Some brief consideration has been given to debates which relate to practice. Theory is an important underpinning of all aspects of mental health promotion – from analysis of situations through to evaluation of programmes designed to enhance mental health. Introduction to the breadth of theory available to mental health promotion practice has been provided and subsequent chapters will illustrate the use of these in practice.

Box 3.5 Some summary questions for reflection

1 What ideas about the nature of health promotion and mental health promotion do you encounter in the practice situations with which you are familiar?

2 What model(s) of health promotion inform mental health promotion activities that you are involved in or observe?

3 What mix of values and principles would you wish to adopt in your current (or future) practice. If you are involved in practice at the present time are there any constraints on working in accordance with your chosen principles?

4 Where do you stand on the various debates outlined? What views on the debates do you identify in the contexts of practices in which you work? Are there any ways in which your views are at variance with those of the context in which you work?

5 What specific mental health promotion policies exist in the country in which you live or work?

6 To what extent are the mental health implications of general policy areas made explicit?

7 How do you use theory in your work? What theories do you draw on and how do you decide which to use?

8 Identify one or more mental health promotion issues that you are likely to work on in the near future. What theories and models might you draw on in analysing the issue and planning some activity in response?

References

Acheson, D. (1998) *Independent Inquiry into Inequalities in Health.* London: The Stationery Office.

Adams, J. and White, M. (2005) Why don't stage based activity promotion interventions work? *Health Education Research*, 20(2): 237–43.

Albee, G.W. and Ryan Finn, K.D. (1993) An overview of primary prevention, *Journal of Counselling and Development*, 72(2): 115–23.

Barry, M. (2001) Promoting positive mental health: theoretical frameworks for practice, *International Journal of Mental Health Promotion*, 3(1): 23–34.

Beattie, A. (1979) *Models of Health Education.* London: Health Education Council.

Beattie, A. (1991) Knowledge and social control in health promotion: a test case for social theory and social policy, in J. Gabe, M. Calnan and M. Bury (eds) *Sociology of the Health Service*. London: Routledge.

Bennett, P. and Murphy, S. (1997) *Psychology and Health Promotion.* Buckingham: Open University Press.

Bronfenbrenner, U. (1979) *The Ecology of Human Development: Experiments by Nature and Design.* Cambridge, MA: Harvard University Press.

Canadian Public Health Association (1996) Proceedings of a workshop on mental health promotion, Toronto, Canada, June 20–1. Available at: www.cpha.ca/english/natprog/menthlth.htm (accessed 18 March 2006).

Caplan, R. and Holland, R. (1990) Rethinking health education theory, *Journal of Health Education*, 49(1): 10–12.

Connor, M. and Norman, P. (1995) *Predicting Health Behaviour*. Buckingham: Open University Press.

Da Silva, M.J., McKenzie, K., Harpham, T. and Huntly, S.R.A. (2005) Social capital and mental illness: a systematic review, *Journal of Epidemiology and Community Health*, 59: 619–27.

DHSS (Department of Health and Social Security) (1976) *Prevention and Health: Everybody's Business*. London: HMSO.

DHSS (Department of Health and Social Security) (1977) *Prevention and Health*. London: HMSO.

DoH (Department of Health) (1992) *The Health of the Nation*. London: HMSO.

DoH (Department of Health) (1998) *Our Healthier Nation: A Contract for Health*. London: HMSO.

DoH (Department of Health) (1999a) *The Mental Health National Service Framework*. London: The Stationery Office.

DoH (Department of Health) (1999b) *Saving Lives: Our Healthier Nation*. London: The Stationery Office.

DoH (Department of Health) (2001a) *Tackling Health Inequalities: Consultation on a Plan of Delivery*. London: The Stationery Office.

DoH (Department of Health) (2001b) *From Vision to Reality*. London: The Stationery Office.

DoH (Department of Health) (2001c) *National Service Framework for Older People*. London: The Stationery Office.

DoH (Department of Health) (2004a) *The Children's National Service Framework*. London: The Stationery Office.

DoH (Department of Health) (2004b) *Choosing Health: Making Healthy Choices Easier*. London: The Stationery Office.

DoH (Department of Health)/Welsh Assembly (2005) *Shaping the Future of Public Health. Promoting Health in the NHS: Delivering Choosing Health and Health Challenge, Wales*. London: The Stationery Office.

Donaldson, M. (1978) *Children's Thinking*. London: Fontana.

Downie, R.S., Fyfe, C. and Tannahill, A. (1990) *Health Promotion: Models and Values*. Oxford: Oxford University Press.

Ewles, L. and Simnett, I. (2001) *Promoting Health: A Practical Guide*. London: Bailliere-Tindall.

Freudenberg, N. (1981) Health education for social change: a strategy for public health in the US, *International Journal of Health Education*, 24(3): 1–8.

Friedli, L. (2001) Promotion drive, *Community Care*, 3–9 May, pp. 26–7.

Glanz, K. and Rimer, B.K. (1995) *Theory at a Glance: A Guide for Health Promotion Practice*. Bethesda, MD: National Cancer Institute.

Green, A. (1987) Is there primary health care in the UK? *Health Policy and Planning*, 2(2): 129–37.

Green, L.W., Glanz, K., Hochbaum, G.M., Kok, G. and Kreuter, M.W. (1994) Can we build on, or must we replace the theories and models in health education? *Health Education Research*, 9(3): 397–404.

Herrman, H., Saxena, S., Moodie, R. and Walker, L. (2004) Introduction: promoting mental health as a public health priority, *Promoting Mental Health: Concepts, Emerging Evidence, Practice*. A report from the World Health Organization in collaboration with the Victoria

Health Promotion Foundation and the University of Melbourne. Geneva: World Health Organization.

Hunter, D. (2003) *Public Health Policy*. Oxford: Polity Press.

Jones, S.C and Donovan, R.J. (2004) Does theory inform practice in Australia? *Health Education Research*, 1: 1–14.

Kaprio, L.A. (1979) *Primary Health Care in Europe*. Copenhagen: WHO Regional Office for Europe.

Lalonde, M. (1974) *A New Perspective on the Health of Canadians*. Ottawa: Government of Canada.

Macdonald, G. and O'Hara, K. (1998) *Ten Elements of Mental Health, Its Promotion and Demotion: Implications for Practice*. London: Society of Health Education and Promotion Specialists.

Mann, M., Hosmans, C.M.H., Schaalma, H.P. and de Vries, N.K. (2004) Self-esteem in a broad spectrum approach to mental health promotion, *Health Education Research*, 19(4): 357–72.

McKeown, T. (1979) *The Role of Medicine: Dream, mirage or nemesis*, 2nd edn. Oxford: Basil Blackwell.

McKinlay, J.B and McKinlay, S.M. (1977) Medical measures and the decline or mortality, *Millbank Memorial Fund Quarterly/Health and Society*, Summer, pp. 405–28.

McLeroy, K.D., Bibeau, D., Steckler, A. and Glanz, K. (1988) An ecological perspective on health promotion programs, *Health Education Quarterly*, 15(4): 351–77.

Mentality (2005) How does mental health promotion work? Available at: www.mentality.org.uk (accessed 8 October 2005).

Mrazek, P.J and Haggerty, R.J. (eds) (1994) *Reducing Risks for Mental Disorders: Frontiers for Preventive Intervention Research*. Washington, DC: National Academic Press.

Mull, J.D. (1990) The primary care dialectic: history, rhetoric and reality, in J. Coreil and J.D. Mull (eds) *Anthropology and Primary Health Care*. Oxford: Westview Press.

Naidoo, J. and Wills, J. (2000) *Health Promotion: Foundations for Practice*, 2nd edn. Edinburgh: Bailliere Tindall.

NHS Centre for Reviews and Dissemination (1996) *Undertaking Systematic Reviews on Research and Effectiveness: CRD Guidelines for those Carrying Out and Commissioning Reviews*. York: University of York.

Nutbeam, D. (2001) Getting evidence into policy and practice to address health inequalities, *Health Promotion International*, 19(2): 137–40.

O'Brien, M. (1993) Social research and sociology, in N. Gilbert (ed.) *Researching Social Life*. London: Sage Publications.

Orford, J. (1993) *Community Psychology*. Chichester: John Wiley and Sons.

Patton, G., Olsson, C. and Toumbourou, J. (2002) Prevention and mental health promotion in Australia: the evidence, in L. Rowling, G. Martin and L. Walker (eds) *Mental Health Promotion and Young People: Concepts and Practice*. Sydney: McGraw-Hill.

Pawson, R. and Tilley, N. (1997) *Realistic Evaluation*. London: Sage Publications.

Prochaska, J.O., Redding, C.A., Evers, K. and DiClemente, C.C. (1997) The transtheoretical model and stages of change, in K. Glanz, F.M. Lewis and B.K. Rimer (eds) *Health Behavior and Health Education: Theory, Research, and Practice*, 2nd edn. San Francisco: Jossey Bass.

Raeburn, J. (2001) Community approaches to mental health promotion, *International Journal of Health Promotion*, 3(1): 13–19.

Raeburn, J. and Rootman, J. (1998) *People-Centred Health Promotion*. Chichester: John Wiley and Sons.

Rodmell, S. and Watt, A. (eds) (1986) *The Politics of Health Education: Raising the Issues*. London: Routledge and Kegan Paul.

Rogers, A. and Pilgrim, D. (1996) *Mental Health Policy in Britain. A Critical Introduction*. Basingstoke: Macmillan Press.

Rychetnik, L. and Wise, M. (2004) Advocating evidence-based health promotion: reflections and a way forward, *Health Promotion International*, 19(4): 247–58.

Scanlon, K. (2002) A population health approach: building the infrastructure to promote mental health in young people, in L. Rowling, G. Martin and L. Walker (eds) *Mental Health promotion and Young People: Concepts and Practice*. Sydney: McGraw-Hill.

Secker, J. (1998) Current conceptualizations of mental health and mental health promotion, *Health Education Research*, 13(1): 57–66.

Sheeran, P. and Abraham, C. (1995) The health belief model, in M. Connor and P. Norman (eds) *Predicting Health Behaviour*. Buckingham: Open University Press.

SHEPS (Society of Health Education and Health Promotion Specialists) (1998) *Health Promotion Specialists in the NHS*. Glasgow: SHEPS.

Tilford, S., White, M., Godfrey, C., Nicholson, F. and South, J. (1998) *Evidence Based Health Promotion: Commissioning Interventions for the Prevention of Smoking in Young People*. Leeds: Centre for Health Promotion Research, Leeds Metropolitan University.

Tilford, S., Green, J. and Tones, K. (2003) *Values, Health Promotion and Public Health*. Leeds: Centre for Health Promotion Research, Leeds Metropolitan University.

Tones, B.K. and Tilford, S. (2001) *Health Promotion: Effectiveness, Efficiency and Equity*. Cheltenham: Nelson-Thornes.

Tones, B.K. and Green, J. (2004) *Health Promotion: Planning and Strategies*. London: Sage Publications.

Trifiletti, L.B., Gielen, A.C., Sleet, D.A. and Hopkins, K. (2004) Behavioural and social science theories and models: are they used in unintentional injury research, *Health Education Research*, 20(3): 298–307.

Tuckett, A. (2006) Is lifelong learning going to be just a pipe dream? *Guardian: Education Guardian*, 23 May.

Tudor, K. (1996) *Mental Health Promotion*. London: Routledge.

United Nations (2000) *The Millennium Development Goals*. Geneva: United Nations.

Weare, K. (2004) The International Alliance for Child and Adolescent Health in Schools (INTERCAMHS), *Health Education*, 104(2): 65–7.

Whitelaw, S., Baldwin, S., Bunton, R. and Flynn, D. (2000) The status of evidence and outcomes in stages of change research, *Health Education Research*, 15(6): 707–18.

WHO (1978) *Declaration of Alma Ata, International Conference on Primary Health Care*, Alma Ata, 6–12 September. Geneva: WHO.

WHO (1984) *Health Promotion: A Discussion Document on the Concept and Principles*. Copenhagen: WHO Regional Office for Europe.

WHO (1986) *Ottawa Charter for Health Promotion, International Conference on Health Promotion*, Ottawa, 17–21 November. Copenhagen: WHO Regional Office for Europe.

WHO (1988) *Healthy Public Policy. Strategies for Action: The Adelaide Recommendations*. Geneva: WHO.

WHO (1991) *Sundsvall Statement on Supportive Environments for Health*. Geneva: WHO.

WHO (1997) *The Jakarta Declaration of Leading Health Promotion into the 21st Century*. Geneva: WHO.

WHO (1998a) *Fifty-First World Health Assembly (WHO/47): Health Promotion*. Copenhagen: WHO.

WHO (1998b) *Health Promotion Evaluation: Recommendations for Policymakers*. Geneva: WHO. Available at http://www.who.dk/document/e60706.pdf (accessed 20 March 2006).

WHO (2000) *Report of the Technical Programme: Fifth Global Conference on Health Promotion: Bridging the Equity Gap*, Mexico, 5–9 June. Geneva: WHO.

WHO (2001) *Mental Health: Strengthening Mental Health Promotion*, Fact sheet 220. Geneva: WHO.

WHO (2003) *Bangkok Charter for Health Promotion in a Globalized World*. Geneva: WHO.

Wight, D., Abraham, C. and Scott, S. (1998) Towards a psychosexual theoretical framework for sexual health promotion, *Health Education Research*, 13(3): 317–30.

4 Infancy and childhood (0–5 years and 6–12 years)

Sylvia Tilford

Editors' foreword

According to Article 24 of the United Nations Convention on the Rights of the Child 'health is the basis of a good quality of life and mental health is of overriding importance in this' (United Nations 1989). This chapter will consider the important task of promoting mental health in the first phase of the lifespan. In addition to its importance for childhood itself clear associations have been demonstrated between mental health in childhood and adulthood (Rutter 1996). The division between this chapter and Chapter 5 is broadly in line with the age of transfer, in many countries, from primary to secondary education. Three special issues have been selected for this phase of the lifespan. The first is inequalities in child mental health, the second concerns childhood itself and the way that societal conceptions of children influence the development of mental health and the third is the promotion of mental health of children experiencing major life events.

Introduction

The chapter will begin with comment on the nature of children and childhood followed by discussion of the determinants of mental health and the identification of vulnerable populations. Children's perceptions of mental health will be noted prior to reviewing the evidence on the effectiveness of activities designed to promote mental health for the pre-school years (0–5 years) and the primary school years (5–12 years). The chapter will conclude with a consideration of policy measures to support the promotion of child mental health; some examples of good mental health promotion practice; and an assessment of the extent to which theory and principles inform current mental health promotion practice.

The nature of children and childhood

According to the Convention on the Rights of a Child (United Nations 1989) anyone under the age of 18 is described as a child. Many statements on childhood designate it as the period prior to achieving the maturity to take on adult responsibilities, although there is no consistency either within or between countries in denoting adult status for differing areas of life. In most Western societies adolescence is designated as a period between childhood and adulthood. There have been debates about whether the period of childhood has always been recognized or whether it is essentially a modern concept (Aries 1962; Pollock 1983 in Hunt 2005: 85). In general there is now broad support for the view that there are differing ideas of children and childhood across cultures, and that ideas have changed over time.

Contrasting ideas of the essential nature of a child as either 'good' or 'evil' have run through Western cultures (Stainton-Rogers 2001). Where the child was seen as 'good', childhood was a period of innocence in which children developed self-knowledge and needed an environment offering protection against the wider world in which to grow and develop. Childhood was important in its own right, not simply a period of pre-paration for adult life. These ideas have influenced much pre-school education where children are encouraged to express themselves through free play and creative work within a facilitating and protecting environment. While the general need for protec-tion of young children would not be challenged, questions can be asked about the nature and degree of protection that they need and the appropriate balance between protection and gradual exposure to risks.

Contrasting conceptions of the child as 'evil', 'wicked' or 'naughty' have influenced views on the purpose and process of socialization. In enabling the child to become 'socialized' or 'saved' (within a religious perspective) discipline and punishment were seen as essential to the process. By the nineteenth century, children were more likely to be described as 'naughty' rather than as 'evil', but the emphasis on discipline prevailed (Stainton-Rogers 2001). The idea of the 'naughty' child, often in opposition to the 'good' one, continues to be a feature of popular discourse on children and evidence can also be seen in the media and children's literature.

Childhood in the disciplines of psychology and sociology

Concepts and theories from the various schools in psychology and sociology are continuing influences on thinking and practice in mental health promotion. From psychology there are, for example, theories on the ways that children learn and their role in the learning process; how their understanding of the world develops; and how they develop emotionally and socially. Theories of development have addressed cogni-tive (Piaget, in Grieve and Hughes 1990: 26–50); moral (Kohlberg 1963, in Danziger 1971: 97); and socio-emotional (Erikson 1963; Bowlby 1971) aspects with **critical periods** identified for some of them. Attachment theory which focused on the devel-opment of emotional attachments through the process of bonding has had a strong influence on thinking about early mental health (Winnicott 1964; Bowlby 1971). The process was seen as important not only for mental health in childhood, but also as a foundation for relationships throughout life. There are a number of questions which have run through developmental psychology:

- Is the child active or passive in the development process? In contrast with the relatively passive conceptions held by the behaviourists others such as the social interactionists depicted the child as an 'active agent'.

- Should the developmental process be seen as universal or as particularistic. Much early psychology paid relatively little attention to differences across cultures or even gender. Theories have been tested out in diverse cultures but critiques that psychological ideas are dominated by Western thinking continue to be offered (Burman 1997; Moghaddan and Studer 1997).
- What should be the relative emphasis on the individual versus the collective? The dominant emphasis of psychology for much of its history has been on the individual with little, if any, reference to social context, although there were exceptions, such as Bronfenbrenner (1979).

In sociological analysis the focus is less on the individual child and more on the relationships between childhood and society. Conceptions of this relationship have differed within the various schools of sociology. Of particular relevance to this chapter is what is described as a 'new **paradigm** of the sociology of childhood' which draws heavily on **social constructionism**. The new paradigm proposes that the diversity of ideas about childhood across cultures and contexts should be recognized. Aspects of this paradigm fit neatly with core principles of health promotion. For example:

- Children are, and must be, seen as active in the construction and determination of their own social lives; of the lives of those around them; and of the societies in which they live. They are not simply the passive subjects of social structures and processes.
- Children have a voice of their own and should be listened to, and involved in democratic dialogue and decision-making. They have cultures of their own, independent of the perspective and concerns of adults.
- Relationships between adults and children involve the exercise of power (as well as the expression of love). It is necessary to take account of the way in which adult power is maintained and used, as well as the children's resilience and resistance to that power.

(Prout and James 1990; Dahlberg et al. 1999)

Mental health of young children

Data describing the mental health of children is less easy to obtain than data on risk factors and ill health. To describe positive mental health holistic measures can be used with psychological well-being and emotional literacy often used as a proxy for mental health. More commonly a reductionist approach is adopted where attributes linked to positive mental health are measured including self-concept, self-efficacy, self-esteem, resilience, empowerment and coping skills. Indicators for some of these attributes are better developed than for others and it has been observed that indicators of positive mental health in children need further work (Maher and Waters undated, in Zubrick and Kovess-Masfety 2004: 59). They reported on work to develop indicators at individual, community and organization and societal levels. Box 4.2 lists the types of indicators they suggest for the three levels.

In many countries children in the pre-school age group come into contact with health services which offer developmental checks and provide opportunities for record-

---

Box 4.1   Summary points on children and childhood

- A focus on mental health in childhood is important for childhood itself as well as building a foundation for the whole of the lifespan.
- There are historical and contemporary differences in conceptions of the nature of children and childhood.
- A number of disciplines, including psychology and sociology have contributed to the theory of childhood.
- A balance has to be reached between meeting the protection needs of children and allowing the development of autonomy.
- There is some commonality between key concepts of the 'new paradigm' of childhood and health promotion.

Box 4.2   Some suggested indicators of positive child mental health

Individual and family

- *Individual*: sense of belonging; self-esteem; engagement, self-determination; control and quality of life; resilience; empowerment.
- *Family*: parental mental health; freedom from violence; family cohesion; parent–child attachment; use of appropriate parenting practices; providing safe, secure environments.

Organizational and community

Safe supportive environments; quality of social and learning environments to enhance development of self worth and skills; children's rights met; presence of policies to promote equity and justice, ensure child protection and minimize violence and bullying.

Societal indicators of positive child mental health

- *Resource poor countries*: access to essential requirements of water, adequate food and safe shelter; primary education and primary health care; protection against conflict and violence.
- *Countries with basic resources*: equity and social participation for parents; societal valuing and protection of children; integrated and supportive child public health policy; strong legislative platform for child mental health issues; adequate resource allocation for child mental health.

(Maher and Waters, in Zubrick and Kovess-M 2004: 159)

---

ing positive health. The main emphasis is typically on the early identification of issues placing mental and physical health at risk. In children of school age, although countries differ, there is little that might be identified as regular monitoring and recording of holistic mental health, either by health or education services. *Bright Futures* (Mental Health Foundation 1999) called for measures of school performance in the UK to include social and emotional well-being and inclusion practices for children and young people experiencing emotional and behavioural difficulties. Given the shortfalls in data a superficial answer to the question about the extent of mental health in children would be to say that those children who are not identified as having mental health problems are healthy. There are some large scale general health surveys within, and across countries which can throw some light on positive mental health although these tend to focus more on later childhood and adolescence than on the earlier period.

When it comes to mental ill health the WHO quantifies this at a global level while individual countries publish information derived from routine statistics and from surveys. Given the differences in what is categorized as a mental health problem and the differing age ranges for which figures are provided data are not easy to compare. The WHO (2001) estimates that about 10 percent of children experience mental health problems. At the national level the Health Survey for England (DoH 1998) also reported a figure of 10 percent for those aged between 0 and 15 years. A later survey (Melzer et al. 2000) reported data for over 10,000 children between 5 and 15 years for three main childhood disorders: conduct disorder; hyperactivity; and emotional disorders as defined in the International Classification of Diseases (ICD). Five percent had clinically significant conduct disorders, 4 percent had emotional disorders and 1 percent were hyperactive. This survey reported on the associations between the presence of a disorder and a range of variables and data are drawn on in the following discussion of mental health determinants.

Many commentators have come to the conclusion that the extent of mental health problems in children is on the increase but any such conclusions have to be tentative given the problems of definition, the measurement problems, variations in applications of ICD categories, changes in readiness to bring difficulties to the attention of services and changes in what is defined as a mental health problem. At the same time the responses in the UK to the latest 2004 survey have been cautiously optimistic (Ward 2005). After a period of 25 years over which figures on problems had risen, they now appeared to have stabilized. The charity Young Minds welcomed the fact that problems had not increased since the 1999 survey and noted that the Government had made significant investments in improving child mental health (Ward 2005).

Special issues for consideration in this chapter

Three special issues were selected for this chapter. The first is inequalities in mental health particularly those arising from socio-economic, gender and ethnicity differences, and the ways that these can be reduced. Attention to inequalities is necessary throughout the lifespan but especially so during childhood because of the significance of early experience for the rest of life. The second issue concerns childhood itself, how it is conceived and the implications this has for the way that mental health is promoted. Ideas held will, for example, influence the voice that children are allowed to have in the decisions that affect them as they progress through childhood and govern the balance that is achieved between promoting autonomy and providing protection. The third issue is the promotion of the mental health of children who are experiencing major changes in their lives from the impact of conflict and violence; the loss of parents through relationship breakdown or illnesses such as HIV/AIDS; or the effect of natural disasters. While children in all countries experience changes the life situations of children in some parts of the world pose very considerable challenges to the development of mental health.

Determinants and influences of child mental health

Chapter 2 considered determinants of mental health and these can be categorized in various ways (Lalonde 1974; Bronfenbrenner 1979; Dahlgren and Whitehead 1991). The ecological model in Figure 4.1 will be used as a framework for the discussion. It shows that factors are multiple and interacting.

Environmental factors: socio-economic, cultural, natural and built

The evidence base on the links between specific factors and health differs although certain factors have been cited as particularly powerful in their impact on mental health as explained in Chapter 2 (Albee and Ryan Finn 1993).

Socio-economic and cultural factors

Economic influences
Regardless of whether definitions are used of **absolute** or **relative poverty**, children experiencing poverty are more likely to have risk factors for mental ill health or to

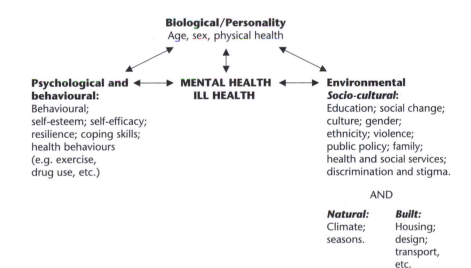

Figure 4.1 Model of influences on health

experience ill health outcomes (Patel 2001). The State of the World's Children Report (Bellamy 2005) estimated that there are one billion children worldwide living in poverty, with some regions having a higher incidence than others. In Sub-Saharan Africa, for example, the percentage of the population living on less than US$1 a day over the period 1990 to 2002 was 43 percent compared to 21 percent in the rest of the world. While there are countries and environments where virtually all children experience poverty, in others it is commoner for a proportion of the child population to experience it. For example, in the UK there is a strong link between poverty and social class, with 16 percent of children between 5 and 15 years of age in the lowest income groups with mental health problems compared with just under 6 percent in the highest income groups (Melzer et al. 2000). The complex impact of poverty on children's lives and the potential impact on mental health can be suggested as illustrated in Figure 4.2.

Education
While informal education in family and community contexts promotes mental health, it is widely recognized that lack of participation in formal education is associated with a whole range of poorer outcomes, including poorer mental health (Bellamy 2001). UNICEF reported in 2005 (Bellamy 2005) that 114 million children of primary school age are not enrolled in school. Although the figures for enrolment are now high in most parts of the world they remain relatively low, and persistently so, in others. In Sub-Saharan Africa, for example, the figure for the period 1998–2003 was 58 percent compared with 80 percent worldwide (Bellamy 2004). Fall out rates are also important since failure to complete school is associated with poorer health outcomes (Patel 2001). There is still a gender gap for recruitment to school and for total years in primary school with retention rates generally better for boys. In those countries where all children have the opportunity to go to school for the full legal period there are some whose attendance is low and there is evidence that they also experience poorer mental health (Melzer et al. 2000).

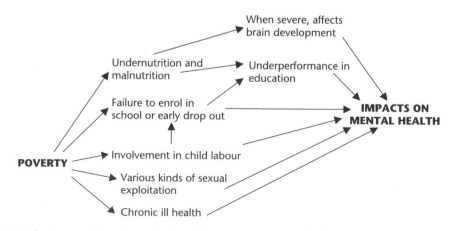

Figure 4.2 Some relationships between child poverty and mental health

Culture and ethnicity
Culture refers to the whole way of life of a population group including health related beliefs and values. Many countries are multi-cultural and likely to contain differing and conflicting ideas about children and the nature of childhood as well as about the mental health of children. Explaining mental health differences with reference to culture alone can be problematic since socio-economic factors can also play a significant role. To seek to change aspects of culture alone as a solution to problems would therefore be described as victim blaming.

When so much theory pertaining to mental health is derived from Western culture it can be easy to apply this without consideration of transferability to other cultures. For example, Zubrick and Kovess-Masfety (2004) emphasize the need to apply the concept of resilience with care. They drew on a study by Rousseau of unaccompanied children from Somalia who are often considered to have a high risk of mental ill health. Using ethnographic data Rousseau showed that the children were protected by the meaning attributed to separation within their nomadic cultures and through the establishment of continuity through lineage and age group structures.

Figures by ethnicity for the 5–15 year age range in Melzer et al.'s (2000) UK survey showed some interesting differences in relation to ethnicity. Ten percent of white, 12 percent of black children, 8 percent of Pakistani and Bangladeshi and 4 percent of the Indian samples were reported as having a mental health problem.

Social and family structures
Children grow up in different types of family and extended kinship structures. When these are put under strain or break down it becomes more difficult for children to achieve mental health. Major causes of disruption are relationship breakdowns, the impact of armed conflict and of major physical health problems. For example, 13 million children in the world had lost one or both parents to AIDS by 2001, with 90 percent of these children being in Sub-Saharan Africa; approximately 10 percent of children in some African countries were HIV/AIDS orphans (Bellamy 2001). As the resilience literature shows, many children do maintain positive health in difficult family circumstances, in part because protective factors can be identified.

Melzer et al. (2000) reported on child mental health in relation to a number of family variables. Sixteen percent of children living with lone parents were recorded as having problems compared with 8 percent living with married or cohabiting couples. Prevalence of disorder increased with a decrease in educational qualification of parents and was closely linked with family employment and household income. Children living with parents who were experiencing mental ill health also had higher rates of problems. Between one-third and two-thirds of children who have a mentally ill parent will develop problems themselves. Rates were also higher for children of refugees and migrants, children experiencing discrimination and children experiencing violence.

Gender
From birth children's experiences are influenced by their biological labelling as male or female. Different cultural expectations of female and male children, although of varying strengths, are characteristic of virtually all societies and are powerful influences in

the development of gender identity. Different patterns of socialization for boys and girls can impact on various indicators of mental health such as self-esteem, identity, resilience and empowerment. Where societies discriminate on the basis of gender, negative impacts on mental health are to be expected.

Data from a number of countries show mental health problems in young children as being more prevalent with boys than with girls. For the ages 4 to 15 years the Health Survey for England (DoH 1998) survey reported 12 percent of boys and 8 percent of girls with problems. Figures have to be interpreted with care since some specified mental health problems are related to conduct behaviours where there may be a greater readiness to ascribe problems to boys than to girls. In the Melzer et al. (2000) survey gender differences were found for two out of the three categories of disorder examined (conduct and hyperactivity), with little difference for emotional disorders. Gender socialization in childhood may continue to influence patterns of behaviour and mental health throughout life.

Violence and conflict

Children in all countries can be exposed to violence within their homes and in their immediate communities. Added to this there is exposure to the violence associated with conflict and war situations which can result in the loss of family members, loss of home, physical trauma and even recruitment to active participation in warfare.

In the domestic context children can observe violence and also experience various types of abuse themselves. Many parts of the world lack systems of child protection and a great proportion of violence to children goes unrecognized and even where systems do exist it can be under-recognized. In the case of infants, Jaffe et al. (1990, in Humphreys 2001: 147) reported that babies under the age of 1 who witness violence have poorer health, poor sleeping habits and are prone to excessive screaming. According to Hughes (1988, in Humphreys 2001: 146) the pre-school age group registers the highest levels of behavioural disturbances of any age of children in response to domestic violence. While physical abuse, when there are visible consequences, may come to the attention of others, emotional abuse is less likely to do so. Emotional abuse is under-recognized and the true incidence, according to Mind (2005), could make it the commonest form of maltreatment rather than the least common, as recorded on child protection registers. In South Africa, where many children live in situations of severe disadvantage, it has been estimated that 20 percent of children suffer from a mental illness due to high levels of violence and family problems (Johnson 2005). At the same time a number of writers have pointed out the resilience of some children who experience violent situations (Jaffe et al., in Humphreys 2001: 147). Moore and Pepler (1998, in Humphreys 2001: 147), in a study of 113 children of mothers in a women's refuge and a control group of 100 children in two parent, non-violent families, found that the mother's behaviour and mental health played a key role in children's adjustment. Children whose mothers were able to maintain positive parenting strategies, even in the context of very violent situations, showed the most positive adjustment.

UNICEF has stated (Bellamy 2001) that on any given day more than 20 armed conflicts are being fought round the world, most of them in poor countries. The 'State of the World's Children' report (Bellamy 2005) estimated that 1.6 million children have been killed in conflicts since 1990, and 20 million children have been forced by conflicts or human rights violations to leave their homes. For children exposed to conflict there can be both immediate and long-term psychological consequences, not only from the direct effects on the conflict but also from the disruption of families and communities and impact on educational opportunities. There are very particular concerns for the mental health of young children who are recruited to active roles in warfare. Damaging methods are used to socialize them into killing and the long-term consequences have yet to be fully elucidated.

A particular aspect of violence is bullying within the school setting and it is seen as a significant threat to the development of children's (and adolescents') well-being. This includes bullying of children by other children and by adults. Studies of the prevalence of bullying have been undertaken in a number of countries and figures vary from 8 percent to 46 percent for regularly bullied children and between 5 percent and 30 percent for those who actively bully on a regular basis. The form of bullying behaviours differs between boys and girls, but boys and girls are bullied equally often (Fekkes et al. 2005). Fekkes et al. also questioned children about a number of aspects of bullying and its management in schools and reported that pupils did not perceive teachers as dealing effectively with many incidents of bullying. They called for a whole-school approach to bullying prevention.

Work

It is accepted that work is an important determinant of mental health in adults but not so readily seen as an influence in the 0–12 year age group. In pre-industrialized countries children have contributed to the activities which form the basis for family survival – herding, growing crops, water carrying, caring for younger children and so on. In the nineteenth century the earliest countries to industrialize made extensive use of child labour until legal changes were initiated. Nonetheless many children continued to work within informal settings in order to support families. Countries that are currently industrializing are making significant use of child labour. According to UNICEF (Bellamy 2005) 97 percent of child labourers work in developing countries. In Sub-Saharan Africa 41 percent of children aged 4 to 14 are involved in what are described as the worst forms of child labour. In Asia one in five children under 14 are working, and because of the large numbers involved this adds up to 60 percent of the child labour market internationally. Although there are powerful reasons for protecting children from involvement in formal work situations their exclusion is not necessarily straightforward. UNICEF (Bellamy 2005) has emphasized that many children are heading up households and need to work. If prevented from doing so they can be forced into more dangerous situations of prostitution. Involvement in work can impact directly on mental health or, indirectly, through influencing school attendance and other determinants of health.

Discrimination

Children who are in refugee families, asylum seekers, children from some minorities, children who are homeless or maintaining very slender links with homes, and children with disabilities can all experience discrimination which can impact negatively on mental health. While it is usual to think about age related discrimination as more applicable to later stages of the lifespan, children can also be discriminated against simply because of their age. The survey by Melzer et al. (2000) reported higher levels of problems for children experiencing discrimination.

Social responsibilities
Many children take on care responsibilities for sick parents, grandparents or for siblings. Developing a sense of the numbers involved in caring is difficult since there are problems of definition and in identifying those involved – especially in those countries where many children drop out of school early. In the UK the strategy document *Caring for Carers* (DoH 1999) estimated that there are between 20,000 and 50,000 young carers many of whom received no support at all from statutory or voluntary services. Ten thousand children were estimated to have parents who suffered from mental illness.

Worldwide, large numbers of children are providing care in families experiencing AIDS related illness or where one or both parents have died from the illness. In addition to the strains on mental health imposed by the illness or the loss of parents a high proportion of such households are experiencing serious levels of poverty which also has consequences for mental health. Carers in such situations are more likely to be girls and unable to stay in school, and it may also be difficult for any younger siblings to continue in school because of the financial situation. Even in countries with well developed social and education provision, young people who are providing major support can be unrecognized. They may be reluctant to talk about family situations even though changes in school attendance and performance may give some hints of difficulties. While children may gain positively in a number of ways from caring, many negative effects have been identified from research:

- problems at school;
- isolation from children of the same age and other family members;
- lack of time for play, sport or other leisure activities;
- conflict between the needs of persons being helped and their own needs, leading to feelings of guilt and resentment;
- feeling that there is no one there for them, that professionals do not listen to them;
- lack of recognition, praise or respect for their contributions;
- feeling that they are different from other children and unable to be part of groups;
- feeling that no one else understands their experience.

(DoH 1999: 76, 78)

The additional problems experienced by young carers from ethnic minorities included:

- families are less likely to contact social services for fear that children will be taken away;
- they are more likely to be excluded from school;
- they are often expected to take responsibility for interpreting for the person being cared for regardless of whether they understand the issue or whether it is appropriate for their age.

Physical environmental influences

These include the prevailing geographical and natural influences and also those aris-ing from disasters, whether or not these are naturally caused. In the case of the former there are factors associated with urban or with rural living. In Western coun-tries there has been some tendency to idealize rural living and to see negative influ-ences as more associated with urban living. Children living in rural communities can be socially isolated from a great deal and as noted from Zambia orphan children in rural areas are less likely than those in urban ones to be enrolled in school (Bellamy 2001).

While access to water and sanitation may not immediately appear to be related to mental health it can be argued that they do play an important role. In those countries where water has to be fetched, often from significant distances, young children can be involved in the task alongside their mothers. This can take away opportunities for play and also can impact on school attendance or the capacity to benefit from it when tired. Lack of regular sources of clean water and sanitation facilities are related to higher levels of diarrhoeal and other diseases which can, if experienced frequently, impact on children's capacities to learn.

The influence of the built environment on health is discussed fully in Chapter 5 and that discussion is relevant to this chapter. We can specially note the importance of traffic which places barriers to children's capacity to play except in designated play-grounds and parks. Article 31 of the Convention on the Rights of a Child requires that governments recognize the right of children to 'engage in play and recreational activ-ities'. As Tranter and Doyle (1996: 86) remind us 'the highest justification of play is the joy of the spirit. It requires no extrinsic justification'. It is also seen as vital to early child development and mental health.

Individual factors

These include biological and congenital factors, physical health, specific competencies and behavioural determinants. Physical health is intimately related to mental health throughout life. Before birth there is evidence that the foetus responds to what is hap-pening to the mother and this, together with the birth experience, can impact on the infant's earliest interactions with the world. Children who have congenital disorders or who develop early physical health problems may not be able to interact optimally in the first stage of life, which impacts on early attachments. Prolonged malnutrition in childhood has been shown to be a risk factor for psycho-social development as well as for physical health (WHO 1999). Children with long-lasting physical health problems are especially vulnerable. In 2001 it was reported that 1.3 million children under the age of 15 years were living with HIV/AIDS (Bellamy 2001). In some countries such children are subject to severe discrimination and social isolation, increasing the challenges to their mental health.

Models of mental health typically include specific attributes of people which act as determinants of mental health including self-concept and self-esteem, coping skills and resilience. Self-esteem is the value placed on the self-concept. High self-esteem according to Mann et al. (2004), who have reviewed fully the links between self-esteem and mental health, is not only a key dimension of mental health but also acts as a protective buffer against negative influences. Young children can experience a full range of life events – bereavement; parental separation and divorce; transition to school; serious illness; and movements from one country to another. Such changes can all present challenges to achieving and maintaining mental health, with some children being more resilient than others.

Various lifestyle behaviours such as exercise impact on mental health. In infancy and earliest childhood behaviours are governed to a great extent by others but gradually the child has some control. Compared with later periods in life there are fewer factors to consider, although diet, physical activity and early encounters with drugs and alcohol are relevant as childhood progresses. Arguably the most important behaviour in infancy and early childhood is that of play, through which there is the potential for the child to build mental health.

Box 4.3 Summary points on determinants of health

- Determinants operate at differing levels: individual; family; community; societal.
- Determinants interact in such a way as to enhance or to reduce mental health.
- The relative impact of individual determinants differs. Poverty and its consequences is generally agreed to be a major determinant.

Evidence on mental vulnerability in childhood

While the majority of children are mentally healthy, an important percentage have one or more mental health problems and a large number of children live in situations which pose considerable challenges to the achievement of mental health, as described in the previous section. They can become vulnerable as a result of a very specific circumstance such as bereavement, or through the prevailing experience of living with one or more of the many challenges to mental health. In adopting a public health approach to mental health consideration of whole populations is necessary to identify those parts of the population who are relatively well protected as well as those groups who are relatively vulnerable. There are also individual children outside specific vulnerable groups who, for various reasons, are placed in vulnerable circumstances and whose situations also need to be recognized by relevant services.

All children experience vulnerability at some time or other, while some can be said to be vulnerable for most of their childhood. Individuals, or groups of children who are defined as vulnerable, rarely have one area of vulnerability. Choosing the most appropriate way to designate vulnerable groups is not easy. Broad categories such as children experiencing social inequalities can be used or more specific categories such as children acting as carers or experiencing violence. In commenting on any designated groups of children the full complexities of their situations have to be borne in mind.

Whether or not children in vulnerable situations develop positive mental health depends to some extent on the presence of protective factors. In challenging circumstances many children's mental health is protected. Key protective factors have been identified. For example, License (2005) reports the evidence for the following factors (based on *Bright Futures* (Mental Health Foundation 1999) and the Wells et al. (2001) review):

- individual emotional resilience;
- confidence in individual sense of personal value;
- supportive relationships within the family and in the wider community;
- social inclusion;
- a healthy social and economic environment;
- the existence of at least one good parent–child relationship and affection within the family; and
- authoritative discipline.

Children's views on mental health and well-being

Taking children's views into account is a general principle of health promotion and is recognized in Article 12 of the Convention on the Rights of the Child (United Nations 1989), which 'States parties shall assure to the child who is capable of forming his or her own views the right to express those views freely in all matter affecting the child, the views of the child being given due weight in accordance with age and maturity' (Flekkøy and Kaufman 1997: 150). While there are differences of views about when children have achieved adequate maturity for such participation it can be argued that some exploration of children's ideas is possible, using appropriate methods, at least from the age of language development, if not earlier. Although there is a growing literature which reports on dialogue with children about health very little has focused on what we can broadly describe as mental health. The *Bright Futures* report (Mental Health Foundation 1999) involved children in an inquiry which focused on mental health problems rather than positive mental health with 400 submissions obtained from children under 10 years. Evaluations of the UK Healthy School Award included information from interviews with primary age pupils on health, including mental health (Warwick et al. 2005). Children understood health to include physical and emotional well-being and healthy schools were places in which there was a non-bullying environment and there are people to talk to about problems. In addition to understanding how children conceptualize mental health, their views on the physical and social aspects of the environment which affect their health are also important.

Evidence of effective mental health promotion interventions: 0–5 and 6–12 years

This division of discussion into two age bands broadly mirrors the pre-school and formal education years while recognizing that the precise age for entering formal education differs between countries. Evidence has been drawn from systematic reviews, other commentary reviews and from individual studies which have been evaluated carefully. Programmes and activities which have been less fully evaluated but which indicate areas of good mental health promotion practice are discussed in a later section.

From 0 to 5 years

Ensuring the promotion of mental health of children in this age group cannot take place in isolation from the promotion of the health of parents and others who are involved as major caregivers. Activities to prepare parents for childbirth and the post-natal period are designed to promote adult mental health and also to enable parents to promote the mental well-being of their children. These programmes are also discussed in Chapter 6 and references in this chapter are mainly to child health outcomes. Much of the published evidence in this age group is drawn from studies of children who could be described as vulnerable, with fewer studies reporting on the promotion of positive mental health in children in more advantaged situations. Many of the evaluated studies were carried out in the USA and involved at-risk groups rather than population groups.

Community wide programmes

The UK Sure Start programme is a major UK Government programme designed to support families with children under 4 years and their communities in disadvantaged areas (Sure Start 2005). It includes 524 individual programmes each designed to be autonomous with services owned and determined by local communities. It drew on the positively evaluated Headstart programme in the USA (Schweinhart and Weikart 1980). Sure Start takes an holistic approach to child health and integrates early education, play, child health care, family support and preparation for parental employment. Parents can participate fully in developing the goals and activities within local Sure Start programmes. An illustrative account of one programme is provided in Box 4.4.

Box 4.4   Case study: a Sure Start programme in Leeds, UK

Situated in inner city Leeds the programme focused on tackling the housing issues facing young families. Fortnightly drop-in sessions were arranged for parents to meet with housing staff, to discuss a range of issues from completion of housing forms to housing improvements. One particular issue which emerged was the provision of fencing to secure play areas for young children, and necessary changes were implemented. Housing staff also held monthly walkabout sessions giving families an opportunity to draw attention to environmental problems such as litter, rubbish tipping or inadequate lighting. Families' sense of self-esteem, social participation and mental well-being were promoted through helping to resolve some local environmental health issues.

Social isolation and loneliness are factors influencing mental health addressed by the programme. Sure Start also works with individual parents on an outreach basis and this work is evolving to include work with asylum seekers. It may be the first contact that asylum seeker families experience in the UK, other than meetings with the Home Office or other authorities. The Sure Start team has been able to make a unique contribution to families' lives. It has promoted mental health through developing trust, responding flexibly to needs and beginning to address the social alienation that 'hard to reach' families can experience.

> In common with other Sure Start programmes parents are involved at many levels within the organizational structure of the programme. This strong involvement has taken time to establish but has enabled parents not only to make sure that appropriate services are developed but also increased confidence and assertiveness and opened up job opportunities within the local area. Outcomes, identified from a comprehensive evaluation of the programme, include aspects of parents' mental health which may impact on children's mental health development. Long-term outcomes are unknown at this early stage.
>
> (*Joy Walker, 2005 Leeds Metropolitan University* 2005)

Extensive national and local levels evaluation of Sure Start have been carried out. The first reports from the national evaluation were available at the end of 2005. Only a limited impact of Sure Start was detected and this was often restricted to specific sub-populations (Ward 2005). Children of teenage mothers and from one parent households or workless households scored lower than in the control areas. It was possible, the evaluators concluded, that the utilization of the Sure Start services by those with greater human capital left others with less access to services than in non-Sure Start areas. Concerns have been expressed about the early findings and the contrast with positive reports emerging from local evaluations. Issues have also been raised about the difficulties of evaluating this type of programme and generating the hard evidence that some people require. The local evaluations combining qualitative and quantitative data provide a richer insight into the impact of Sure Start on children and their families and communities. The results from the ongoing national evaluations will be watched with interest.

Preparation for parenting

Infants need food, shelter, opportunities for social interaction and the formation of strong emotional bonds. It is the role of parents and other caregivers to provide these. Programmes offering preparation for the transition to parenthood and the care of infants are promoted widely. In addition there are programmes for parents who are seen to be vulnerable or parenting in difficult circumstances. It would be good health promotion practice to identify and respond to parents' expressed needs in designing programmes but they are frequently professionally determined and do not always accord with expressed needs (Crowley 2005).

Programmes have been widely implemented in many countries and can be provided in community locations, through home visiting or combinations of the two. Some have been rigorously evaluated and participants followed up over for several years – even to early adulthood. They have involved low income mothers, families with a first child, teenage mothers, families where there are health problems or other risk situations such as the likelihood of abuse. Many well publicized programmes have used health professionals but others have used mothers from the local community. Activities include various kinds of education and training, counselling, support and health monitoring. One example of a home-based programme is a two year programme which provided education and support for disadvantaged adolescents in a first pregnancy, and involved home visits by trained nurses (Olds et al. 1988, 2002). Participants and their children showed a range of positive outcomes compared with those in a control group. This programme has been replicated elsewhere in the USA and in other countries.

The California Abecedarian Project (Ramsey et al. 1998) was a centre-based day care programme for children between the ages of 0 and 5 years in high risk families defined by low education and income and a history of family and psychological difficulties. The programme focused on language, cognitive, perceptual–motor and social development, and nutrition. Compared with children in a control group the IQ scores in the intervention group were at normal levels. Impact on primary school performance also occurred, up to the age of 12 years, following the extension of the intervention into school age.

The American High/Scope Perry Preschool Project (Schweinhart and Weikart 1998) is a well publicized project for children beyond infancy involving Afro-American children between the ages of 3 and 4 from disadvantaged backgrounds. It has been used in many Headstart programmes. It combines a weekly half day pre-school intervention and home visits over a two year period. Long-term follow ups into early adulthood have been reported with positive impacts in comparison with a control group, on cognitive development, school achievement and completion and fewer conduct problems and arrests. This project has provided good evidence on the long-term impact of early and appropriate intervention.

A number of parenting programmes, support mechanisms and pre-school programmes have demonstrated success in higher income countries in reducing violence towards infants and children. There is, to date, a lack of strong evaluations of interventions in low income countries. Some USA studies have also shown that parenting support programmes can be cost-effective if they involve children in disadvantaged families or with special needs.

The above programmes used professionals but others have drawn on community resources. A good example is the Community Mothers' Programme in the Republic of Ireland, discussed more fully in Chapter 6. The children of the participants in the community mothers' programme were likely to have received all their immunizations; to have been read to daily; to have played more cognitive games; and to have been exposed to more nursery rhymes (Johnson et al. 1993). In a follow up study after 7 years (Johnson et al. 2000), a number of positive outcomes were reported and the conclusions were that the intervention improved several aspects of childrearing in the first year, the benefits were not only to intervention children but also to subsequent ones and some benefits were sustained over several years.

Physical health

Programmes which address physical health can be measured by mental health as well as physical health outcomes. Activities which address the nutritional needs of vulnerable children are important since malnutrition is a risk factor for physical and mental health. Programmes in various parts of the world have used low cost community health workers recruited locally and combined nutritional and educational advice. The Integrated Child Development Scheme in India has reached 17 million children since it was set up in 1975 (Patel et al. 2004). This is a holistic early childhood and development programme addressing the inter-related needs of children and adolescent girls and women from disadvantaged communities. The greatest impact has been achieved through interventions combining nutritional and psycho-social elements. In many countries the provision of breakfast for children should also be evaluated in mental health as well as physical health terms.

Box 4.5   Summary points on interventions with 0–5-year-olds

- There is good evidence of effective outcomes from parenting programmes with at-risk children, including some evidence of cost-effectiveness in US studies.
- Home visiting programmes have been implemented in a number of countries and are effective when community volunteers are used.
- Community wide programmes in disadvantaged communities of the Sure Start type are evaluated well by users but the evidence is not yet available of their impact on the communities where they are implemented.

6–12 years

The school is widely seen as a major way to reach children in this age group, while at the same time the mental health promotion needs of children unable to enrol in school must not be overlooked. Theoretically health promoting schools include the building of links between schools and communities and should therefore reach out of school children. In general, however, most 'out of school' children are more likely to be reached through other community activities. Settings in which children can also be involved include places of religious worship, health centres and, in many countries, the workplace.

Environmental actions to facilitate mental health promotion in this age group

Creating environments that promote all aspects of health is one of the five pillars of the Ottawa Charter. Evidence of the impact of environmental health changes on health is less developed than that for some other aspects of health promotion. In many countries children have participated in projects designed to enable them to highlight issues about their environments and to identify appropriate actions in response. Such participation has been identified with mental health gains. A good example of such projects is 'Growing up in Cities', a participatory action research project which involved children between 10 and 15 years in low income environments in a number of countries. Griesel et al. (2004) reported on the evaluation of the project in two areas of Johannesburg (see Box 4.6). Through a multi-method approach the project evaluation sought to examine the claims in the literature (Hart 1997) that active participation of children is associated with gains in self-esteem; locus of control and self-efficacy; increased sense of responsibilities for communities; improved communication and problem-solving skills; and awareness and appreciation of democratic processes. The evaluation aimed to measured impacts on self-esteem, locus of control and self-efficacy, and to gather qualitative information from children and parents. The qualitative results demonstrated that children had benefited from the programme as seen from their own and their parents' perspectives. They had an enhanced awareness of their environment and a greater sense of rights and abilities to express views and take actions to improve living conditions. However, these benefits were not matched by changes on the psychometric measures. In addition to questioning the reliability of the measures used the cultural relevance of the concepts was queried.

Box 4.6   Growing up in cities

The Project worked in two areas of the city: Canaan, an urban squatter camp, and Ferreirasdorp, a high rise complex inhabited mostly by Indian families. In both areas children participated in a number of activities:

- drawing their homes and neighbourhoods;
- walks to show researchers aspects of their environments;
- role plays;
- group activities to identify problems and propose changes;
- songs and games.

The outcomes of their work were presented to city officials and action plans developed. Before plans for Canaan could be implemented the community was forcibly evicted and relocated to open land 40km away. The project continued to work with the children and a children's centre and playground were developed in response to their expressed needs.

There are growing concerns in some countries about environmental safety leading to reduced opportunities for children to experience play outside the home and to learn to cope with risks. As Colin Ward (1990, in Tranter and Doyle 1996: 81) said: 'One should be able to play everywhere, easily, loosely and not forced into a playground or "park". A truly child friendly city should be one big playground'. The city of Munich has attempted to respond in stating that it should be a 'playable city' where the entire environment is conducive to children's play rather then simply in playgrounds (Moore 1986). Across Europe there have been many initiatives to reclaim streets as play areas along the lines of the Home Zone project described below. Providing safe walking routes to school; opportunities for safer cycling; play areas which are perceived to be safe; and immediate environments where traffic hazards are reduced have all been identified as necessary. Home Zones is a widespread movement in the Netherlands, Denmark and Germany (Biddulph 2001) that has more recently been introduced into the UK and is one response to the need for social spaces, which fits with health promotion principles. The description of an example of a Home Zone programme can be seen in Box 4.7.

Box 4.7   Living in a Home Zone and children's mental health

The Methleys is an inner city neighbourhood in a northern city in England and one of nine national pilot Home Zone schemes created in the UK. Home Zones are part of the UK Government's policy to ensure the road space is shared between drivers and other road users with the wider needs of residents in mind, including children's play and those who walk and cycle in the area (DTLR 2001a, b). The aim of creating a Home Zone is to change the way that streets are used and to improve the quality of life in residential areas by making them greener environments and places where people, rather than traffic, have priority. This was important in the Methleys' neighbourhood, which mainly consists of dense housing with very small gardens or yards and little space in which children can play. Children have participated actively throughout the creation of the Home Zone, expressing views on how the area should look and creating artwork for street signs and bricks used in the streetscape. They have lobbied MPs in Westminster; undertaken a fact finding visit to Home Zones in Holland; and even threatened to take the city council to court if they failed to provide a safer environment in which to live. The social cohesion in the community has given local children a stake in their area, as one 7-year-old girl living in the neighbourhood said: 'I think the Home Zone is good . . . and I like my street. I've got lots of friends here. I like riding my roller blades'.

   The Home Zone has altered children's perceptions of how their street can be used. The green spaces help provide traffic calming and a safer environment permitting a wider range of activities and play. Improving the quality and attractiveness of an environment where children live and play can potentially promote mental health by adding to their sense of positive well-being. One 11-year-old boy summed up the mental health benefits felt by children: 'It's really peaceful around here and you don't get any hassle'.

   (Joy Walker, Leeds Metropolitan University. Further reading and weblinks: http://www.homezones.org/homeZUKmethleys.htm http://www.methleys.org.uk)

Community programmes

Child to Child

This programme straddling school and community, has been implemented in more than 80 countries and involves health and education workers in partnership. Initially it was set up in developing countries to enable young children aged 7 to 10 years with caring responsibilities for their siblings to do this in health protective and health promoting ways. It was embedded in the concept of primary health care (see Chapter 3), the idea of children as agents of change, and the importance of partnerships for health. According to Pridmore and Stephens (2000) a delicate balance was sought between encouraging children's altruism and exploiting their roles as parent substitutes although this had not always been achieved. The early focus of the programme on the education of siblings broadened to recognize the power of children to influence their peers, their families and the community. Evaluation was not a major element in the early years but has now increased (Pridmore and Stephens 2000). The reports on specific mental health have been limited but one evaluation study carried out in Uganda indicated that Child to Child was successful in developing self-concept and children's behaviour towards each other.

School-based programmes

The school's role in the promotion of health initially focused on education for health and in offering health services. With the development of the health promotion movement the school as key health promoting setting has been widely communicated and programmes have been set up across the world (WHO 1993, 1996, 1997). A health promoting school constantly strengthens its capacity as a healthy setting for living, learning and working (WHO 1997). Health promoting schools focus on policies, the school environment, the formal and informal curriculum, **hidden curriculum** and school–community partnerships. Some countries have developed Healthy Schools Awards where schools can set goals and chart their progress towards the achievement of health promoting schools. A specific aspect of health such as mental health can be chosen as a starting point for developing a health promoting school or all aspects of health can be addressed from the outset. Figure 4.3 illustrates the various elements of mental health promotion within a health promoting school.

Not all evaluations of health promoting schools (HPSs) have provided specific reports on mental health outcomes. One which did was the HEA European Network of Health Promoting Schools evaluation study (Jamison et al. 1996). Levels of self-esteem rose in most schools but more in primary than secondary schools with some pilot schools showing greater gains than the reference schools. Pupils in pilot schools

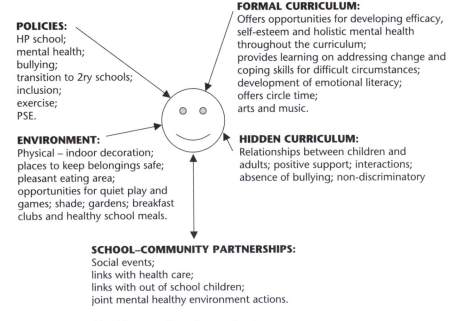

POLICIES:
HP school;
mental health;
bullying;
transition to 2ry schools;
inclusion;
exercise;
PSE.

FORMAL CURRICULUM:
Offers opportunities for developing efficacy, self-esteem and holistic mental health throughout the curriculum; provides learning on addressing change and coping skills for difficult circumstances; development of emotional literacy; offers circle time; arts and music.

ENVIRONMENT:
Physical – indoor decoration; places to keep belongings safe; pleasant eating area; opportunities for quiet play and games; shade; gardens; breakfast clubs and healthy school meals.

HIDDEN CURRICULUM:
Relationships between children and adults; positive support; interactions; absence of bullying; non-discriminatory

SCHOOL–COMMUNITY PARTNERSHIPS:
Social events;
links with health care;
links with out of school children;
joint mental healthy environment actions.

Figure 4.3 A mental health promoting primary school

were less likely to be bullies. Simple changes which involved pupils in planning and development had a significant impact on pupil behaviours and self-esteem.

More recently results from the UK National Healthy School Standard (NHSS) evaluation have been reported (Schagen et al. 2005; Warwick et al. 2005). The programme is aimed at all schools and local education authorities are accredited to take part. It is based on the philosophy of the health promoting school and has three main aims:

- to reduce health inequalities;
- to promote social inclusion; and
- to raise levels of pupil achievement through school improvement.

Schools can participate at three levels of intensity, each of which is certificated. The evaluation compared schools who had achieved Level 3 with comparison schools using national data sets from the Health Related Behaviour Questionnaire (HRBQ) (Balding 2002) and school inspection (Ofsted) data. The HRBQ showed that pupils in primary schools at Level 3 differed in only two respects from comparison schools, one of which was mental health related. Children were less likely to be afraid of school due to bullying. No significant difference was found on the self-esteem scores. Ofsted data are derived from school inspections where all aspects of school life are assessed on 11 seven point scales. The scales included to a number of social inclusion indicators relevant to the NHSS, in particular emotional well-being, behaviour and participation. On the basis of data from 7666 primary schools, one-third of which were at Level 3, a significant relationship was found between being at Level 3 before inspection and scores on 10 of the 11 scales with a particularly strong relationship with the provision of personal, social and health education (PSHE).

In an Australian study, Stewart et al. (2004) reported on the success of health promoting primary schools in developing resilience. Children at ages 8, 10 and 12 years in 20 schools were studied as part of a three year multi-strategy health promotion project in low socio-economic catchment areas. Data were also collected from staff and parents. Resilience was measured by use of a modified version of the California Healthy Kids Survey which asks questions about feelings at home and school. Parents and caregivers provided information about school and family climates and school staff reported on organizational factors relevant to the HPS approach. The results of the study suggested that the development of student resilience; feelings of connectedness to adults and teachers; having good peer relationships and a strong sense of autonomy and self-capacity; and parental recognition of a supportive school environment were influenced by the degree to which schools supported and applied a 'health promoting school' environment and approach.

Most commentators argue for whole-school approaches to mental health promotion whether or not these are part of designated health promoting schools or Healthy School Award schemes (Weare 2004). If a number of aspects of school experience act to reduce mental health the introduction of projects specifically designed to enhance it in one part of the curriculum cannot be expected to have major impact. Nonetheless much of the evidence on school mental health promotion comes from studies outside the context of health promoting schools or whole-school approaches.

There has been a series of systematic reviews of mental health promotion in schools and Green et al. (2005) have also drawn together the 322 studies included in eight previous reviews (Hodgson et al. 1995; Durlak and Wells 1997; Tilford et al. 1997; Haney and Durlak 1998; Lister-Sharp et al. 1999 (two reviews); Wells et al. 2001; CASEL 2003). All reviews included primary school children alongside older groups. Green et al. (2005) noted that the majority of interventions in the reviews were classroom-based studies implemented from single schools through to a national basis. Programmes focused on a variety of outcomes including: problem-solving skills; promotion of self-esteem; bullying and violence prevention; reduction of aggressive behaviours; and coping with stressful experiences and educational transitions. Some were specifically designed for children at high risk of poor social and emotional health. Whole-school approaches and family community partnerships were in the minority in the studies reviewed. Green et al. (2005) reported that the eight reviews concluded that school-based mental health promotion interventions can be effective and individual reviewers had commented on various characteristics of effective interventions:

- aimed at the promotion of mental health as opposed to the prevention of mental illness (Wells et al. 2001);
- aimed at promoting positive mental health and involving changes in the school climate rather than brief class-based and person-centred programmes (Durlak and Wells 1997; Wells et al. 2001);
- were implemented continuously for more than a year (Wells et al. 2001);
- went beyond practice in the classroom and created consistent opportunities for applying the learned skill (CASEL 2003);
- replicated positive behavioural implementations in different sites and sustained them over time (CASEL 2003);
- adopted a health promoting schools approach (Lister-Sharp et al. 1999).

Culturally relevant programmes

Many mental health promotion programmes have been developed without any particular reference to their cross-cultural relevance. *Zippy's friends* is an example of a project designed to be relevant to young children in differing countries and cultures (Bale and Mishara 2004). Designed for all 6–7-year-olds, not just at-risk populations, the programme teaches coping skills on a one hour a week basis over 24 weeks. Children are taught to deal with everyday difficulties; identify and talk about feelings; and role play dealing with situations. The programme emphasizes children's abilities to learn, adapt and improve skills and to be helpful and supportive of others. As Bale and Mishara point out, this contrasts with the individualistic focus of those programmes that emphasize personal competence over collective involvement. Evaluations from Lithuania and Denmark report that children in the programme compared with those not involved used more, and more effective, coping strategies; had improved social skills; and exhibited less problem behaviours. Teachers report positive impact on classroom environments and improved student–teacher relationships. They also report that children become better at dealing with conflicts.

Anti-bullying interventions

There have now been a variety of such programmes and they have been included in both systematic and commentary reviews of mental health promotion. Twenty-three model interventions were reviewed by Roberts and Hinton-Nelson (1996, in Stevens et al. 2001: 156) who identified characteristics of good model programmes:

- they should be founded on a theoretical framework or guiding philosophy which provides theoretical evidence on how the programmes can improve situations;
- those which recognize the social environments of children are more successful than those focusing only on individual determinants;
- they should include intensive collaboration with specialized services and make efforts to reduce barriers to access for children at risk;
- they should provide detailed information about monitoring and outcome data;
- they can be replicated or adapted to other settings.

An example of a whole-school Bullying Prevention Programme which was developed in Norway and replicated in other countries is that of Olweus (1989, 1993). Designed for children between 6 and 15 years the study is also relevant to the following chapter. It was designed to reduce problems both within and outside the school, prevent new problems occurring and reduce opportunities and rewards for bullying. Significant reductions in reported bullying and victimization and antisocial behaviour and an improved social climate were achieved.

Children experiencing major life events

Some countries have developed programmes for children experiencing difficult life events, especially divorce. One carefully evaluated programme in the US was organized in small mixed sex groups over 10 weeks and focused on the expression of feelings and sharing of experiences, cognitive skill building, and anger expression and control. Positive outcomes for programme children when compared with controls were recorded: decreases in anxiety; increase in competencies; and less negative self-attitudes (Pedro-Carroll et al. 1992). This study demonstrated that positive gains can be achieved through specially targeted programmes. Recent meta-analyses of programmes for children experiencing divorce also concluded that the various programmes have reported positive outcomes (Durlak and Wells 1997; Stathakos and Roehrle 2003). According to Stathakos and Roehrle best results were obtained from programmes initiated within two years of a divorce, with no more than ten sessions of 60–75 minutes and medium sized groups tended to be more effective than small ones. Rather than targeted programmes for at-risk children the preferred school-based approach in some countries would be for a whole-school programme to develop general coping strategies for life events with such programmes complemented by additional pastoral support, as needed.

Children in health care settings

The impact of physical health problems on mental health was discussed earlier. Parallel to the idea of health promoting schools is that of health promoting hospitals. Such a hospital will address mental and physical health through all its dimensions. Evaluations of initiatives to develop such hospitals have been produced although the evidence in relation to child mental health is limited. Within health services there has been a greater readiness to involve children in the decisions relating to their health even at ages where cognitive development theorists might challenge their capabilities to do so. As Thurston and Church stress (2001: 229) a new pragmatic approach is needed towards how we view children and childhood. The emphasis on protecting the child from responsibility and maintaining dependence has to be questioned.

Box 4.8   Summary of evidence for the age group 6–12 years

- There has been widespread adoption of the health promoting school settings approach and evidence that such schools can impact positively on mental health.
- There is evidence what whole-school approaches to mental health promotion are the most effective.
- Efforts to promote positive mental health such as competence enhancement and resilience development can be effective.
- Various programmes with at-risk children experiencing life events such as divorce have been shown to be effective.
- To date, a relatively small part of research evidence has come from low income countries.

International and national policy impacting on child mental health

In theory virtually all areas of public policy can impact in some way on the mental health of children whether or not the links are made explicit. Policies specifically labelled as mental health and originating mainly from the health sector frequently tend to focus on illness rather than on positive mental health. In order to make a sustained effect on mental health the relevant policy areas need to work in partnership.

International

Policies which explicitly address mental health of children as well as those which address its social determinants are relevant. The World Health Organization is a major international influence on specific health policy. Its statements are not binding but it can influence dialogue and the development of policy within countries. It regularly examines all aspects of child health and its promotion, including mental health. More recently statements on mental health have secured greater prominence. Where school age children are concerned the WHO has called on all countries to take up the Health Promoting Schools concept and it is reasonable to assume it has influenced the take up by countries worldwide. A recent initiative has seen the publication of a number of documents on mental health which set an agenda and provide a summary of the evidence of mental health promotion interventions.

Given the links between social disadvantage and mental health indicators, strategies to reduce disadvantage and achieve greater equity are of major importance. Strategies proposed to reduce poverty include various types of debt release tied to specific actions within countries and more and better aid and efforts to increase the fairness of world trade. The millennium goals listed in Chapter 3 provide a point of reference for countries although progress towards them is slower than projected.

Policy which addresses the rights of children is an important influence on many activities which bear on children's mental health. The key document is the United Nations Convention of the Rights of the Child (United Nations 1989) which is legally binding and to which 102 countries were signatories by 2003. It addresses conventional issues relating to children such as welfare and protection but also focuses on less usual ones such as participation and citizenship rights. While widely supported it has also been criticized for assuming the 'universality of a free-standing, individual child who is to be protected and socialized into a culture according to liberal democratic principles' (Stevens 1995, in Griesel et al. 2004: 282). An alternative document has been produced for Africa, the *African Charter on the Rights and Welfare of the Child*, which takes into consideration both rights and responsibilities and came into force in 2000.

National

Parallel with the international domain there are policies specifically designated as mental health plus other policies which impact directly or indirectly on children's mental health. Policy actions can be designed to influence the mental health of all children or vulnerable groups. Aynsley-Green et al. (2000) have said that there is an urgent need for children and adolescents to be explicitly recognized at all levels of health policy. In all aspects of health promotion there have been comments about the lack of active involvement of children in identifying needs and planning initiatives. As noted by Hart-Zeldin (1990, in Kalnins et al. 2002: 224), 'policy documents typically address the health needs of children in terms of directives of what must be done *for* children, not *with* children'.

In the UK it is the Children's National Service Framework which is most relevant to this chapter (DoH 2004). This sets out a vision and 11 national standards designed to lead to general health improvement, redress health inequalities and improve the quality of services for children. Standard 9 specifically focuses on mental health and ill health although most of the other standards can be linked, in some way, to mental health. The Framework is a ten year programme which requires substantial changes in various areas of practice. It provides evidence-based guidelines for practice which will require multi-agency responses.

Given the very strong links between social inequalities and mental health major emphasis is required on policies designed to achieve greater equity and reduction of inequalities. Countries will differ on what are seen to be key areas for action. In the UK the Government since 1997 has made efforts to reduce child poverty setting a goal of halving child poverty by 2010 (where poverty is defined as children living in households earning less than 60 per cent of median income). While there is evidence that child poverty has been reduced the target has not been fully reached (Ward 2006). In South Africa considerable importance is attached to policies which redress the inequities associated with apartheid history which will, of course, include policy designed to reduce child poverty (Johnson 2005).

There are other policy areas that are important for promoting mental health. Opportunities for one or both parents to spend time with their children, especially in infancy have been seen as important. Workplace policies to support maternity and paternity leave and financial arrangements which adequately provide for such leave are needed to allow one or both parents to have time with children in the earliest months. Many countries in the world have no such provision to support early parenthood but there are systems in place in others. In higher income countries an increasing proportion of women either wish to return promptly to the workplace after childbirth or are forced to do so through economic circumstances. Where there is a lack of high quality affordable child care available to support working parents the promotion of child mental health becomes more difficult. In the case of young teenage mothers who want to return to school, educational policy on this, together with appropriate childcare support, is needed. In low income countries there is often no choice about whether to work after childbirth, and little or no formal childcare support.

There has been a long-term recognition that many children arrive at school with limited experiences of those aspects of early learning seen as important for engagement in primary school. Education policy in many countries recognizes the importance of pre-school education and widening access to this but globally large numbers of children still have no access. Programmes of the UK Sure Start type, incorporated within public health policy, are potentially an important contributor to efforts to redress disadvantage. Other policies, if implemented adequately, can support parents in promoting early mental health: play, transport, public libraries, workplace and so on.

Good practice examples

In this section we will describe a few interventions that have not been subjected to the same degree of evaluation as studies discussed earlier. This may be because they are innovative projects and implemented on a small scale to date or from contexts where the resources have not been available for detailed evaluation. To be designated as good practice it is expected that projects recognize health promotion principles and are implemented with care and incorporate some critical reflection. The examples chosen are intended to be illustrative and they have been selected from a number of countries.

A media culture in the Maldives: for and about children

The Early Child Development Project used a multi-media approach to reach households across the 1200 islands of the Maldives. The aim was to create a media culture where children would be told they were valued; would see themselves regularly on the media; would be encouraged to express themselves; and would have their expressions valued from infancy. Following a survey of existing knowledge attitudes and practices materials were developed for children and their caregivers. They integrated child rights, with a focus on developing confidence and self-esteem, and on gender issues, including the use of reverse gender stereotypes, and the use children with disabilities in all materials (Bellamy 2001).

Effective parenting in Turkey

A mothers' training programme works in 24 provinces with mothers. Fathers, older siblings and grandparents join in the play activities for younger children. As a result of all family members contributing to an interactive and stimulating environment, children score better in language and development tests. Family environments are enhanced and one mother said: 'Now I am not hitting my child anymore. My husband is not hitting me either' (Bellamy 2001).

Working with refugees in the former republic of Macedonia

Children of pre-school refugee families from Kosovo were helped through a joint project between UNICEF and the Albanian League of Women: 150 volunteers were trained in community work, family visits, groups meetings and child development issues; 6500 families with 9000 children were reached with messages and materials about parenting under crisis. The emergency project improved the care and attention children were receiving in a difficult situation and also helped to identify children needing counselling. When the refugees returned to Kosovo the programme was adapted for the local rural Macedonian communities. In addition to gains for the children the project was seen to empower women as active decision-makers in the family and community – and so thereby enabling them to promote children's mental health (Bellamy 2001).

Community-based rehabiliation (CBR) programmes

Children with disabilities meet challenges in achieving mental health. CBR programmes in many low income countries have worked to change attitudes to disability and provided help and support through volunteers working with parents and teachers. In Jordan, for example, the CBR project works to change attitudes towards disabilities encouraging parents to recognize disabilities and seek help. The project is a part of a national effort to improve parenting in the home and uses young women volunteers who work closely with young children. The knowledge and skills of all caregivers concerning child rights and the physical, emotional and psychological needs of children are increased. Significant changes in areas where the project is working have been recorded: parents seek assistance; children are integrated into schools; and local attitudes towards the rights of people with special needs have changed (Bellamy 2001).

Books for young children

Making books available to children from infancy onwards is important – not simply for developing literacy. For younger children sharing the activity of looking at a book with another person can be important in relationship building. Stories can allow children to be exposed to experiences and the ways to cope with them. This can develop understanding of others who may be having such experiences – loss, new brother or sister, divorce of parents, etc. and provide some preparation for similar experiences. A new scheme in the UK is to provide all pre-school children with a small selection of books. The child to child readers mentioned earlier are an example of making books available to young children.

Training of teachers

For teachers to be able to promote mental health they may need further training. In South Africa with especially high levels of gender-based violence (GBV) a pilot project was developed to incorporate work on gender-based violence in the primary school curriculum. The project was evaluated in five schools within Cape Town. Teachers attended eight 2 hour sessions and received classroom materials. Two training models were used: a whole-school approach where staff across the school were involved in the training; and a train the trainers model where those initially trained went on to train colleagues. The training focused on identifying and challenging teachers' knowledge and attitudes on gender and GBV, reflections on the messages they were giving out to pupils and developing strategies for addressing the issue in schools. The programme was initially evaluated at teacher level. After the training teachers demonstrated a positive change in attitudes to gender and GBV; a greater appreciation of the role of schools in addressing it; and increased confidence to undertake relevant teaching in the classroom. The whole-school approach to training was more effective than the 'train the trainer' (Dreyer et al. 2001).

The application of health promotion theory and principles to mental health promotion practice

In the previous chapter we outlined a number of health promotion principles including active participation of communities and individuals in the setting up and implementation of programmes, redressing inequalities and developing empowerment. We will comment on each in turn as they relate to mental health promotion in childhood.

In infancy and very early childhood there are constraints associated with stage of development which impose limits on active participation in decision-making about activities. At the same time adults have particular responsibilities in ensuring that the rights to participate in line with capacity are fostered from the earliest age. Of particular importance, therefore, are those interventions in the antenatal and postnatal period which ensure that parents and other major caregivers gain understanding of the child as an active participant in the developmental process and seek to support this. Some mental health promotion programmes do facilitate the active participation of children while others can be top–down and involve relatively low levels of participation. In a high proportion of the evaluation studies meeting criteria for inclusion in systematic reviews programmes have been professionally determined with little reported involvement of children in setting them up. In many instances it is probably appropriate to conclude that no dialogue with children took place. Mayall (2001: 198), in reflecting on schools, challenges us to think more fully about this process of participation:

> A healthy school would be one in which children acted as participants in the continuous process of improving the learning, social and physical environment. This approach differs from that proposed in some of the health promotion literature, in which damaging assumptions about children's immaturity, lack of knowledge and self esteem colour the discourse.

Reduction of health inequalities is a priority for health promotion. Significant and lasting effects require both international and national policy actions. Actions to reduce poverty are arguably the most urgent and securing full enrolment in education and attendance for the defined years also of great importance. While there is recognition of policy needs and examples of appropriate responses across countries can be listed the need continues for more action in order to begin to make a significant impact on health inequalities in children. Programmes such as the US Headstart, UK Sure Start and Healthy Promoting Schools programmes, which can be implemented widely across populations, have the greatest potential to make significant contributions to this goal if complemented by other healthy public policies.

Empowerment, as an outcome and as a process is a key principle of health promotion. Within the health promoting school health education in the curriculum should be consistent with this principle and also focus on positive health. In practice the goals of educational activity tend to be a mix of positive mental health outcomes plus those linked to primary and also secondary prevention, and the approaches adopted can be a mix of empowerment and preventive approaches.

There is a particular shortcoming of health education interventions which take place outside the context of a 'health promoting schools' or 'whole schools approach', namely that contextual influences may be insufficiently taken into consideration. Too often the achievement of mental health or the prevention of problems is located within the child rather than addressed within an eco-holistic framework.

Basing practice on evidence and theory is essential in enhancing mental health promotion. Earlier sections have illustrated the range of evidence available. Where theory is concerned, the situation is more complex. Many systematic reviews have made a point of recording the theory base of interventions but reviewers have also made the general point that too frequently there is little reporting of the theoretical underpinnings of an intervention. The theory used in a selection of interventions referred to in the book is specified in Appendix 1. Earlier we raised questions about applying theory developed in Western contexts across the world. There is a greater sensitivity to this as an issue and efforts are being made to develop culturally appropriate theory and practice but much progress has still to be made.

Conclusions

In this chapter we hoped to emphasize universal interventions focused on positive mental health and undertaken, where possible, in the context of health promoting settings. At the same time, in recognition of the variety of practice and the evidence available from evaluations we have included activities focusing on aspects of mental health that have not been undertaken within the context of settings or whole-school approaches. Some have been universal, but others were directed towards children who have been designated 'at risk'. Interventions have ranged from those which clearly applied key health promotion principles to those with a narrower health education focus.

Societies are increasingly multi-ethnic and multi-cultural and it has to be recognized that conceptions of mental health in childhood will differ and these differences will need to be understood and acknowledged in developing mental health promotion activities. At the same time difficult questions can arise in pluralist societies about values and practices in some groups which might be considered to place the mental health of children 'at risk'.

This chapter has considered the evidence for effective programmes in childhood. There is evidence from activities implemented on a universal basis as well as evidence for programmes with vulnerable groups. Although active efforts are being made to bring evidence together from countries across the world it is still the case that most disseminated evidence is drawn from programmes in a small number of higher income countries. We raised a few special issues for the chapter at the outset and can provide closing comments on these. In the case of inequalities in mental health the extent and nature of the problems is widely acknowledged and many proposals made for redressing problems at the global level. Although there have been improvements in some countries the inequities across the world remain large. Within specific countries there have been initiatives that have illustrated a commitment to improve mental health of disadvantaged children. At the outset we commented on the competing ideas about children and childhood some of which were very much in tune with empowerment models of health promotion. There are a growing number of policies and activities that now make tangible efforts to give children a participatory role in decisions about situations which affect them. At the same time there are many situations where the approach to children is top-down and authoritarian and their active involvement is not encouraged. In all parts of the world very large numbers of children are experiencing adverse circumstances which are barriers to achieving mental health. Many demonstrate high levels of resilience in the face of these circumstances but others are vulnerable to mental ill health or are experiencing problems. There is an urgent need for national and international action to improve the health of all the world's children.

Box 4.9   Questions to reflect on when considering mental health promotion for young children

- What images of children are presented in contemporary media? Are they consistent?
- To what extent are neighbourhoods with which you are familiar child friendly and contain the elements of a mental health promoting environment?
- What is effective parenting of small children?
- Why are schools so important in the promotion of the mental health of children between 6 and 12 years?
- What examples of efforts to involve young children as active partners in decision-making do you observe? What are the arguments for and against promoting such partnerships?
- What are the strengths and weaknesses of programme that adopt a risk reduction approach?
- Using the model of a mental health promoting school as a guide what would be present in a 'mental health promoting hospital for children'?
- Why are whole-school approaches to mental health recommended?
- Why is play so important in the life of young children?
- How would you draw on Piaget's theory of cognitive development in planning health promotion activities for young children?

References

Albee, G.W. and Ryan Finn, K.D. (1993) An overview of primary prevention, *Journal of Counsellng and Development*, 72(2): 115–23.

Aries, P. (1962) *Centuries of Childhood*. Harmondsworth: Penguin.

Aynsley-Green, A., Barker, M., Burr. S. et al. (2000) Who is speaking for children and adolescents and for their health at the policy level? *British Medical Journal*, 3231: 229–32.

Balding, J. (2002) Young people in 2001. 15,881 young people tell us about what they do at home, at school and with their friends, *Education and Health*, 20: 59–67.

Bale, C. and Mishara, B. (2004) Developing an international mental health promotion programme for young children, *International Journal of Mental Health Promotion*, 6(2): 12–16.

Bellamy, C. (2001) *The State of the World's Children 2000*. New York: UNICEF.

Bellamy, C. (2004) *The State of the World's Children*. New York: UNICEF.

Bellamy, C. (2005) The State of the World's Children. New York: UNICEF.

Biddulph, M. (2001) *Home Zones: A Planning and Design Handbook*. Bristol: Policy Press.

Bowlby, J. (1971) *Attachment and Loss*, Vol. 1. Harmondsworth: Penguin.

Bronfenbrenner, U. (1979) *The Ecology of Human Development: Experiments by Nature and Design*. Cambridge, MA: Harvard University Press.

Burman, E. (1997) Developmental psychology and its discontents, in D. Fox and I. Prilleltensky (eds) *Critical Psychology: An Introduction*. London: Sage Publications.

CASEL (2003) *Safe and Sound: An Educational Leader's Guide to Evidence Based Social and Emotional Learning Programs*. Chicago: The Collaborative for Academic, Social and

Emotional Learning (CASEL) in Cooperation with the Mid-Atlantic Region, University of Illinois in Chicago.

Chambers, R. and License, K. (2005) *Looking after Children in Primary Care*. Abingdon: Radcliffe Publishing.

Crowley, M. (2005) Working with parents, in R. Chambers and K. License (eds) *Looking After Children in Primary Care*. Oxford: Radcliffe Publishing.

Dahlberg, G., Moss, P. and Pence, A. (1999) *Beyond Quality in Early Childhood Education and Care: Postmodern Perspectives*. London: Falmer Books.

Dahlgren, O. and Whitehead, M. (1991) *Policies and Strategies to Promote Social Equity in Health*. Stockholm: Institute of Futures Studies.

Danziger, K. (1971) *Socialisation*. Harmondsworth: Penguin.

DoH (Department of Health) (1998) *Health Survey for England: The Health of Young People, 95–97*. London: The Stationery Office.

DoH (Department of Health) (1999) *Caring for Carers: A National Strategy for Carers*. London: The Stationery Office.

DoH (Department of Health) (2004) *Core Document, National Service Framework for Children, Young People and Maternity Services*. London: HMSO.

Dreyer, A., Kim, J. and Schaay, N. (2001) *What do We Want to Tell Our Children About Violence Against Women*. Johannesburg: Open Society Foundation for South Africa.

DTLR (Department for Transport Local Government and the Regions) (2001a) *Home Zone: Challenge, Guidance to Prospective Bidders*. London: HMSO.

DTLR (Department for Transport Local Government and the Regions) (2001b) *Home Zones and Quiet Lanes: Consultation on Statutory Guidance and Regulations*. London: HMSO.

Durlak, J.A. and Wells, A.M. (1997) Primary prevention mental health programs for children and adolescents: a meta-analytic review, *American Journal of Community Psychology*, 25(2): 115–38.

Erikson, E. (1963) *Childhood and Society*. New York: Norton.

Fekkes, M., Pijpers, F.I.M. and Verloove-Vanhorick, S.P. (2005) Bullying: who does what, when and where? Involvement of children, teachers and parents in bullying behaviour, *Health Education Research*, 20(1): 81–91.

Flekkøy, M.G. and Kaufman, N.H. (1997) *The Participation Rights of the Child. Rights and Responsibilities in Family and Society*. London: Jessica Kingsley Publishers.

Green, J., Howes, F., Waters, E., Maher, E. and Oberklaid, F. (2005) Promoting the social and emotional health of primary school aged children: reviewing the evidence base for school based interventions, *International Journal of Mental Health Promotion*, 7(3): 30–6.

Griesel, D., Swart-Kruger, J. and Chawla, L. (2004) Children in South Africa can make a difference: an assessment of 'Growing Up in Cities' in Johannesburg, in V. Lewis, M. Kellett, C. Robinson, S. Fraser and S. Ding (eds) *The Reality of Research with young People*. London: Sage Publications with The Open University.

Grieve, R. and Hughes, M. (1990) *Understanding Children*. Oxford: Basil Blackwell.

Haney, P. and Durlak, J. (1998) Changing self-esteem in children and adolescents: a meta-analytic review, *Journal of Clinical Child Psychology*, 27(4): 423–33.

Hart, R.A. (1997) *Children's Participation*. London: Earthscan Publications.

Hodgson, R., Abbasi, T. and Clarkson, J. (1995) *Effective Mental Health Promotion: A Literature Review*, Technical Report 13. Cardiff: Health Promotion Wales.

Humphreys, C. (2001) The impact of domestic violence on children, in P. Foley, J. Roche and S. Tucker, (eds) *Children in Society*. Basingstoke: Palgrave in association with The Open University.

Hunt, S. (2005) *The Life Course: A Sociological Introduction*. Basingstoke: Palgrave Macmillan.

Jamison, J., Ashby, P., Hamilton, K. et al. (1996) *The Health Promoting School: Final Report of the ENHPS Evaluation Project in England*. London: European Network of Health Promoting Schools, Health Education Authority.

Johnson, B. (2005) Mental health promotion in schools: an exploration of factors relating to risk, resilience and health promoting schools in order to enhance the wellbeing of our youth. Unpublished PhD thesis, University of the Western Cape.

Johnson, Z., Howell, F. and Molly, B. (1993) Community Mothers Programme: randomized controlled trial of non-professional intervention in parenting, *BMJ*, 306: 1449–52.

Johnson, Z., Molly, B. and Scallen, E. et al. (2000) Community Mothers Programme: seven years follow up of a randomized controlled trial of non-professional intervention in parenting, *Journal of Public Health Medicine*, 22(3): 337–42.

Kalnins, I., Hart, C., Ballantyne, P. et al. (2002) Children's perceptions of strategies for resolving community health problems, *Health Promotion International*, 17(3): 223–33.

Lalonde, M. (1974) *A New Perspective on the Health of Canadians*. Ottawa: Government of Canada.

License, K. (2005) Supporting parenting: the evidence, in R. Chambers and K. License (eds) *Looking After Children in Primary Care*. Oxford: Radcliffe Publishing.

Lister-Sharp, D., Chapman, S., Stewart Brown, S. and Sowden, A. (1999) Health promoting schools and health promotion in schools: two systematic reviews, *Health Technology Assessment*, 3(22): 1–207.

Mann, M., Hosman, C.M.H., Schaalma, H.P. and de Vries, N.K. (2004) Self-esteem in a broad-spectrum approach for mental health promotion, *Health Education Research*, 19(4): 357–72.

Mayall, B. (2001) Children's health at school, in P.T. Foley, J. Roche and S. Tucker (eds) *Children in Society*. Basingstoke: The Open University in association with Palgrave.

Mental Health Foundation (1999) *Bright Futures: Promoting Children and Young People's Mental Health*. London: Mental Health Foundation.

Meltzer, H., Gatward, R., Goodman, R. and Ford, T. (2000) *The Mental Health of Children and Adolescents in Britain*. London: Office for National Statistics Her Majesty's Stationery Office.

Mind (2005) *Children and Young People*, Fact sheet. London: Mind.

Moghaddam, F.M. and Studer, C. (1997) Cross-cultural psychology: the frustrated gadfly's promised, potentialities and failure, in D. Fox and I. Prilleltensky (eds) *Critical Psychology: An Introduction*. London: Sage Publications.

Moore, R.C. (1986) Munich: becoming a playful city, *Playright* (IPA Journal), 15: 9–11.

Olds, D.L. (2002) Prenatal and infancy home visiting by nurses: from randomized trials to community replication, *Prevention Science*, 3(3): 153–72.

Olds, D.L., Henderson, S.R., Tatelbaum, R. and Chamberlin, R. (1988) Improving the life-course development of socially disadvantaged mothers: a randomized controlled trial of nurse home visitation, *American Journal of Public Health*, 78: 1436–44.

Olweus, D. (1989) Bully/victim problems among schoolchildren: Basic facts and the effects of a school based intervention program, in K. Ruben and D. Heppler (eds) *The Development and Treatment of Childhood Aggression*. Earlside, NJ: Erlbaum.

Olweus, D. (1993) *Bullying at School: What We Know and What We Can Do*. Oxford: Blackwell.

Patel, V. (2001) Poverty, inequality and mental health in developing countries, in D. Leon and G. Walt (eds) *Poverty, Inequality and Health*. Oxford: Oxford University Press.

Patel, V., Swartz, L. and Cohen, L. (2004) The evidence for mental health promotion in developing countries, *Promoting Mental Health: Concepts, Emerging Evidence and Practice*. Geneva: WHO.

Pedro-Caroll, J.L., Gillis, L.J. and Cowen, E.L. (1992) An evaluation of the efficacy of a preventive intervention for 4th–6th grade urban children of divorce, *Journal of Primary Prevention*, 13(2): 115–30.

Pridmore, P. and Stephens, S. (2000) *Children as Partners for Health*. London: Zed Books.

Prout, A. and James, A. (1990) A new paradigm for the sociology of childhood? provenance, promise and problems, in A. James and A. Prout (eds) *Constructing and Deconstructiing Childhood: Contemporary Issues in the Sociological Study of Childhood*. London: The Falmer Press.

Ramsey, C.T., Bryant, D.M., Campbell, F.A., Sparling, J.J. and Wasik, B.H. (1988) Early intervention for high risk children: the Caroline Early Intervention Programme, in R.H. Price, E.L. Cowen, R.P. Lorion and J. Ramos-McKay (eds) *14 Ounces of Prevention: A Casebook for Practitioners*. Washington, DC: American Psychological Association.

Rutter, M. (1996) Connections between child and adult psychopathology, *European Child Adolescent Psychology*, 5(supp.1): 4–7.

Schagen, S., Blenkinsop, S., Schagen, I. et al. (2005) Evaluating the impact of the National Healthy School Standard: using national datasets, *Health Education Research*, 20(6): 686–96.

Schweinhart, L.J. and Weikart, D.P. (1980) *Young Children Grow Up: The Effects of the Perry Pre-School Project on Youths Through 19*. Ypsilanti, MI: High Scope Educational Research Foundation Press.

Schweinhart, L.J. and Weikart, D.P. (1998) High/Scope Perry Preschool program effects at age twenty seven, in J. Crane (ed.) *Social Programs that Work*. New York: Russell Sage Foundation.

Stainton-Rogers, W. (2001) Constructing childhood, constructing childhood concern, in P. Foley, J. Roche and S. Tucker (eds) *Children in Society, Contemporary Theory, Policy and Practice*. Milton Keynes: The Open University.

Stathakos, P. and Roehrle, B. (2003) The effectiveness of intervention programmes for children of divorce – a meta-analysis, *International Journal of Mental Health Promotion*, 5(1): 31–7.

Stevens, V., de Bourdeeaudhuij, I. and van Osst, P. (2001) Anti-bullying interventions at school: aspects of programme adaptation and critical issues for further programme development, *Health Promotion International*, 16(2): 155–67.

Stewart, D., Sun, J., Patterson, C., Lemerle, K. and Hardie, M. (2004) Promoting and building resilience in primary school communities: evidence from a comprehensive 'health promoting school' approach, *International Journal of Mental Health Promotion*, 6(3): 26–33.

Sure Start (2005) The Sure Start principles. London: Department for Education and Skills and Department for Work and Pensions. Available at http://www.surestart.gov.uk/aboutsurestart/about/thesurestartprinciples2/ (accessed 25 June 2005).

Thurston, C. and Church, J. (2001) Involving children and families in decision making about health, in P. Fole, J. Roche and S. Tucker (eds) *Children in Society: Contemporary Theory, Policy and Practice*. Basingstoke: Palgrave in assocation with The Open University.

Tilford, S., Delaney, F. and Vogels, M. (1997) *Effectiveness of Mental Health Promotion Interventions*. London: Health Education Authority.

Tranter, P.J. and Doyle, J.W. (1996) Reclaiming the residential street as play space, *International Play Journal*, 4: 81–97.

United Nations (1989) *The Convention on the Rights of the Child*. Geneva: UN.

Walker, J. and Walker, R. (2002) Home zones: child health benefits from neighbourhood action and subsequent policy change, *ChildRIGHT*, 184: 18–19.

Ward, L. (2005) Child mental illness 'now stable at one in 10', *Guardian*, 1 September.

Ward, L. (2006) Sure Start sets back the worst placed youngsters, study finds, *Guardian*, 1 December.

Warwick, I., Aggleton, P., Chase, E. et al. (2005) Evaluating healthy schools: perceptions of impact among school-based respondents, *Health Education Research*, 20(6): 697–708.

Weare, K. (2004) Editorial: the international alliance for child and adolescent mental health and schools, *Health Education*, 104(2): 65–7.

Wells, J., Stewart-Brown, S. and Barlow, J. (2001) *A Systematic Review of the Effectiveness of School Mental Health Promotion Interventions*. Oxford: Health Services Research Unit.

WHO (World Health Organization) (1993) *The European Network of Health Promoting Schools*. Copenhagen: WHO European Region.

WHO (World Health Organization) (1996) *Promoting Health Through Schools: WHO's Global Initiative*. Geneva: WHO.

WHO (World Health Organization) (1997) *Promoting Health Through Schools: Report of a WHO Expert Committee on Comprehensive School Health Education and Promotion*. Geneva: WHO.

WHO (World Health Organization) (1999) *A Critical Link: Interventions for Physical Growth and Child Development*. Geneva: WHO.

Winnicott, D.W. (1964) *The Child, the Family and the Outside World*. Harmondsworth: Penguin.

Zubrick, S.R. and Kovess-Masfety, V. (2004) Indicators of mental health, *Promoting Mental Health: Concepts, Emerging Evidence and Practice*. Geneva: WHO.

5 Adolescence and emerging adulthood (12–17 years and 18–24 years)

Louise Rowling

Editors' foreword

The position of young people is rapidly changing across the globe. As this chapter notes, young people on the verge of adulthood are less homogenous than those of school age, but also they are less homogenous as a group than in the past. Transition into adulthood, is as the author points out, a period which is determined by a range of factors, and consequently it is variable in different cultures, in different socio-economic groups and so on. This chapter explores some of the distinct factors that impact on the mental health of adolescents and young adults. Importantly, it considers issues such as violence and grief, which are not always recognized at policy level. Different transition phases, such as school to work are explored and the role of mental health promotion is considered in relation to these stages, drawing strongly on resilience research. The role of the built environment in supporting the development of social networks is also highlighted. An important point, from a global perspective, is the impact on young people's mental health of environmental change through major life transitions, such as forced migration or family changes. Evidence in relation to the determinants of mental health and a useful and thorough section of examples of good practice from a wide range of settings is provided.

Introduction

The term 'mental health promotion' has been interpreted by the World Health Organization (WHO) to have two meanings – aiming to raise the position of mental health in individuals, families and societies so that decisions of government and business improve, rather than compromise, the population's mental health; and improving the mental health state of populations by reducing disease through prevention, treatment and rehabilitation (WHO 2001). Underlying these two meanings is the presumption that mental health and mental illness differ in degree of health/illness rather than having a qualitative difference in conceptualization (Rowling 2002a). This limited conceptual clarity is overcome by Hosman and Jané-Llopis's (1999) more positive definition where mental health promotion is viewed as the creation of individual, social and environmental conditions that enable optimal psychological and psycho-physiological development. This definition is about positive mental health rather than the opposite of mental illness and is the conceptualization adopted in this chapter.

The young people who are the focus of this chapter can be grouped as 12–17-year-olds (adolescents)[1] and 18–24-year-olds (young adults). However, there can be variations to this classification determined by social conditions such as engagement in education, paid work, family formation or unemployment and lack of connection to family and social institutions. These groups of young people face demands, expectations and challenges which are more numerous and carry larger risks than those experienced by young people only a generation ago (Zubrick et al. 1997). It is a time of major life changes in physical and sexual development, social relations, identity as well as shifting dependence/independence and significant educational demands. These changes apply to both the 12–17-year-old, adolescent, group, and the emerging adulthood, 18–24-year-old, group. The experiences of these age groups can trigger mental health problems, create vulnerabilities and exert particular constraints on their access to resources. Several disorders are identified as having their onset at this age, including depression, schizophrenia and substance abuse (WHO 2001).

Worldwide it is estimated that one in twenty young people experience developmental, emotional or behavioural problems and one in eight have a mental disorder (WHO 2004a, 2005) while in Britain in the 11–16 age group, 12 percent of boys and 10 percent of girls have a diagnosable mental disorder (Green et al. 2005). In terms of prevalence in Australia it is estimated that two in every five young people in the community suffer from a depressed mood in any six month period (NHMRC 1997). The measurement differences between countries confuse intercountry comparisons. However research does reveal that a significant minority of children and particularly adolescents in Australia, experience depressive and anxiety symptoms with 4 percent of 12–16-year-olds showing evidence of depression and anxiety when rated by parents and teachers (Zubrick et al. 1995). This is consistent with international epidemiological data from child and adolescent populations, of 3–30 percent (Verhulst and Koot 1992).

In Australia, the population with the highest prevalence of mental health problems and illnesses of 27 percent is young adults aged 18–24 years (Andrews et al. 1999). A study of 15–24-year-olds (Donald et al. 2000) explored mental health problems and illnesses through measuring depression. Their survey used adverse life changes to study mental health. The indicators were identified as psychological distress, suicide attempts and ideation, and depressive symptomatology. They focused on life transitions identified as national priority targets (CDHAC 2000a) because they have the potential to have detrimental consequences for young adults' well-being. The study found that nearly 40 percent of 18–24-year-olds had experienced distress as a result of a relationship break-up (Donald et al. 2000).

A recent (2005) UK report, *Transitions: Young Adults with Complex Needs*, noted that up to 20 percent of all 16–24-year-olds have a mental health issue and suicide is the cause of a quarter of all deaths among 16–24-year-old men (Social Exclusion Unit (2005). These mental health issues/disorders have the potential for a broad impact due to the developmental disruption and disabling effect arising from the concomitant life transitions. Reinherz et al.'s (1999) research indicates that the experience of depression in the transition to adulthood compromises the choices and decisions young people make, and therefore represents a risk for continued impairment and future disorder. As will become clear in the descriptions through this chapter, attention in mental health research, policy and practice is only now being turned to the 18–24 age group but concerted action is still in its infancy. This is disturbing given the high rate of mental disorders for the emerging adult group.

Special mental health issues

A major mental health issue for young people is experiencing bullying and harassment. Research has repeatedly attributed depression and depressive symptoms to harassment or bullying both as a result of being a victim or a bully (Olweus 1993; Bond et al. 2000; Rigby 2003). For many young people it is the school setting where this occurs. As this is a key environment where young people develop their social skills and interact with peers and adults, negative experiences not only affect their mental health and academic achievement, but limit their capacity to acquire the skills to feel confident in interpersonal interactions. The impact of victimization varies across individuals and environments.

In Australia, from a mental health perspective, the life events involving loss and bereavement are recognized as a priority mental health target and young adults, as a priority target group (CDHAC 2000b). Using loss and change as an indicator, identifying young adults as a priority target is supported by research from the US where numerous studies have identified that about a quarter of college students are in their first 12 months of a bereavement following the death of family and friends or a broken love relationship (Brown and Christiansen 1990; Balk 1997). Loss may interfere with the natural progression of intellectual-emotional-psychological growing up (Kastenbaum 2001). For this age group major life changes are occurring that have significant impact at the time and into adulthood in all developmental domains (social, emotional, physical and cognitive).

Discrimination and social exclusion in varying forms are highly correlated with mental health problems. Higher suicide rates among Australian Indigenous and same sex attracted young people have been attributed, in part, to discrimination on the grounds of race and sexual preference respectively (Department of Health and Family Services 1997). In the United Kingdom much of the variation in rates of hospital admissions can be accounted for by variations in unemployment, poor housing, homelessness and law and order (Kings Fund 2000). But policy change is occurring. The new National Service Framework (1999), particularly Standard 1 on mental health improvement, should help address disparities, with partnerships highlighted as a requirement between health agencies, schools, workplaces and people and organizations in neighbourhoods.

In addressing mental health the focus needs to be on the individual and their environment, that is young people not only acquiring the skills to be in position to take advantage of opportunities particularly for the 18+ age group, but also where environments are created so young people feel understood and supported. The environmental focus is also about changing the language, culture and practice principles in organizations and thereby enhancing an organization's capacity to work in an effective and sustained way with young people (Victorian Health Promotion Foundation 2003).

Special mental health considerations

There are a number of special considerations that need to be taken into account in examining the mental health of adolescents and young adults. First is the influence of prevention research. A great deal of research on the adolescent group about creating positive mental health through weakening risk factors or strengthening protective factors has occurred, particularly in the United States, under various labels of youth development, assets and strengths and social emotional learning. A major problem is the limited dissemination of models used in this research and their adaptation to various conditions (Greenberg and Weissberg 2003). So although there are solid research findings they have not been well used in practice.

Another special consideration is the focus needed for mental health promotion. Many of the issues that impinge on young people's mental health are outside the responsibility of the health sector. The need to have a joined up approach has been recognized in a report from the United Kingdom Department for Education and Science (DfES 2004) on Children and Adolescent Mental Health Services (CAMHS) services. In this report Tier 1 services for mental health improvement focus on those professionals who are not mental health specialists. A range of strategies are needed for the health sector to cooperate and influence other sectors (CDHAC 2000b; Rowling and Taylor 2005), the purpose being to build the capacity of sectors and organizations connected to young people to acknowledge and address mental health issues.

A third special consideration relates to the role of risk factors in conceptualizing mental health promotion. Understanding of risk provides insight into resilience and positive mental health, but over-emphasis in prevention research on risk has resulted in policy makers and researchers viewing young people negatively through the lens of risk. Brown (2004) argued that this had a destructive effect on young people's lives. In the United States a diagnosis of risk was necessary to gain access to treatment, popularly known as the 'diagnosis for dollars' phenomenon. For young people this contributed to their cognitive dissonance about school and society, that is believing schools should be supporting young people not only seeking their problems. This they resolved by a reduction in adult credibility (Brown 2004). Unfortunately this loss of faith in systems, and the adults that are part of them, begins at a time when young people need to feel connected to adults and social institutions.

A fourth special consideration is a growth in anxiety among young people. Jean Twenge has conducted meta-analyses of American children and college students from the 1950s to 1990s (Twenge 2000). She found rising anxiety in young people and talks about its occurrence in terms of free floating anxiety and argues that anxiety is more commonplace than depression. Her conclusion is that it is the lower sense of control over their lives and loss of connectedness that is contributing to rising anxiety in young people. Their experience of too much freedom can lead to poor outcomes, in which young people are anxious and paralysed by their choices and blame themselves when things do not go well. The two forces impacting on increased anxiety of this age group, low social connectedness and high environmental threat, pointing to the importance of social bonds and cognitive skills to effectively appraise threat. Increased anxiety is a cause for concern because it tends to predispose individuals to depression (Twenge 2000).

A final consideration flows through this chapter. It is the stigmatizing that occurs when young people are solely viewed through the lens of risk and problems. Care is needed so that focusing on the determinants of mental health and mental illness, such as economic or social disadvantage, does not highlight the possibility of failure. Rather that the agency of young people achieving success is the theme, looking at success and variations in the strategies young people use to manage threat and challenge in an active way.

Box 5.1   Summary points for mental health, adolescents and young adults

- One in twenty young people worldwide experience developmental, emotional or behavioural problems.
- Young adults have particularly high levels of mental health problems and illnesses.
- Viewing young people through the lens of risk limits mental health promotion action.
- Intersectoral action is crucial for mental health promotion for young people.
- Labelling young people in terms of risk and problems can be stigmatizing.

Theories and frameworks related to adolescents and young adults

Risk factor research currently predominates for young people skewing the focal point to mental health problems. The orientation of most interventions is individuals, risk behaviours, and problems such as poor social skills and low self-esteem. Judging an individual's mental health by absence of risk factors and problems of individuals is a narrow approach. A challenge is the conceptualizing of positive mental health for these age groups focusing on contexts and process such as school connectedness, whole populations such as the school community, and organizational change that creates supportive environments. This is a 'population health' approach which involves 'simultaneous consideration of the needs and goals of population groups inhabiting the community, and the examination of the conditions of life that enhance or impede their health or the health of the community' (McMurray 1999: 9).

One current popular theoretical framework is resilience, used as a descriptor for positive mental health and well-being. It has been conceived and described in different ways that focus on individual traits and supportive environments, and on the outcome and process of resilience (Olsson et al. 2003). Consideration of resilience and young people has emerged from observation and research that indicates that a proportion of young people have positive outcomes despite having faced diverse potentially harmful life experiences. The early resiliency research arose from phenomenological descriptions of the characteristics of young people who survived adversity while living in high risk environments (Werner and Smith 1982). From this research resilient qualities of individuals and the support conditions that predicted personal and social success were identified leading to a focus on protective factors, assets and strengths (Benard 1995; Benson 1997). Summarizing this work Richardson (2002: 310) states: 'The list of traits, states, characteristics, conditions and virtues in the literature is exhaustive; and the resulting paradigm shift from the identification of risk factors to the nurturing of personal strengths has been significant'.

These various findings were reduced to lists of characteristics – a 'checklist approach' and adopted as a guide for the teaching of skills deemed necessary for the development of resilience. But this reductionist approach often occurred in the absence of the theoretical understanding of the process of how people acquire resiliency skills (Richardson 2002) and with little appreciation for the context of young people's lives. A more comprehensive approach was provided by Kumpfer (1999). She used a social ecology or person-process-context approach where stressors or challenges were filtered through an environmental context of risk and protective factors, a person–environment transactional process, internal resiliency factors and resiliency processes for resilient and maladaptive outcomes. This echoes Benard's (1995) emphasis on protective processes. The process of fostering resilience is long-term and developmental, where children are viewed through strengths rather than risks and deficits, and where there is action to change systems, structures and beliefs as well as the development of personal skills (Benard 1999). Many later researchers have moved on from a focus on protective factors to examining the underlying processes and mechanisms.

To summarize the components of resilience, it is a holistic process involving positive mental health of young people within the context of their lives, shaped by their varying skills and the environment, contributing to a hopeful future in the face of adversity. In a general transactional model the interaction of young people and adults in the context of wider society is an essential component in resilience: how young people feel, relate to the world and are shaped by it is important, as well as what they think.

Along with resilience another conceptualization of positive mental well-being comes from a focus on social and emotional learning (for example, see Antidote 2003; CASEL (collaborative for academic, social, emotional learning) in Greenberg and Waissberg 2003; and SEBS (social emotional behavioural skills) in Weare and Gray 2003). Also linked are emotional literacy (Weare 2003) and emotional intelligence (Goleman 1996). Weare and Gray (2003), in their research on children's emotional and social competence and well-being, commented on this wide range of terms and the need for a common language. They recommend 'emotional and social competence' and 'emotional and social well-being' as being straightforward and non-specialist. The use of the term 'competence' implies knowledge, attitudes and behavioural components, which make the term particularly appropriate for use in school and other settings (Weare and Gray 2003: 15). Social and emotional competence is defined as 'the ability to understand, manage and express emotional aspects of one's life in ways that enable the successful management of life tasks such as learning, forming relationships, solving everyday problems, and adapting to the complex demands of growth and development' (Elias and Zing 1997: 2). A problem with the focus on social and emotional learning or competence, however, is that it is focused on the individual and as this chapter illustrates the factors that impact on young people's mental health are often outside the individual's control involving social and environmental conditions. Weare and Gray (2003) acknowledge this by suggesting that a broad range of research and practice should be drawn upon and integrated into frameworks to maximize positive outcomes for young people.

The critical role of the impact of context is evident in an analysis of what makes safe environments. Safe social environments such as local communities, schools and families can contribute to young people's mental health. Violent behaviour inside the school and from the surrounding community (see section on built environments) impacts on young people in schools, environments once considered protective locations. Developing a sense of safety both physical and psycho-social has become increasingly important. Intervention points for promoting well-being in young people need to be focused on peers, schools and families. Witnessing parental domestic violence has emerged as the strongest predictor of perpetration of violence in young people's own intimate relationships (Indermaur 2001). However the concept of a 'cycle of violence' presents a fatalistic few of possible outcomes. The majority of those who have grown up in violent homes do not go on to be violent in their relationships because the link between witnessing and perpetrating is complex and mediated by a number of social and situational factors (Indermaur 2001).

The need for the proposed paradigm shift from risk to positive mental health is not easy to address. Talking about strengths and human capacity to rebuild is difficult territory for those trained in pathology and **DSM IV** (APA 1994) paradigms. The challenge involves a re-orientation of practice to focus on resourcefulness, success, capacity, hope and competence and a reconceptualization of what created positive mental health.

Box 5.2   Summary of theories and frameworks related to adolescents and young adults

- Risk factor research has focused mental health on problems rather than strengths and positive outcomes.
- Reframing mental health through focusing on resilience can be useful but often is individualistic in focus and ignores the social context.
- Synthesizing research drawn from a broad range of research will advance practice.
- Research on gender, in the areas of violence and loss, highlights the importance of research that aims to understand young people's current life worlds.

Determinants of, and influences on, mental health

The influences on mental health are, as outlined in other chapters, multiple, interacting and operating at different levels. Factors can be grouped in different ways but the broad division into personal and environmental divided into social, cultural and economic and the natural plus built environments is followed (see Chapter 4, Figure 4.1).

Personal

As indicated previously a concentration of the early research was on the characteristics of individuals that put them 'at risk'. This resulted in a focus on ameliorating these deficits, often by teaching skills. However the risk factor research emanating principally from the United States has an emphasis on individual volition and personality turning attention away from socially structured inequalities related to race, class and gender (Settersten et al. 2005).

Researchers from various perspectives are questioning current conceptualizations of young adults' educational, social and personal lives after compulsory schooling. They advance new perspectives on the altered life trajectories of choice and complexity now experienced by school leavers. A consistent theme is the changed nature of young adults' lives, reflecting social and economic pressures on educational, work and personal life goals (Rowling et al. 2005).

Pais (2000) contends that young adults are on individualized time dimensions in transitions, past time influencing the present and future time involving aspirations and plans. The experience has been described as the 'in between' period, as a 'butterfly's flight', stopping nowhere for long (Pais 2000: 220), with a reality status of 'no-longer-but-not-yet' (Beck 2000: 213), and 'invisible early twenties' (Social Exclusion Unit 2005: 9).

Jeffrey Arnett (2004) argues that becoming an adult is a much longer process than in previous generations and asserts that the developmental markers for adulthood now consist of accepting responsibility for oneself, making independent decisions and achieving financial adequacy. These are all conceived of as gradually attained rather than viewed as distinct discrete markers characteristic of past lifespan psychiatrists such as Erikson (1965). Sociologists (Furstenberg et al. 2003) maintain that the traditional markers of marriage and parenthood are no longer seen as necessary for the attainment of adult status. They argue that the changed life course in becoming adult results from the economic and social conditions that have an impact on the age group. That is, social conditions are reshaping young adults' lives and a young person's aspirations for the future shape their life plan directing the shift from school to further study, family formation and/or paid work. Families, educational and social institutions have been slow to recognize and accommodate these changes, with resultant adverse outcomes reflected in mental health morbidity and youth suicide rates. It should, however, be noted that this research is mostly based on young people in Western cultures, and that the transitional phase may be quite different for the same age group in other cultures and societies.

Social

Within this section a broad view of social factors is taken. Consideration is given to the interpersonal interactions as well as the social institutions and wider social forces (linked to economic factors) that impact on young people's well-being. These forces include the rising individualism, consumerism and materialism linked to anxiety and social exclusion (Eckersley 2002). Consumerism contributes to the breakdown in community and social life with too much pressure on families and working hours being too long, factors all linked to economic growth (Eckersley 2004). Anxiety is an adaptive response to social exclusion, a key factor in determining mental health.

The market economy and globalization have created social conditions that have impacted on the lives of 18–24-years-olds in Western societies. As already noted, the

research on this group and their mental health is not as extensive as for early adolescence. Young people on the verge of adulthood are far less homogenous than a
school age group. In Western societies they are taking longer over the transition to
adulthood. However for others the transition may be accelerated. Age boundaries in
policy and service provision do not recognize these changes (Social Exclusion Unit
2005).

Impact of gender

Gender roles and their impact on mental health will be examined through two life
experiences of young people: violence and harassment, and loss and grief.

For adolescents and young adults interpersonal violence and harassment is the
source of significant mental health problems. The World Health Organization identified three types of violence: self-directed, interpersonal and collective (WHO 2002a).
While self-directed violence, in particular self-harm and suicide, are important mental
health problems, interpersonal violence is the focus here. This involves family/partner
and community violence. The WHO report uses an ecological model to frame discussion consisting of four levels: individual, relationship, community and society. Youth
violence includes aggressive acts including bullying and harassment, intimate partner
physical aggression, sexual coercion, psychological abuse and controlling behaviours
(WHO 2002a). Gender is an important factor in relationship violence for young people.

In Australian research 42 percent of 19–20-year-old women who have had a
boyfriend admitted they experienced physical violence from the boyfriend at least once
(Indermaur 2001). For male victimization, the rates appear similar. However the experiences of victims are different. Almost one-third (30 percent) of 19–20-year-old women
reported they had been frightened or hurt, whereas this was reported by only one in
eight (12 percent) of 19–20-year-old men. The experience of fear is taken as the key
characteristic of domestic violence for most victims. Half of female victims experienced
fear where only 11 percent of males did. The gender disparity commonly recognized in
domestic violence, and reflected in criminal statistics, is revealed by the subjective
experience of the aggression: girls are at least four times as likely as boys to have been
frightened by an episode of intimate aggression (Indermaur 2001).

The operation of a cycle of violence together with social marginalization has the
potential of concentrating violence in certain disadvantaged areas. The implication is
that strategies to prevent domestic violence must have particular relevance to disadvantaged communities, and their effectiveness must be evaluated in terms of the
differences they make to those communities suffering the most violence (Indermaur
2001).

In relation to life changes, coping styles and loss, a review from the Health Development Agency (2001) on young men's health identified a gap between the health of
young men and women and the impact of gender roles in the experience and expression of mental distress. Female adolescents grieving the death of a sibling report lower
self-esteem and higher anxiety/insomnia than male counterparts (Fleming and Balmer
1996). This could be interpreted as young men not experiencing the same impact, or
being more concerned about possible vulnerability created because of social sanctions
that such reporting would induce (Fleming and Balmer 1996). The experience of loss

and grief exemplifies different coping styles and while these differences are along gender role lines, care is needed in attending to the differences.

For young males who may be uncomfortable with verbal expression, options that need to be sanctioned include diversion and reflection; processing by action rather than verbally expressing feeling; and by thinking an event through rather than talking (Martin and Doka 2000). These are all characteristic of what Martin and Doka (2000) call instrumental coping. Another style involving more verbal expression and feelings-based experience of grief is labelled intuitive coping. What is needed are environments that validate the varying ways of expressing grief, sanctioning options for young males of diversion and reflection processing by action rather than verbally expressing feeling; by thinking it through rather than talking (Rowling 2003). The gender role for female grievers is also restricted. Those who do not express their grief through verbalizing are seen to be hard and not grieving.

Environments that validate the varying ways of expressing grief, for young males of diversion and reflection (Martin and Doka 2000), processing by action rather than verbally expressing feelings, and by thinking it through rather than talking are needed. This is particularly important as a strategy to help address the high suicide rate among young males, whose coping styles are often limited and self-destructive, and whose socialization can limit beneficial help seeking.

Action that would address issues around violence, gender and coping styles needs to focus on different levels. For young people individual approaches could be through psycho-education about healthy relationships and negotiation skills. However this approach has its limitations when the determinants are social and structural. For example incentives to complete school and vocational training for marginalized young people could have longer term outcomes on young people as perpetrators and victims of violence. Also structured school environment programmes to address bullying, intimidation and sexual harassment that include individual and school policy and practice have had positive outcomes (Olweus 1993).

Examining violence and harassment and loss and grief among young people illustrates two key issues. First, that there is a need to understand the life worlds of adolescents and young adults from the perspective of how they experience events. Second, to avoid stereotyping individual behaviour as male or female and educate young people about the options there may be for coping with life changes they may experience as threatening.

Education

Another determinant of mental health is education in terms of both achievement – the long- and short-term impact of success and failure in academic study; and the role educational institutions as social environments play in young people's lives. Young people who have a good experience at school regardless of whether they were high achievers, are more likely to belong to the 'can-do group', in other words those children with high self-esteem (Mental Health Foundation 1999).

Involvement in education and academic success directly and indirectly impacts on mental health. The report, *Bright Futures* (Mental Health Foundation 1999), concludes that children whose emotional needs are being met are more able to apply themselves to learning. This assertion is important in that it acknowledges that for schools, achieving educational outcomes are the key drivers that maintain schools' involvement in mental health activities. Schools are often the sites for implementing mental health programmes, but mental health activities are prioritized against the many competing demands made on limited school time. Hence research that links mental health to learning is vital. There is overwhelming evidence that young people who leave school early with low levels of educational attainment are at higher risk of experiencing social exclusion as young people and throughout their lives (Social Exclusion Unit 2005).

Two recent reports have identified the critical role of teaching in mental health promotion. In their evaluation of the UK Healthy Schools programme Warwick and colleagues (2005) identified the importance of teaching in Personal and Social Education (PSE) for the students. Students reported they valued the active involvement in these lessons as it helped them gain new understandings about their lives and the lives of others. They also valued the different teaching style whereby they were 'being informed' rather than 'being told'. A report form the National Institute for Health and Clinical Excellence (NICE) draws together evidence from a number of recent evaluations of National Healthy School Standards (Cole 2004). In particular, an examination of Ofsted inspection reports revealed that Level 3 primary schools scored higher than the norm on measures including personal development and PSHE provision. Findings were not so strong for secondary schools but these schools did receive positive feedback on PSHE and standards of care. The role of the standards of care, points to the importance of the whole-school environment being welcoming, showing respect and being committed to the well-being of young people.

Rutter et al.'s seminal work (1979) identified the important role of the school as a social institution – as being a supportive or a threatening environment. The importance of having positive experiences in school was highlighted by Resnick et al. (1993). They identified that what was significant for young people was that they felt part of the school, were close to others and perceived they were treated fairly, in other words, that they experienced 'connectedness'.

The role of educational institutions in mental health

Along with the connection between mental health and educational success, schools and higher education institutions play important roles in young people's lives. Brown (2004) cites evidence from studies in the American Child Development Program that shows the promise of resilience constructs in interventions that take a whole-school approach (involving educators, administrators, counsellors and community). These studies showed positive effects on school related attitudes (liking school), social attitudes, skills and values (concern for others) and improvement in academic achievement.

Along with adopting a whole-school approach, another area is the building of personal caring relationships, the welfare/pastoral care structures and practices in the school. Action to enhance relationships involving students and staff is supported by the research evidence that indicates the importance of adults in keeping young people connected to school. Seligman (1995) asserts that teacher qualities of being student centred, building on student's interests, goals and dreams as a starting point for learning, build motivation for learning as well as strengths.

While caring relationships and classroom teaching contribute to the development of resilience so does the wider school environment and the climate within the school. Henderson and Milstein (1996) articulate six conditions that describe schools that build resiliency. They are schools that provide opportunities for meaningful participation, increase pro-social bonding, set clear consistent boundaries, teach 'life skills', provide caring and support, and set and communicate high expectations. These conditions go further than building skills of adolescents as individuals and include the characteristics of the environment that can support young people. Administrators have a vital role to play in creating a supportive environment for students and for staff. McLaughlin and Talbert (1993) articulate three conditions that achieve this. Administrators can:

1 Demonstrate positive beliefs in their staff
2 Set expectations and trust teachers and
3 Provide ongoing opportunities for teachers to reflect, talk and make decisions together.

The importance of this wider school role is echoed in the UK Healthy Living Blueprint for Schools (DfES 2004). Attention is drawn to factors that promote health including ethos and environment of the school (leadership; involving pupils in decision-making; good quality professional development; close links with parents and the community) and whether the curriculum is used flexibly to promote pupils' health related understandings and practices.

In the last decade the global development of 'health promoting schools' or 'healthy schools' has reflected the shift in how to influence a range of health behaviours including enhancing mental health through school processes and structures. Rather than having a sole focus on prevention of specific health problems through teaching, or for mental health through short-term interventions for at-risk young people, school health promotion in recent years has come to focus on the whole-school community. This is operationalized as a 'settings' approach to health promotion, namely health promoting schools (WHO 1998), and healthy schools (DfEE/DoH 1999). The importance of a whole-school approach is evident in addressing well-being which involves 'mapping the whole of life and considering each life event or social context that has the potential to affect the quality of individual lives or the cohesion of society' (Trewin 2001: 6). The whole-school context approach is supported by current educational quality practice: 'Context is all-important in emotional and behavioural development – the social context of the school; the learning and social context provided in the classroom; the context formed by the pattern of relationships in which pupils find themselves' (QCA 2001: 2). If we translate this to apply to schools, we are concerned about measuring individual factors and the social context – the school community. Previous activity in healthy schools presents a strong foundation on which to build work in school mental health promotion. The *National Healthy Schools Standards* (DfEE/DoH 1999) includes mental health in addressing social exclusion aiming to reduce health inequalities and raise pupil achievement. Emotional health and well-being are included in the standards. Mental health is further elaborated in 'Promoting children's mental health within the early years and school settings' (DfES 2001).

Work on school mental health promotion reinforces the orientation that the social organization and structure of schools needs to be the starting point. If we take this route then we are working for all not selecting out a group. From an educational perspective there are four elements that need to be combined to effectively develop an educational resilience paradigm. First a positive culture, a school climate that enhances connectedness, through norms, structures and processes is required. Second there needs to be a positive relational context of adult/young person interactions. Third, the educational processes need to be building young people's critical solutions-based thinking. The fourth element involves a focus on teachers/educators mental well-being.

While academic success for young people is important the role of staff morale and performance is vital (Mental Health Foundation 1999). Schools are working environments as well as learning environments. If the focus is on the school context as the entry point then interventions will be multi-strategic and dynamic and they will meet educational needs as well as health needs. So for school mental health promotion the morale of teachers and communication within the school community will be just as important as a focus on mental health issues for students. Teacher morale is a mental health issue. Low morale is a major concern for teachers themselves and for the well-being of students because teachers who feel unsupported and under pressure are more likely, through their disciplinary and control techniques, to use shouting and humiliation (Lister-Sharpe et al. 1999).

As a young person moves through adolescence the consequences of what happened in earlier schooling become important. Early school career, a family's attitude as well as teacher expectations can dictate outcomes for young people so that they leave education at the first opportunity (Schoon and Bynner 2003), limiting their chances of success in their lives.

One of the challenges students entering higher education encounter, is creating a new identity as a learner. In making the transition to higher education they initially encounter identity discontinuity and displacement in negotiating this new and different learning context. Weiss (1990, in Mackie 2001) found that students rapidly need to establish social contacts and relationships in order to build a new sense of self within the new learning environment. It is students with a sense of connectedness, in other words those who have established interpersonal relations and communicate effectively with other students and educators and who identify with the values of the institution who, Lawrence (2003) suggests, reap the most benefits from the unfamiliar learning situation.

As mentioned previously, higher education institutions have been slow to focus on the supportive role they can play other than through the provision of counselling and health services and first year experience programmes. During the 1990s the concept of 'health promoting universities' with support from WHO (Tsouros et al. 1998) was gaining credence particularly in the United Kingdom (Dooris 2001). There is now activity in many parts of the world: China (www.cuhk.edu.hk/healthpromotion); Canada (www.healthyconference.ualberta.ca); the US (www.ahcnet.org); and Ireland (www.tcd.ie/College.Health/healthpromotion). However practice is not consistent. Some activity is driven by university health services or by nursing faculties, others are linked to healthy city projects. They vary in focus from policy development to implementation of workplace programmes for staff or health campaigns for students.

School to university transition

For 18–24-year-olds whose life opportunities include further career development the focus is not just on academic study but also on vocational choices. Linking learning with career and life options creates a different context than that which exists for schooling. Linking future career with growing independence in life and learning results in a complex interaction of influencing factors. From a mental health perspective it is easy to see why this complexity creates the milieu for a high incidence of mental health problems and illnesses. Additional evidence indicates that young adults experience challenges and risk conditions including becoming autonomous learners, developing and maintaining intimate relationships and establishing a sense of direction (Balk 1997; Hemmings et al. 1997). A paradox for this age group is that their developing independence may preclude students disclosing to academic advisors personal factors (such as adverse life changes) that impact on their studies (Rowling et al. 2005). Additionally they may be distant from supportive networks and environments.

There is an absence of attention to affective components such as control and anxiety within current first year experience programmes. Most attention is focused on student identity, academic integration and identifying with the university. The absence of affective areas is significant given that the major reason students cite for considering deferment is 'emotional health' (McInnis et al. 2000). Most universities now have specific programmes targeting first year students and there is considerable research on these programmes (for example, First Year Experience Centre at the university of South Carolina: http://www.sc.edu/fye/), research that principally focuses on the learning environment. Much of this research does not account for the personal and social issues of life transitions that have the potential to impact on students' adjustment and learning and mental health.

School to work transition

Another group of young adults, who may range in age from 15–19, are those who make a transition from school to work. A poor transition, that is leaving school with limited educational attainment and experiencing periods of unemployment (Dusseldorf Skills Foundation 2005) is associated with missed opportunities for the development of skills for employment. This is the experience for many young people in those countries where school attendance is limited. Decisions made during this transition about areas, such as further education and employment, have far reaching consequences. Disadvantaged young people can be the least equipped to make these decisions. Leaving school before the minimum age (where such exists)[2] and entering the workforce is far more disadvantaging than it was in previous generations. These young people leave themselves vulnerable to unemployment, insecure or badly paid work, early family formation (for example, young age pregnancy) and social exclusion when they are unable to be self-supporting (Social Exclusion Unit 2005).

A study using two cohorts of British children, one born in 1958 and a comparable group born in 1970, provides evidence that the experience of disadvantage weakens individual adaptation (Schoon and Bynner 2003). Subsequent experiences of adversity exacerbates a young person's well-being and negatively impacts on their staying on at school. Social class impacts on whether young people stay on at school, but these researchers found that, along with middle class parents, working class parents had aspirations for their children to succeed. They suggested that strengthening parental aspirations through the medium of teacher–parent interaction could support young people's aspirations for staying on at school. They argued that a resilience framework should therefore be harnessed to draw on the strengths and high aspirations of less privileged parents for their children's welfare and development.

Data from the British National Child Development Study (Bynner et al. 2002) from two cohorts of young people provides an indication of the impacts of a poor school to work transition. Compared to the 1958 cohort, for those born in 1970 there were fewer job opportunities and more stayed at school longer, but a higher number completed school and gained degree qualifications. Despite higher educational attainment overall, more of the school to work group reported feelings of depression, particularly young women. Greater experience of unemployment was posited by the researchers as a reason for the higher incidence of depression. Young people with university degrees were a third less likely to report symptoms of depression than those with no higher education qualifications (National Child Development Study, Bynner et al. 2002). These findings provide the evidence that educational achievement is supportive of mental health and well-being and that for those who left at a minimum age, had low prestige training and experienced unemployment there were adverse mental health outcomes. It could also be argued that being employed in a workplace setting like educational settings provides some form of structure and meaning for those young adults who make the transition between school and work.

Box 5.3   Summary points on educational determinants of mental health

- The life trajectory for young adults is not as predictable or as homogeneous as in previous generations.
- Young people whose emotional needs are met are more likely to apply themselves to learning.
- Research that links mental health and learning is vital.
- Young people who leave school early are at higher risk for social exclusion.
- Four elements are necessary: a positive school culture; a positive relational context between adults and young people; educational processes building critical solutions-based thinking; and teachers'/educators' well-being needs being considered.
- Young adults entering post-compulsory educational environments need to develop new identities as learners.

Economic

A key factor that underpins the occurrence of mental disorders is the experience of relative social disadvantage (Desjarlais 1997). Poor mental health is linked to limited access to important resources such as income, employment and education (Wilkinson and Marmot 1998). Economic factors that create social disadvantage inter-relate with other resource bases. Poverty is linked to low academic achievement and leaving school early, thereby limiting participation in the labour market and access to meaningful jobs. Being unemployed increases anxiety for children and young people as well as for adults (Twenge 2000).

Wilkinson (1997) suggests that economic and social inequality undermine broader social cohesion and, thus, negatively impact on social connectedness and community safety. This is important for future outcomes for young people. For those leaving school early who are in casual part-time employment; who are not connected to social institutions such as religious, sports or arts groups; and whose communities are fragmented, the conditions for promotion of mental health and support are limited. For the emerging adulthood group the changed work environment, particularly the casualization of the workforce and uncertainty of employment after training, restrict opportunities for socialization, adult identity growth and the development of a sense of a future.

Young people from socio-economically disadvantaged backgrounds are more likely to experience difficulties such as low academic achievement that influence attainments into adulthood (Bynner et al. 2000). The experience of disadvantage does not necessarily occur immediately, vulnerabilities may only emerge later and persistent socio-economic disadvantage has stronger effects than intermittent adversity (Schoon and Bynner 2003).

In its plan for addressing the economic participation of young people, the Victorian Health Promotion Foundation (2003) identifies the following factors as important:

- access to work and meaningful engagement;
- access to education;
- access to adequate housing; and
- access to money.

A research study in rural Scotland (Pavis et al. 2002) provides evidence of how the inter-relationship of these factors impacts on young people's well-being. Many of these factors echo discussion in previous sections about key transitions in young adults' lives. Employment provides the resources for becoming independent, not only financially but also for psychological and geographic distance from family. Employment is a key factor in identity formation and provides young people with a sense of purpose and a structure to the day (Jahoda 1988, in Pavis et al. 2002: 3). These researchers found that place of employment and low wages limited the housing options of young people in rural areas. Often affordable accommodation was sub-standard and lacked basic facilities. From a mental health promotion perspective, labour market participation can promote social cohesion and integration (Pavis et al. 2002). This social well-being outcome supports a holistic approach to the complex needs of young adults in that they experience life as a whole, while also at particular times encountering difficulties in specific life domains (employment, housing, family relationships, community integration).

The complexity of factors impacting on young people is exemplified in the study's finding that rural isolation exerts both positive and negative influences depending on life stage, being enhancing in childhood because of the freedom, and constraining during adolescence and young adulthood due to limited access to public leisure facilities and other social experiences. Acknowledgement of this complex interaction of factors led the researchers to conclude that 'concepts such as well-being and quality of life make sense only when they are grounded within specific cultural contexts and individual biographical experiences' (Pavis et al. 2002: 12).

Social exclusion due to low income, unemployment, poor housing and living in a disadvantaged area as a young person can move social exclusion from one generation to the next, particularly through conception at a young age and youth offending (Social Exclusion Unit 2005). Opportunities are needed to help them negotiate the transitions to adulthood in ways that can lift them out of the cycle of disadvantage. The recognition of the multiplier effect of social exclusion and economic disadvantage on young people's physical, social and mental health is reflected in the work of the UK Social Exclusion Unit 'neighbourhood renewal' projects as described in the next section.

Built environment

The human built environment involves buildings, open spaces and a 'sense of place', a feeling of attachment or belonging to a physical environment and the sense of personal and collective identity that comes from this sense of belonging (Butterworth 2000). That is, places have meaning and resonance for people and symbolize people's personal histories, interpersonal relationships and shared events in relationships, families and communities. Boyd and colleagues (1997) identified the built environment as being a source of stress and impacting on people's social networks and supports. Lack of social support and social interaction, particularly support through adversity, is linked with poor mental health outcomes (Social Exclusion Unit 2005).

Built environments that promote social interaction and participation support the development of social networks, social support, sense of community, community competence and a sense of place – all important determinants of community mental well-being. For example, young people need places where they can meet, places which provide recreation and learning opportunities. They also need to feel included and welcomed in public places such as shopping malls. Positive interactions in such places provide opportunities for different age groups to meet, breaking down generational barriers, encouraging young people to take on adult roles and enhance their social skills (Butterworth 2000). Such encounters build a sense of place and community through feelings of belonging as well as a sense of personal and collective identity that comes from these connections. Educational institutions also provide a sense of place for young people, where identities as learners, achievement of success in a range of ways and opportunities for social support from peers and adults exist.

The built environment includes not only the physical environment but how it *feels* to be in that space. As well as providing opportunities for building young people's competence, it can limit their socialization and negatively impact on their well-being.

Concerns for personal safety can restrict young people's mobility. The sources of their fear can be many: their lived experiences; for marginalized young people, harassment and policing by regulatory agencies; parents projecting fears as a mechanism for scaring young people and thereby physically containing their socializing; media sensationalizing problems; and young people being stereotyped as perpetrators of violence.

Young people who lose treasured places, such as those who are new arrivals or those who become homeless due to domestic violence and abuse, may experience loss of fundamental trust and security in the predictability of relationships as well as loss of identity that comes with connection to a community. From a mental health promotion perspective actions to support communities and create a sense of community have the potential to have important outcomes. As mentioned at the beginning of this section empowerment processes and outcomes are essential strategies for working with communities. Empowerment for individuals involves gaining access to and control over resources which include participation in community organizations. The outcomes of these processes include perception of having control over certain situations and areas in their lives and competence in participating in the decisions that shape their lives (Perkins and Zimmerman 1995, in Butterworth 2000: 21).

Empowerment processes exist in the community development aspect of arts-based programmes. Mental health outcomes of involvement in community arts activities include increased competence, self-esteem, social inclusion and sense of well-being (Matarasso 1997). A feeling of competence builds from successful experiences of interacting with, and having an impact on, other people. Feeling competent is essential for positive mental health. In contrast feeling powerless is damaging for individuals and communities. Competence is created through such processes as groups being supported to determine their own stories and communicate them through music, song, dance and theatre (Rowling and Taylor 2005). The use of theatre to engage marginalized young people is accepted globally as an important and culturally appropriate contributor to their involvement in the process of articulating their mental health concerns. This practice is respectful and valuing of young people and provides opportunities to gain insight into their lived experiences. It also provides the opportunity to include young people from disadvantaged backgrounds whose literacy skills may preclude their involvement in traditional programmes. Being respectful of members of communities that are excluded either socially or economically from full participation in society builds the capacity and competence of both the community and its individual members (Rowling and Taylor 2005). Research indicates that communities with high rates of participation in community activities have better health outcomes than those with low levels of civic engagement (Marmot 2000).

Organized sport is a significant feature of the lives of many thousands of young people, offering opportunities to form lasting friendships and learn social values and organizational skills that are transferable to other areas of their lives. Sporting activities are an important vehicle through which migrant, refugee and marginalized young people can build competence, supportive relationships and a sense of identity, thereby enhancing their mental health and well-being. Programmes can enhance young people's physical and mental health by building social connectedness, through organized sporting clubs, and contribute to reducing racism and discrimination in sporting environments.

Barriers to involvement in sport and its mental health benefits exist for young women of different ethnic origins. Many come from cultures where women and girls are socialized to play a more passive role and participation in sport may conflict with values held by both their families and women themselves. New arrival families may also hold particular fears for the safety of young women in an unfamiliar country and hence be less inclined to grant them the freedom and independence available to boys. In some cultures it may be unacceptable for young women to participate in a mixed gender sporting environment.

Other social environments such as youth and religious groups can also provide opportunities for young people to take leadership responsibilities or have their varying contributions acknowledged and valued. This facilitates the development of feelings of competence and connectedness to the varying communities, and builds identities as learners and leaders among younger age children. Providing a range of opportunities for different experiences in schools and local neighbourhoods may be particularly important for those who are educationally disadvantaged (Resnick et al. 1993).

Box 5.4   Summary of the impact of the economic and built environments

- Leaving school early without access to full time work can lead to disconnection economically and socially and failure to develop a sense of the future.
- Young adults not in full-time work or education have complex needs, for example they face sub-standard housing, and a lack of opportunities for developing independence and social engagement.
- Support is needed that encapsulates their lived experience resulting in integrated service provision.
- The built environment plays a central role in mental health.
- Absence of connection and/or identification with a place has a broad impact on mental health.
- Building a sense of community or identification with a group is an important mental health promotion action.
- Empowerment processes and outcomes are central health promotion strategies in creating connections to 'place'.

Summary comments on the determinants of mental health

Twenge's analysis of over 60 years of research (Twenge 2000) provides a useful overview of the inter-relationships between the determinants of mental health. She found increasing anxiety in young people. The factors articulated as impacting on this provide strong support for the need to address all the determinants of mental health. Her work examines two types of anxiety: trait anxiety (a relative stable individual difference in anxious predispositions), and state anxiety (a transient emotion in a particular situation). Importantly, she described three ways of examining this:

- Overall threat, where anxiety increases as the environmental threat increases.

These threats can be physical or psychological. The individual appraisal of threat is also important.

- Economic conditions, here anxiety increases as economic conditions deteriorate. This accounts for why poverty is an important factor for mental health.
- Social connectedness, where anxiety increases as social bonds weaken. Young people's anxiety strongly effects what is happening in society at large.

Two forces were identified that most affected this increase in anxiety: low social connectedness and high environmental threat (Twenge 2000). In our culture of fear, young people have limited sense of future (Furedi 2002). It is therefore important for young people to develop the cognitive skills to effectively appraise threat and for families, social institutions and the wider society to enhance social bonds and connectedness.

The known mental health 'vulnerability' of this group

The vulnerability of adolescents and young adults can be looked at in two ways. First the absence of attention to the needs of particular groups who fall into a gap in accessing mental health services because of their age. They often can no longer use CAMHS services, but may not be eligible to use Adult Mental Health Services (AMHS). They may also encounter professionals in either service who do not want to consider the complex needs of young adults (Social Exclusion Unit 2005; Young Minds 2005a). As a group, society has not created a supportive environment for them in terms of access to help. A second source of vulnerability is life circumstances that create adversity. For example 24 percent of 13–15-year-olds who had emotional difficulties had had a broken love relationship (Meltzer et al. 2000). The gap in services exacerbates the challenges in the life worlds of specific groups such as same-sex attracted young people, young parents, new arrivals to the country, those leaving care or those who have been excluded from school, those in the criminal justice system, the homeless and those who are carers, especially of a parent with a mental illness (Young Minds 2005b).

Three of these vulnerable groups will be examined here: young parents, same-sex attracted young people and young carers. The focus for young parents in this chapter is their mental health, the impact of their parenting is discussed in Chapter 6. In a UK study parenthood at a young age was associated with high level mental health problems with significantly higher level of depression in the medium term postpartum (Liao 2003). Lower educational attainment and disrupted employment create economic hardship, possibly compounded by lower educational attainment and interrupted employment, leading to depression (Ross and Huber 1985, in Liao 2003: 3).

A range of the determinants of mental health already discussed are triggered by early parenthood. Liao (2003) in reviewing research identified that most of the adverse health consequences of young parent childrearing is a result of social and economic factors rather than young age. Educationally girls may leave school before the minimum leaving age or delay or interrupt the completion of high school, entry into university or completion of university. The need for new mothers, who have a job or still go to school, to care for a young baby/child may create a strain because of the conflicting demand in time and energy due to the two sets of roles of being a mother and of being an employee (or student). Social exclusion is experienced as a result of discrimination (exclusion from school) and demeaning labelling such as 'pregnant girl' or 'teenage mum'. Preferable language is 'young women' or 'young parents'.

Young mothers' programmes have been implemented in many schools to assist young pregnant women. Strategies implemented include promoting awareness of key support staff who can help them; informing them of the full range of options to complete their education; providing them with access to information about local community services such as child care and health care; and involving them in the development of flexible school strategies which reflect and support their needs.

Another group, young gay, lesbian, bisexual and trans-sexual people, face particular challenges. Coming to terms with their sexuality can be extremely stressful, lonely and involve alienation from family. There can be high levels of verbal and physical harassment at school and in the wider society. This can contribute to depression, drug and alcohol use, fear and anxiety. The needs of this group are of particular concern in relation to suicide (National Institute for health and Clinical Excellence (NICE), Crowley et al. 2005). Developing mental health promotion strategies for same-sex attracted (SSA) young people is not easy given the stigma and fear associated with 'coming out'.

The third vulnerable group are young carers, particularly those caring for a parent with a mental illness. Dearden and Becker (2004) have conducted research on the needs of several thousand young carers at three time periods: 1995, 1997 and 2003. The existence of a child as a carer may be hidden in families and schools. Families may minimize a child's caring role and the child will collude with this due to family loyalty. This 'family secret' may also be hidden from schools and other educational institutions. Information about their relative's illness may be withheld from younger adolescents creating anxiety and misunderstanding.

Young carers too have reported anxiety, depression and illness as a result of emotional distress. The responsibility of caring has accelerated the transition from childhood to adulthood for many young carers (Dearden and Becker 2004), making them 'wise beyond their years'. A 'normal' childhood may be difficult to achieve as social interaction with peers (for example friends coming to their home) and balancing education/paid work and caring is challenging.

The meaning of mental health to young people

An Australian study asked young people themselves about what they thought promoted their mental health, which was framed as resilience and well-being (Fuller et al. 2002). Results identified that they perceived three factors to be important: feeling loved and connected to the family; peer connectedness and fitting in at school; and having a good teacher. In relation to their families the positive aspects they cited were support, love, security and belonging. They had different expectations of mothers and fathers, the former were seen as the emotional bedrock and the latter the guide.

A qualitative study, *Listening to Children*, explored the attitudes and perceptions of young people (aged 12–14 years) across socio-economic and ethnic groups in Scotland about mental health and mental illness (Armstrong et al. 1998). Factors reported as promoting mental health were family, friends, personal achievements, feeling good about yourself, having people to talk to, pets, presents and having fun. Factors which caused people to feel mentally unhealthy were identified as death of a family member, friends or pets, break up of relationships, peer pressure, falling out with friends, divorce or parents fighting, and boredom. More activities were seen as a way of attaining positive mental health and adult interventions of various types were seen as important in helping young people feel physically and emotionally safe. Young people's knowledge about mental health and illness came from the media, especially the TV. School and parents did not seem to have played a formal role in developing the attitudes of the young people.

Evidence of effective mental health promotion with adolescents and young adults

Much of the research base for health promotion arises from US prevention science and a risk and problem orientation. Prevention science has made significant advances in understanding the malleable risk and protective factors for the onset of mental health problems (WHO 2004b). But the mental health prevention activity has focused on reducing risk factors in individuals and families especially those affecting young people – home-based, individually focused intervention programmes being complemented by school focused interventions that most frequently target individuals 'at risk'. There is now a growing emphasis on strengths, social and emotional learning and positive youth development.

Wells et al. (2002, 2003) reported on a systematic review of mental health promotion interventions in schools conducted in 1999. Most of the 17 studies were American, but the conclusion about elements of programmes that create a positive impact was clear:

- they adopt a whole-school approach;
- they are implemented continuously for more than a year;
- they involve changes to the school climate; and
- they are aimed at the promotion of mental health compared to the prevention of mental illness.

(Wells et al. 2002: 197)

There was evidence that programmes which promote emotional and social competence can contribute substantially to emotional well-being.

There are efforts in place to strengthen the evaluation of health promoting schools in countries which, to date, have reported few, if any studies. Mūkoma and Flisher (2004) reported from a systematic review of health promoting schools that they were unable to find any evaluations from Africa. Their review arose from the need to develop a framework for evaluating health promoting schools in South Africa. The criteria used for inclusion in the review overlapped those of Lister-Sharp et al. (1999) but also differed in some respects. Nine studies were included in the review from European countries, Australia and the US. They reported positive developments from process evaluations but did not comment specifically on mental health outcomes. In reflecting on the challenges for evaluating complex initiatives of the health promoting schools type they stressed the need for further research on evaluation methodologies for health promoting schools. In developing a framework for evaluation for South Africa, they recommended the use of quantitative and qualitative methodologies to comprehensively evaluate process, intermediate and long-term outcomes.

A review by the CASEL (Collaborative for Academic, Social and Emotional Learning) group of school-based prevention and youth development programmes concluded that these interventions are most effective when they simultaneously target both student's personal and social strengths and the school environments (Greenberg and Weissberg 2003).

However, these reviews do not provide evidence on some important health promotion characteristics. In a UK review on mental health and young people in England which mainly involved American studies, Harden and Rees (2001) reached the conclusion that although involvement of young people is seen as a key part of health promotion practice, only 7 per cent of the studies reviewed provided a role in the intervention development for young people. They concluded that this represents a conflict with principles of empowerment and partnerships.

MindMatters is a school-based Australian national initiative to promote the mental health of secondary school students. It targets multiple mental health promotion outcomes in the context of a coordinated whole-school approach, focusing on promoting connectedness, the organizational structures, social environment and the individual within this context. MindMatters can be distinguished from prior single topic health education projects because it places mental health within the core educational business of schools rather than identifying it as a health curriculum topic (Sheehan et al. 2002). It also provides a context for the selective inclusion of other targeted programmes and initiatives that address specific aspects of mental health and mental ill health (MindMatters Plus).

The 'content' of MindMatters consists of materials for review and planning for school improvement for mental health, now published as SchoolMatters (Sheehan et al. 2002). This includes practical tools for auditing, planning and managing mental health, and is targeted at school principals and teachers in positions of leadership. Curriculum and whole-school change strategies for selected topics such as bullying and harassment, resilience, stress and coping, help seeking, loss and grief, and mental illness are other components (see MindMatters website: cms.curriculum.edu.au/mindmatters). Community Matters materials were added later to provide for the community context, specific groups of students with high needs, and gathering the student voice. In professional development programmes for teachers the need was identified for material on teachers' mental health. This has resulted in the development of additional MindMatters materials, StaffMatters, available for use in a variety of modes.

There are a number of comprehensive evaluation strategies being utilized for monitoring the process and assessing impacts and outcomes and employing evaluation logic models (Rowling and Mason 2005). The evaluation of the dissemination of materials, the professional development and its impact on schools has been undertaken over a three year period using qualitative and quantitative methods. The

MindMatters dissemination evaluation reveals the complexity of the school site in determining how interventions are actually occurring at school, year level or cohort and classroom levels. This has been echoed by the evaluation of the NHHS (Warwick et al. 2005).

The development of health promoting universities parallels the development of health promoting schools and is being initiated in a number of countries. An initiative in six universities in China set out to create health promoting universities within the Ottawa Charter framework, to improve the supportive environment for health, and empower the university community to improve and sustain their health and that of others. Compared with baseline measures there was a significant increase, after one year in the percentage of students reporting good mental health in the past month. Over three-quarters of students considered the physical environment had improved and over 80 percent reported a good social environment (Xiangyang et al. 2003).

The mental health outcomes from physical activity are increasingly being recognized. A study in a low socio-economic status area of Chile (Bonhauser et al. 2005) evaluated the effects of a school-based physical activity programme on both physical fitness and mental health status of adolescents. The exercise programme was developed by teachers and students who also decided on the mode of implementation. In the intervention group anxiety scores decreased significantly and self-esteem increased but there was no impact on depression scores. The programme achieved high levels of participation.

Across the world many adolescents and young adults have no contact with education services. Large numbers are also not involved in formal workplace settings through which some mental health promotion might take place. Workplace initiatives are discussed in Chapter 6. The most appropriate way to reach these young people is through health services and other community-based activities. In the case of young parents there are programmes in many countries that provide community and home-based support, often using community volunteers (see Chapter 6) and good evidence of effectiveness has been reported.

Box 5.5   Evidence-based principles for implementing quality school mental health promotion

- Take a whole-school approach.
- Use a social competence approach rather than focusing on specific problem behaviours and employ interactive and participatory methodologies.
- Involve planned implementation over a number of years.
- Engage key partners.
- Build core competencies and capacities of participants.
- Utilize comprehensive evaluation strategies that employ evaluation logic models.

(Jané-Llopis et al. 2005: 50–1)

Examples of realistic good practice (national and local) in a variety of cultural circumstances

As in the other lifespan chapters examples of projects and methods are provided which have applied theory and principles of health promotion. They have not always been subject to extensive evaluation.

Developing social, emotional and behavioural skills

Social, behavioural and emotional learning is being piloted in 50 UK schools in contrasting LEAs through the Developing Social, Emotional and Behavioural Skills programme, across the whole school (DfES 2005). The programme is based on a study in 2002 (Weare and Gray 2003) that identified how LEAs viewed problem behaviour as having underlying social and emotional causes which need to be addressed in a holistic, environmental way rather than through approaches which focus on detection, containment, negative reinforcement and punishment. The review included a number of case studies. For example in 1998 the chief educational psychologist in Southampton and the chief inspector for Southampton Education Service embarked on a programme to promote emotional literacy through a range of activities including:

* The development of the emotional literacy of LEA managers through seminars, presentations and publications for headteachers, teachers, governors, parents, pupils, police, colleagues in health and social services, and employers.
* The publication and implementation of a behaviour support plan with emotional literacy as the central focus for the promotion of a pupil inclusion project to reduce exclusions.
* Training and development in anger management and running anger management groups on an apprenticeship cascade model.
* Delivering modular training for senior teachers on behaviour management.
* Delivering anti-bullying training to teachers from 45 schools.
* Devising strategies to combat racial harassment.

The data show that work to promote emotional and social well-being, as well as being successful in its own right, appears to have contributed positively to the LEA's wider strategic aims and educational standards more generally. In 1997 in Southampton LEA there were 113 permanent exclusions. By 2001, this had been reduced by more than 60 percent with no corresponding increase in fixed term exclusions. Most encouragingly, no looked after pupil, the most vulnerable group in the exclusion statistics, had been permanently excluded, and attendance rates had increased (Weare and Gray 2003).

Working with marginalized young people

Young people, particularly young men, marginalized as a result of factors such as unemployment or socio-economic disadvantage, can be difficult to engage in mental

health activities (Turner 2002). Specific practices have been found to aid their participation. These include flexible decision-making processes; being respectful and
non-judgemental of young people; accepting young people for who they are without
stigma and without regard for their past; and investment in the development of relationships between young people and project staff. Positive mental health outcomes of a
participatory approach have been achieved, principally through increased feelings of
self-worth and self-efficacy and of participants feeling more confident to express their
wishes and share their ideas with others (Victorian Health Promotion Foundation
2003). Young people's active participation is a paradigm shift from the risk orientation
of much previous prevention work.

The doing things 'to' young people characteristic of a risk- and problem-based
approach detaches young people from the process and resources. Focus groups with
young people identified how the negative youth at-risk approach reduced adult credibility and young people's faith in schools. Events they experienced resulted in a state
of cognitive dissonance, when action that occurred did not match their expectation,
for example, when a young person was excluded from school because of drug use rather
than being provided with a supportive structure and process set in place to help. This
occurred at a time when the young people, who might be among the most vulnerable,
are excluded from schools which have zero tolerance policies (Brown and D'Emidio-
Caston 1995).

Peer mentoring, peer support and other support structures, together with anti-
bullying strategies, can help promote positive health, including mental health. Making
opportunities for pupils' views to be heard and acted on promotes pupil well-being.
Local Connexions services also work with schools to ensure support and advice for
13–19-year-olds (DfES 2004).

Innovative mental health promotion programmes using the Internet

Three innovative projects in Australia utilize electronic media as a mental health promotion medium with young people. Help-seeking barriers for young people include
reluctance to talking to someone, especially adults such as teachers or parents, about
their problems and concerns, and dissatisfaction with the type and format of information available to them (Harden and Rees 2001). The Internet provides an opportunity to
deliver both mental health information and interventions to young people in an
anonymous way which may overcome some of the barriers to help-seeking, such as lack
of awareness, physical access and stigma associated with help-seeking. Approximately
82 percent of young people aged 14–17 years of age reported using the Internet in 2003
(National Office for the Information Economy 2003) accessed from home, school and
public access points.

Reach Out!

A brief school-based intervention (Nicholas et al. 2004) to encourage adolescents to
seek help via the Reach Out! (http://www.reachout.com.au) website, which provides
information to assist young people in managing a range of difficulties including mental
health problems, found that almost half the students had been to the website following

the presentation and that approximately two-thirds reported that they would use the website to seek assistance if they were having difficulties. Two other Australian Internet interventions, BluePages (bluepages.anu.edu.au), a psychoeducation website providing information about depression, and MoodGYM (moodgym.anu.edu.au) have been shown to be more effective in reducing symptoms of depression than a control intervention using an attention placebo in a community sample (Christensen et al. 2004).

Kids Help Line

The use of the Internet for email contact and web counselling is also proving popular at Kids Help Line, a National Australian Telephone and Online counselling service for 5–18-year-olds (www.kidshelp.com.au). The online service, a recent addition in 2000, continues to expand by 40 percent each year (Kids Help Line 2005). Online counselling and email exceeded telephone counselling in 2004 as the medium of choice for mental health issues (Kids Help Line 2005). Innovative ways such as the use of emoticons and colour to convey moods and feelings are being devised to maximize effective communication. These findings suggest that the Internet may provide some promise in the prevention of depression, particularly in the areas of screening, access to information and help-seeking.

Young Minds

Young Minds is a UK national children's mental health charity which works for a better understanding of the mental health of babies, children and young people and for improved child and adolescent mental health services. In 2004 it initiated the Young Minds SOS (stressed out and struggling) project (www.youngminds.org.uk/sos/) that focuses on 16–25-year-old young people. There are a limited number of projects that focus on this age group. A number of strategies are being employed. There are those focusing on early intervention and treatment, such as commissioning a study to develop guidelines for services, service mapping and a system of Positive Practice Awards. A number of mental health promotion strategies have been implemented. A review of mentoring projects, 'Making mentoring more effective' has been commissioned to develop guidelines for quality practice. The project has found that benefits are modest and that a theorized model for mentoring programmes needs to be developed. A specific focus is on higher education students, particularly international students. Guidance in the published material is aimed at all staff groups in higher education, not just the counselling support services. It exemplifies the advocacy role of the organization, an essential mental health promotion strategy. In this role they have produced responses to a number of government policy documents including the UK Youth Matters Green Paper (Young Minds 2005a). Their response noted:

- High levels of concern regarding financial matters and getting into debt are worrying those who have graduated or who are students and putting some young people off from thinking about going to university. There is some evidence to suggest that financial difficulties affect Higher Education students' mental health and academic performance.

- There is a lack of support, guidance and a general lack of interest in young people who don't want to go to university both from the perspective of careers advice, and interest from teachers.

(Young Minds 2005a)

Building a data resource for mental health promotion

The Health Behaviour in School-aged Children (HBSC) monitoring has been occurring for over 20 years. Across Europe it provides a unique data set. Recently the World Health Organization European Office emphasized the importance of gaining input from young people in defining issues, considering strategies and examples of good practice and debating options and alternative action to enhance their health (Currie et al. 2004). This theme of young people as social actors is echoed by many. It is not merely a strategy for data collection, but rather a key factor in understanding their well-being and in providing the conditions for them to influence policy and programmes that are targeted at them and to build their capacity to alter the circumstances that affect their mental health. This in itself is a positive outcome.

The policy context

In the course of the earlier discussion there have been references to policies which are relevant to the promotion of mental health in adolescents and young adults: such as National Service Frameworks, the Healthy Blueprint for Schools and the Youth Matters Green paper, all in the UK. As in the case of other age groups many policy areas are relevant to the promotion of mental health. Chapter 4 has described policies which relate to the health of young children and many will also be relevant to the period of adolescence. Policies relevant to promoting the health of adults are discussed in some detail in Chapter 6. Readers are recommended to refer to the relevant sections in these chapters.

There is clear evidence of the impact of social policy in relation to the transition of a vulnerable group of young carers into the adult world of employment and training opportunities (Young Minds 2005b). In the UK since the introduction of the Carers and Disabled Children Act (2000) carers over the age of 16 are able to receive an assessment and services, including direct payments, in their own right. This policy shows how the determinants of mental health of a group of vulnerable young people can be addressed both through direct support (Young Carer's Project) and targeted social policy.

The application of mental health promotion theory and principles to mental health promotion for adolescents and young adults

Along with the focus on the policy context for mental health, intersectoral collaboration is a key underlying strategy for mental health promotion. Within this broader perspective, focusing on generic concepts such as social and emotional learning and resilience provide opportunities for a 'joined up' approach to concerns about young people, involving not only mental health and well-being but addressing youth suicide, low self-esteem, poor social skills, low academic achievement, drug abuse and violence. There are some common themes around social and emotional learning and resilience that link these areas, namely social support, connectedness to school and the development of a range of skills including positive coping and thinking patterns, self-efficacy, awareness of and empathy with others, problem-solving, help-seeking skills and conflict resolution (National Crime Prevention 1999). Addressing mental health in this broader orientation involves partnerships across sectors (Rowling and Taylor 2005) and recognizes that focusing on mental health and well-being may impact on educational achievement as well as on mental health and drug use.

Key health promotion processes include advocacy, for example, for a reorientation from problems to positive mental health and well-being, and empowerment through solutions-based thinking. Strengthening the opportunities for enhancing these processes will enable addressing mental health and well-being to shift from a focus of health professionals to being of concern to wider professional and community groups.

Conclusions

Not giving attention to young adults is a serious omission in the provision of services and programmes. Addressing the young adults' needs is vital given the evidence that the developing sense of personal independence may inhibit help-seeking (Donald et al. 2000). This chapter demonstrates how quality mental health promotion practice can address the broad determinants of mental health. Increasing evidence demonstrates how school settings are making a significant contribution to positive mental health for school age young people.

However, it is important that researchers collect data about young people's lives now, that they do not study young people by looking retrospectively at adults' lives. The latter approach ignores the very different complex determinants of mental health that operate for young people in the twenty-first century.

Box 5.6   Questions to reflect on when considering mental health promotion for adolescents and young adults

- Why is a sole focus on risk factor research not conducive to effective mental health promotion for young people?
- How does the concept of resilience or social emotional competence link with a positive view of mental health?
- What are the major differences between adolescents and young adults in the challenges they face that can affect their mental health?
- Is there is a direct link between educational achievement, mental health and success in later life. What areas of mental health policy could acknowledge and address this link?
- How can labour market reforms impact on young adults' mental health?

- How can a mental health promotion project accommodate gender differences in young people's mental health needs?
- How can young-women victims of partner violence be helped, individually, in relationships and the wider community?
- How does education and the educational environment play a critical role in supporting young people's mental health?

Notes

1   For a useful discussion on the term 'adolescent' see, for example, http://www.fao.org/sd/wpdirect/WPan0024.htm
2   For details on young people's rights see, for example, http://www.right-to-education.org/content/age/index.html

References

Andrews, G., Hall, H., Teeson, M. and Henderson, S. (1999) *The Mental Health of Australians*, Report No. 2. Canberra: Mental Health Branch, Commonwealth Department of Health and Family Services.

Antidote (2003) *The Emotional Literacy Handbook: Promoting a Whole School Approach*. London: David Fulton Pub. Available at: www.antidote.org.uk (accessed 10 November 2005).

APA (American Psychiatric Association) (1994) *Diagnostic and Statistical Manual of Mental Disorders*, 4th edn. Washington, DC: APA.

Armstrong, C., Hill, M. and Secker, J. (1998) *Listening to Children*. London: Mental Health Foundation.

Arnett, J. (2004) *Emerging Adulthood: The Winding Road from the Late Teens Through the Twenties*. New York: Oxford University Press.

Balk, D.E. (1997) Death, bereavement and college students: a descriptive analysis, *Mortality*, 2(3): 207–20.

Beck, U. (2000) Risk society revisited: theory, politics and research programmes, in B. Adam, U. Beck, J. Van Loon (eds) *The Risk Society and Beyond: Critical Issues for Social Theory*. London: Sage.

Benard, B. (1995) *Fostering Resiliency in Children*, ERIC document ED 386327. Urbana, IL: ERIC Clearinghouse on Elementary and Early Childhood Education.

Benard, B. (1997) *Turning it Around for All Youth: From Risk to Resilience*, ERIC/CUE Digest No.126. New York: Eric Clearinghouse on Urban Education. Available at: http://eric-web.tc.Columbia.edu/digests/dig126.html

Benard, B. (1999) The foundations of the resiliency framework: from research to practice, in N. Henderson, N. Sharp-Light and B. Benard (eds) *Resiliency in Action: Practical Ideas for Overcoming Risks and Building Strengths – In Youth, Families, and Communities*. Minneapolis, MN: The Search Institute.

Benson, P.L. (1997) *All Kids are Our Kids: What Communities Must do to Raise Caring and Responsible Children and Adolescents*. San Francisco: Jossey Bass.

Bond, L., Thomas, L., Toumbourou, J., Patton, G. and Catalano, R. (2000) *Improving the Lives of Young Victorians in our Community: A Survey of Risk and Protective Factors*. Melbourne, Australia. Centre for Adolescent Health. Available at: www.dhs.vic.gov.au/commcare (accessed 20 May 2004).

Bonhauser, M., Fenandez, G., Püschel, K. et al. (2005) Improving physical fitness and emotional well-being in adolescents of low socioeconomic status in Chile: results of a school based controlled trial, *Health Promotion International*, 20(2): 113–22.

Boyd, W.L., Crowson, R.L. and Gresson, A. (1997) *Neighborhood Initiatives, Community Agencies, and the Public Schools: A Changing Scene for the Development and Learning of Children*. Available at: www.temple.edu/lss/htmlpublications/publications/pubs97–6.htm (accessed 15 January 2006).

Brown, J.H. (2004) Resilience: emerging social constructions, in H.C. Waxman, Y.N. Padron and J.P. Gray (eds) *Educational Resilience: Student, Teacher and School Perspectives*. Connecticut: Information Age Publishing.

Brown, D.E. and Christiansen, K.E. (1990) Coping with loss: emotional acculturation in first semester freshmen, *Journal of the Freshmen Year Experience*, 2(1): 69–83.

Brown, H.H. and D'Emidio-Caston, M. (1995) On becoming at-risk through drug education programs: how symbolic policies and practices affect students, *Evaluation Review*, 19(1): 451–92.

Butterworth, I. (2000) *The Relationship Between the Built Environment and Wellbeing: A Literature Review*. Melbourne: Victorian Health Promotion Foundation. Available at: www.vichealth.vic.gov.au/assets/contentFiles/built_environment.pdf (accessed 10 December 2005).

Bynner, J., Joshi, H. and Tsatsas, M. (2000) *Obstacles and Opportunities on Route to Adulthood: Evidence from Rural and Urban Britain*. London: Smith Institute.

Bynner, J., Elias, P. and McKnight, A. (2002) *Better Educated, More Depressed: How Young People's Lives Have Changed in a Generation*. Available at: www.jrf.org.uk (accessed 13 December 2005).

CDHAC (Commonwealth Department of Health and Aged Care) (2000a) *Promotion, Prevention and Early Intervention for Mental Health: A Monograph*. Canberra: Mental Health and Special Programs Branch, Commonwealth Department of Health and Aged Care.

CDHAC (Commonwealth Department of Health and Aged Care) (2000b) *National Action Plan for Promotion, Prevention and Early Intervention for Mental Health 2000*. Canberra: Mental Health and Special Programs Branch, Commonwealth Department of Health and Aged Care.

Christensen, H., Griffiths, K.M. and Jorm, A.F. (2004) Delivering interventions for depression using the Internet: randomised controlled trial, *British Medical Journal*, 328: 265–70.

Cole, A. (2004) *School Report: Health Development Today*. National Institute for Health and Clinical Excellence (NICE), October. Available at: www.publichealth.nice.org.uk/page.aspx?o=503101 (accessed 24 October 2005).

Crowley, P., Kilroe, J. and Burke, S. (2005) *Youth Suicide Prevention: Evidence Briefing*. National Institute for Health and Clinical Excellence (NICE). Available at: www.publichealth.nice.org.uk/page.aspx?o=503368 (accessed 24 October 2005).

Currie, C., Roberts, C., Morgan, C. et al. (2004) *Young People's Health in Context. Health Policy for Children and Adolescents, No.4*. Copenhagen: World Health Organization.

Dearden, C. and Becker, S. (2004) *Young Carers in the UK: The 2004 Report*. London: Carers UK.

Available at: www.carersuk.org/Policyandpractice/Research/YoungcarersReport2004.
pdf (accessed 15 January 2006).

Department of Health and Family Services (1997) *Youth Suicide in Australia: A Background Monograph*. Canberra: Australian Government Publishing Service.

Desjarlais, R. (1997) *World Mental Health: Problems and Priorities in Low Income Countries*. New York: Oxford University Press.

DfEE/DoH (Department for Education and Employment/Department of Health) (1999) *National Healthy School Standards*. London: Department for Education and Employment. Available at: www.wiredforhealth.gov.uk/PDF/NHSS_A_Guide_for_Schools_10_05.pdf (accessed 15 January 2006).

DfES (Department for Education and Skills) (2001). *Learning to Listen: Core Principles for Involvement of Children and Young People*. Available at: www.everychildmatters.gov.uk/ _files/1F85704C1D67D71E30186FEBCEDED6D6.pdf (accessed 15 January 2006).

DfES (Department for Education and Skills) (2004) *Healthy Living Blueprint for Schools*. Available at: image.guardian.co.uk/sys-files/Education/documents/2004/09/06/ Healthyblueprint.pdf (accessed 10 November 2005).

DfES/DoH (Department for Education and Skills/Department of Health) (2004) *The Mental Health and Psychological Well-being of Children and Young People*. National Service Framework for Children Young People and Maternity services. Available at: www.camhs.net/ files/publications/nsf.pdf (accessed 17 November 2005).

Donald, M., Dower, J., Lucke, J. and Raphael, B. (2000) *The Queensland Young People's Mental Health Survey Report*. Woolloongabba: Centre for Primary Health Care, Princess Alexandra Hospital, University of Queensland.

Dooris, M. (2001) The 'health promoting university': a critical explanation of theory and practice, *Health Education*, 101(2): 51–60.

Dusseldorf Skills Foundation (2005) *How Young People are Faring*. Available at: http:// www.dsf.org.au/papers/180.htm (accessed 13 December 2005).

Eckersley, R. (2002) Taking the prize or paying the price: young people and progress, in L. Rowling, G. Martin and L. Walker (eds) *Mental Health Promotion and Young People: Concepts and practice*. Sydney: McGraw-Hill.

Eckersley, R. (2004) *Well and Good: How we Feel and Why it Matters*. Melbourne: Text Publishing.

Elias, M. and Zins, J. (1997) *Promoting Social and Emotional Learning*. Alexandria, Virginia: ASCD.

Erikson, E.H. (1965) *Childhood and Society*. Harmondsworth: Penguin Books.

Fleming, S. and Balmer, H. (1996) Bereavement in adolescence, in C.A. Corr and D. E. Balk (eds) *Handbook of Adolescent Death and Bereavement*. New York: Springer Pub.

Fuller, A., McGraw, K. and Goodyear, M. (2002) Bungy jumping through life: a developmental framework for the promotion of resilience, in L. Rowling, G. Martin and L. Walker (eds) *Mental Health Promotion and Young People: Concepts and Practice*. Sydney: McGraw-Hill.

Furedi, F. (2002) *A Culture of Fear*. London: Continuum.

Furstenberg, F.F., Kennedy, S., McLloyd, C.C., Rumbaut, R.G. and Setterten, R.A. (2003) *Between Adolescence and Adulthood: Expectations about the Timing of Adulthood*. Research Working Paper 1. Network on Transitions to Adulthood and Public Policy. Available at: www.pop.upenn.edu/transad/ (accessed 10 March 2005).

Goleman, D. (1996) *Emotional Intelligence*. London: Bloomsbury.

Green, H., McGinnity, A., Meltzer, A.H., Ford, T. and Goodman, R. (2005) *Mental Health of Children and Young People in Britain 2004*. Basingstoke: Palgrave Macmillan. Available at: www.statistics.gov.uk (accessed 10 November 2005).

Greenberg, M. and Weissberg, R.P. (2003) Enhancing school-based prevention and youth development through co-ordinated social, emotional, and academic learning, *American Psychologist*, 58(67): 466–74.

Harden, A. and Rees, R. (2001) *Young People and Mental Health: A Systematic Review on Barriers and Facilitators*. London: EPPI-Centre. Available at: eppi.ioe.ac.uk (accessed 15 December 2002).

Health Development Agency (2001) *Boys' and Young Men's Health: Literature and Practice Review*. London: Health Development Agency.

Hemmings, B., Hill, D. and Ray, D. (1997) *First Year University in Retrospect*, ERIC Document ED 429 791. Urbana, IL: ERIC Clearinghouse on Elementary and Early Childhood Education.

Henderson, N. and Milstein, M. (1996) *Resiliency in Schools*. Thousand Oaks, CA: Corwin Press.

Hosman, C. and Jané-Llopis, E. (1999) Political challenges to mental health. *The Evidence of Health Promotion Effectiveness: Shaping Public Health in a New Europe*. Paris: International Union for Health Promotion and Education (IUHPE).

Indermaur, D. (2001) *Young Australians and Domestic Violence: Trends and Issues in Crime and Criminal Justice*, No 195. Canberra: Institute of Criminology. Available at: www.aic.gov.au/publications (accessed 10 November 2005).

Jané-Llopis, E., Barry, M.M., Hosman, C. and Patel, V. (2005) Mental health promotion works: a review, *Promotion and Education*, S2: 9–25.

Kastenbaum, R.J. (2001) *Death, Society and Human Experience*. Boston: Allyn & Bacon.

Kennedy, B., Kawachi, I., Glass, R. and Prothrow-Smith, D. (1998) Income distribution, socio-economic status and self rated health in the United States: multi-level analysis, *British Medical Journal*, 317: 917–21.

Kids Help Line (2005) *Online 2004. Information Sheet 27*. Available at: www.kidshelp.com.au (accessed 20 November 2005).

Kings Fund (2000) *Regeneration and Mental Health program*, Briefing 3. London: Kings Fund. Available at: www.jrf.org.uk (accessed 10 November 2005).

Kumpfer, K.L. (1999) Factors and processes contributing to resilience: the resilience framework, in M.D. Glantz and J.L. Johnson (eds) *Resilience and Development: Positive Life Adaptations*. New York: Kluwer Academic/Plenum Publishers.

Lawrence, J. (2003) The 'deficit-discourse' shift: university teachers and their role in helping first year students persevere and succeed in the new university culture. *UltiBASE*, March, pp. 1–10. Available at: ultibase.rmit.edu.au/Articles/march03/lawrence1.htm (accessed 15 January 2006).

Liao, T.F. (2003) *Mental Health, Teenage Motherhood, and Age at First Birth among British Women in the 1990s*, Working Papers of the Institute for Social and Economic Research, paper 2003–33. Colchester: University of Essex. Available at: www.iser.essex.ac.uk/pubs/workpaps/ (accessed 15 January 2006).

Lister-Sharp, D., Chapman, S., Stewart Brown, S. and Sowden, A. (1999) Health promoting schools and health promotion in schools: two systematic reviews, *Health Technology Assessment*, 3(22): 1–207.

Mackie, S. (2001) Jumping the hurdles: undergraduate student withdrawal behaviour, *Innovations in Education and Teaching International*, 38(3): 265–76.

Marmot, M. (1999) The solid facts: the social determinants of health, *Health Promotion Journal of Australia*, 9(2): 133–9.

Marmot, M. (2000) Social determinants of health, *Medical Journal of Australia*, 172(8): 379–82.

Martin, T. and Doka, K.J. (2000) *Men Don't Cry . . . Women Do: Transcending Gender Stereotypes of Grief*. Philadelphia: Bruner Mazel.

Matarasso, F. (1997) *Use or Ornament? The Social Impact of Participation in the Arts*, Working paper 6. Gloucestershire: CoMedia.

McInnis, C., James, R. and McNaught, C. (2000) *Trends in First Year Experience in Australian Universities*. Melbourne: Centre for Higher Education, University of Melbourne. Available at: www.dest.gov.au/archive/highered/eippubs/eip00_6/fye.pdf (accessed 10 March 2002).

McLaughlin, M.W. and Talbert, J.E. (1993) *Contexts that Matter for Teaching and Learning: Strategic Opportunities for Meeting the Nation's Educational Goals*. Stanford: Stanford University, Centre for Research on the Context of Secondary School Teaching.

McLelland, A. and Scotton, R. (1998) 'Poverty in health', in R. Fisher and E. Nieuwenhuysen (eds) *Australian Poverty: Then and Now*. Melbourne: Melbourne University Press.

McLeod, J., Pryor, S. and Mead, J. (2004) *Promoting Mental Health and Wellbeing through Arts Environment Scheme*. Melbourne: Victorian Health Promotion Foundation. Available at: www.vichealth.gov.au (accessed 2 December 2005).

McMurray, A. (1999) *Community Health and Wellness: A Socioecological Approach*. Sydney: Mosby Publishers.

Meltzer, H., Gatward, R., Goodman, R. and Ford, T. (2000) Mental health of children and adolescents in Great Britain, *International Review of Psychiatry*, 15(1–2): 185–7.

Mental Health Foundation (1999) *Bright Futures: Promoting Children and Young People's Mental Health*. London: Mental Health Foundation.

Mental Health Foundation (2004) *Lifetime Impacts. Childhood and Adolescent Mental Health: Understanding the Lifetime Impacts*. London: Office of Health and Economics. Available at: www.mentalhealth.org.uk/html/content/lifetime_impacts.pdf (accessed 11 December 2005).

Mūkoma, W. and Flisher, A.J. (2004) Evaluations of health promoting schools: a review of nine studies, *Health Promotion International*, 19(3): 357–68.

National Crime Prevention (1999) *Pathways to Prevention: Developmental and Early Intervention Approaches to Crime in Australia*. Canberra: Attorney General's Department.

National Office for the Information Economy (2003) *The Current State of Play: Online Participation and Activities*. Canberra: The National Office for the Information Economy.

NHMRC (National Health and Medical Research Council) (1997) *Depression in Young People Clinical Practice Guidelines*. Canberra: Australian Government Publishing Service.

Nicholas, J., Oliver, K., Lee, K. and O'Biren, M. (2004) Help-seeking behaviour and the Internet: an investigation among Australian adolescents, *Australian e-Journal for the Advancement of Mental Health*, 3(1). Available at: www.auseinet.com/journal/vol3iss1/nicholas.pdf (accessed 15 November 2005).

Olsson, C.A., Bond, L., Burns, J.M., Vella-Broderick, D.A. and Sawyer, S.M. (2003) Adolescent resilience: a concept analysis, *Journal of Adolescence*, 20(1): 1–11.

Olweus, D. (1993) *Bullying at School*. Oxford: Blackwell Publishers.

Pais, J.M. (2000) *Transitions and Youth Culture*. Geneva: UNESCO.

Pavis, S., Platt, S. and Hubbard, G. (2002) Youth employment, psychosocial health and the importance of person/environment fit: a case study of two Scottish rural towns, *Australian e-Journal for the Advancement of Mental Health (AeJAMH)*, 1(3). Available at: www.auseinet.com/journal/vol1iss3/Pavis.pdf (accessed 15 November 2005).

QCA (Qualifications and Curriculum Authority) (2001) *Supporting School Improvement. Emotional and Behavioural Development*. London: Qualifications and Curriculum Authority. Available at: www.qca.org.uk/index.html (accessed 15 January 2006).

Reinherz, H.Z., Giaconia, R.S., Hauf, A.M.C., Sasserman, M.S. and Silverman, A.B. (1999) Major depression in the transition to adulthood: risks and impairments, *Journal of Abnormal Psychology*, 108(3): 500–10.

Resnick, M.D., Harris, L.J. and Blum, R. (1993) The impact of caring, *Journal of Paediatric Child Health*, 29(Supplement 1): S3–S9.

Richardson, G.E. (2002) The metatheory of resilience and resiliency, *Journal of Clinical Psychology*, 58(3): 307–21.

Rigby, K. (2003) Consequences of bullying in schools, *Canadian Journal of Psychiatry*, 48: 583–90.

Rowling, L. (2002a) Mental health promotion, in L. Rowling, G. Martin and L. Walker (eds) *Mental Health Promotion: Concepts and Practice*. Sydney: McGraw-Hill.

Rowling, L. (2002b) Youth and disenfranchised grief, in K. Doka (ed.) *Disenfranchised Grief. New Directions, Challenges and Strategies for Practice*. Champaign, IL: Research Press.

Rowling, L. (2003) *Grief in School Communities: Effective Support Strategies*. Buckingham: Open University Press.

Rowling, L. and Kasunic, V. (in press) Prevention of depression in young people, *Journal of Neuropsychiatry*.

Rowling, L. and Mason, J. (2005) A case study of multimethod evaluation of complex school mental health promotion and prevention: the MindMatters evaluation suite, *Australian Journal of Guidance and Counselling*, 15(2): 125–36.

Rowling, L. and Taylor, A. (2005) Intersectoral approaches to promoting mental health, in H. Hermann, S. Saxena, R. Moodie (eds) *Promoting Mental Health: Concepts, Evidence and Practice*. Melbourne: World Health Organization, Victorian Health Promotion Foundation and the University of Melbourne. Available at: www.who.int/mental_health/evidence/en/promoting_mhh.pdf (accessed 15 December 2005).

Rowling, L., Weber, Z. and Scanlon, L. (2005) Transitions and loss: illuminating parameters of young adult's mental health, *Australian Journal of Guidance and Counselling*, 15(2): 168–81.

Rutter, M., Maughan, B., Mortimore, P., Ouston, J. and Smith, A. (1979) *Fifteen Thousand Hours: Secondary Schools and their Effects on Children*. London: Open Books.

Schoon, I. and Bynner, J. (2003) Risk and resilience in the life course: implications for interventions and social policies, *Journal of Youth Studies*, 6(1): 21–31.

Seligman, M. (1991) *Learned Optimism*. New York: Alfred A. Knopf, Inc.

Seligman, M. (1995) *The Optimistic Child*. Boston: Houghton Mifflin.

Settersten, R.A., Furstenberg, R.R. and Rumbaut, R.G. (2005) *On the Frontier of Adulthood: Theory, Research and Public Policy*. Chicago: University of Chicago Press.

Sheehan, M., Cahill, H. and Rowling, L. (2002) Establishing a role for schools in mental health promotion: the MindMatters project, in L. Rowling, G. Martin and L. Walker (eds) *Mental Health Promotion and Young People: Concepts and Practice.* Sydney: McGraw-Hill.

Silva, R. and Radigan, J. (2004) Achieving success: an agentic model of resiliency, in H.C. Waxman, Y.N. Padron and J.P Gray (eds) *Educational Resilience: Student, Teacher and School Perspective.* Connecticut: Information Age Publishing.

Social Exclusion Unit (2000) *Report of Policy Action Team 8: Anti-social Behaviour.* London: The Stationery Office. Available at: www.socialexclusionunit.gov.uk (accessed 15 December 2005).

Social Exclusion Unit (2004a) *Breaking the Cycle: Summary Report.* Available at: www. socialexclusionunit.gov.uk/downloaddoc.asp?did=263 (accessed 15 December 2005).

Social Exclusion Unit (2004b) *Breaking the Cycle: Summary Report.* Available at: ww. socialexclusionunit.gov.uk/downloaddoc.asp?id=262 (accessed 15 December 2005).

Social Exclusion Unit (2005) *Transitions: Young Adults with Complex Needs.* Available at: www.socialexclusionunit.gov.uk/download.asp?id=785 (accessed 15 December 2005).

Trewin, D. (2001) *Measuring Well Being: Frameworks for Australian Social Statistics.* Canberra: Australian Bureau of Statistics, Commonwealth of Australia.

Tsouros, A., Dowding, G., Thompson, J. and Dooris, M. (1998) *Health Promoting Universities: Concept, Experience and Framework for Action.* Copenhagen: WHO Regional Office for Europe.

Turner, C. (2002) CHAMPS: a case study in youth partnership accountability, in L. Rowling, G. Martin and L. Walker (eds) *Mental Health Promotion and Young People: Concepts and Practice.* Sydney: McGraw-Hill.

Twenge, J. M. (2000) The age of anxiety? Birth cohort change in anxiety and neuroticism, 1952–1993, *Journal of Personality and Social Psychology,* 79(6): 1007–21.

Verhulst, F.C. and Koot, H.M. (1992) *Child Psychiatric Epidemiology: Concepts, Methods and Findings.* Newbury Park: Sage.

Victorian Health Promotion Foundation (2003) *Promoting Young People's Mental Health and Wellbeing through Participation in Economic Activities. Key Learnings and Promising Practices.* Melbourne: Victoria Health Promotion Foundation. Available at: www.vichealth. vic.gov.au/assets/contentsFile/VHP%20youth.pdf (accessed 1 October 2005).

Warwick, I., Aggleton, P. and Chase, E. (2005) Evaluating healthy schools: perceptions of impact among school-based respondents, *Health Education Theory and Practice,* 20(6): 697–706.

Weare, K. (2000) *Promoting Mental, Emotional and Social Health: A Whole School Approach.* London: Routledge.

Weare, K. (2003) *Developing the Emotionally Literate School.* London: Sage.

Weare, K. and Gray, G. (2003) *What Works in Developing Children's Emotional and Social Competence and Wellbeing?* Research report 456. London: Department for Education and Skills. Available at: www.dfes.gov.uk/research/data/uploadfiles/RR456.pdf (accessed 10 November 2005).

Wells, J., Barlow, J. and Stewart-Brown, S. (2002) *A Systematic Review of Universal Approaches to Mental Health Promotion in Schools.* Oxford: Health Services Research Unit, University of Oxford.

Wells, J., Barlow, J. and Stewart-Brown, S. (2003) A systematic review of universal approaches to mental health promotion in schools, *Health Education,* 4: 197–220.

Werner, E. and Smith, R.S. (1982) *Vulnerable but not Invincible: A Longitudinal Study of Resilient Children*. New York: McGraw-Hill.

WHO (World Health Organization) (1998) *WHO's Global School Initiative: Health Promoting Schools*. Geneva: World Health Organization.

WHO (World Health Organization) (2001) *The World Health Report 2001. Mental Health: New Understandings, New Hope*. Geneva: World Health Organization.

WHO (World Health Organization) (2002a) *Regional Strategy for Mental Health*. Manila, Philippines: Regional Office for Western Pacific Region. Available at: www.wpro.who.int (accessed 10 November 2005).

WHO (World Health Organization) (2002b) *World Health Report on Violence and Health*. Geneva: World Health Organization. Available at: www.who.int/violence_injury_prevention/violence/world_report/en/full_en.pdf (accessed 15 December 2006).

WHO (World Health Organization) (2004a) *Prevention of Mental Disorders: Effective Interventions and Policy Options*. Geneva: World Health Organisation, Department of Mental Health and Substance Abuse, in collaboration with the Prevention Research Centre in the Universities of Nijmegen and Maastricht. Available at: www.who.int/mental_health/evidence/en/Prevention_of_Mental_Disorders.pdf (accessed 15 December 2005).

WHO (World Health Organization) (2004b) *Promoting Mental Health: Concepts, Emerging Evidence, Practice*. Geneva: World Health Organisation, Department of Mental Health and Substance Abuse, in collaboration with the Victorian Health Promotion Foundation and the University of Melbourne. Available at: www.who.int/mental_health/evidence/en/promoting_mhh.pdf (accessed 15 December 2005).

WHO (World Health Organization) (2005) *Atlas: Child and Adolescent Resources, Global Concerns Implications for Future Action*. Geneva: World Health Organization.

Wilkinson, R. (1997) Income inequality and social cohesion, *American Journal of Public Health*, 87(9): 591–95.

Wilkinson, R. and Marmot, M. (1998) *Social Determinants of Health: the Solid Facts*. Geneva: World Health Organization.

Wolin, S. (2004) Presenting a resilience paradigm for teachers, in H.C. Waxman et al. (eds) *Educational Resilience*. Connecticut: Information Age Publishing.

Xiangyang, T., Lan, Z., Xueping, M. et al. (2003) Beijing health promoting universities: practice and evaluation, *Health Promotion International*, 18(2): 107–13.

Young Minds (2005a) *Response to Youth Matters Green Paper*. Available at: www.youngminds. org.uk/responses/05_11_04.php (accessed 20 December 2005).

Young Minds (2005b) *Adolescent Mental Health Services*. Available at: www.minds.org.uk/adolescentpolicy/index.php (accessed 20 December 2005).

Zubrick, R., Silburn, S.R., Garton, A. et al. (1995) *Western Australian Child Health Survey: Developing Health and Well-being in the Nineties*. Perth: Western Australia, Australian Bureau of Statistics and the Institute for Child Health Research.

Zubrick, S.R., Silburn, S.R., Gurrin, L. et al. (1997) *Western Australian Child Health Survey: Developing Health and Well-being in the Nineties*. Perth: Australian Bureau of Statistics and WA Institute for Child Health Research.

6 Adulthood: increasing responsibility and middle-age (25–45 years and 45–65 years)

Mima Cattan and Sylvia Tilford

Editors' foreword

Adulthood is a time of major life transitions. This chapter considers the particular issues affecting mental health in adulthood, recognizing that many of these can be equally relevant in early adulthood and in later life. Specific mental health issues discussed here include relationships and parenting, mental health in the workplace, and, for the 45–65 year age group, preparing for retirement. The impact of migration as a global mental health issue is also explored. Many of the examples given are excellent illustrations of multi-agency, multiple methods, mental health promotion interventions, which have long-term impact on communities rather than simply on individuals. Housing, homelessness and work/unemployment are of particular interest with regards to inequalities in (mental) health. This is followed by an exploration of current evidence and examples of good practice. The authors note that there are still major gaps in our understanding of effectiveness in mental health promotion for specific age groups in adulthood. The chapter concludes with a discussion of the application of theory to current practice.

Introduction

Adulthood presents particular demands, responsibilities and achievements. Although the years of economic productivity are not confined to this age group it is the one which makes the major contribution to income generation in societies and to the support of non-productive age groups. Work is a dominant activity through which people make a living and achieve life satisfaction. It is also a period where many have a range of responsibilities for others especially as parents of young children in the earlier years and ongoing parental roles together with degrees of care and support for others, especially in the middle years. In addition there are varying levels of involvement in community activities. There are significant differences between parts of the world in the organization of adult life and the ages at which there is full adoption of adult responsibilities. In some parenting begins from later teenage years and life expectancy is such that many will not have a period of older age, or even middle-age. In the UK the mean age of having children has risen steadily so that active parenting of young children can overlap with support for an older generation. Adulthood is a period of experiencing many life events and transitions. These have the potential to enhance mental health, but also pose challenges which can threaten mental health. While some transitions, such as parenting and bereavement, are almost universal others such as the changes associated with physical disasters, armed conflict and migration affect smaller proportions of people. For most working adults the pre-retirement years are a time when preparation, mentally and in practical terms, is made for life after work. Physical health of adults has consequences for mental health. Globally HIV/AIDS poses significant impact on the mental health of adults as well as the children who may lose one or both parents.

As with other age groups, accounts of the state of mental health frequently start from consideration of its converse – ill health. In 2001 the WHO concluded that mental and behavioural disorders worldwide represented 11 percent of the ill health burden, predicted to rise to 15 percent by 2020. A high proportion of the overall burden is contributed by depression, which is estimated to be rising in high, as well as in middle and low, income countries. There are differences according to income level of countries. Neuropsychiatric disorders accounted for 10 percent of the 'disease' burden in low and middle income countries and 18 percent in high income countries (WHO 2001). Since a great deal of mental ill health goes unrecorded, these figures must be seen as approximate. WHO (2001) concluded that there was a large gap between the increasing burden caused by mental health problems and the resources available to prevent and to treat them.

Suicide is a major contributor to mortality from all causes in some age groups and an important public health concern. According to the WHO (2001) approximately 1 million people died from suicide in 2000 with between 10 and 20 times more people attempting suicide. In all countries suicide is one of the three leading causes of death among people aged 15–34 years. Although rates have typically been higher in older age groups they are now higher in younger adults in about one-third of countries worldwide. Rates vary across world regions and between countries within regions with no data available from some countries, particularly in Africa. Figures across countries have to be interpreted with care since many factors influence the categorization of a death as a suicide. Where suicide carries high stigma alternative causes of death may be recorded.

Special mental health issues

The issues selected for this chapter include some which are particular to the age range and others which, while important for adults, also apply to other life stages. The issues selected are: work; ethnicity, transitions and life events, such as forced migration; conflict and violence. These can impact positively, as well as negatively on mental health and well-being.

Adults typically have a range of responsibilities which can include the bringing up of children, and in some cases grandchildren; caring responsibilities for other family members, especially older ones and those experiencing chronic illness; responsibilities for income generation and those arising from the nature of work undertaken; and community responsibilities. Issues for mental health can arise from any of these individually, and taken together they pose a total level of demand.

Involvement in work is a dominant aspect of adulthood. Mental health can be influenced by access to work; the nature of work and its organization; working environments; remuneration; responsibilities within work; age, sex and racial discrimination; and loss of work. Loss of work can be involuntary and can occur at any time in adult life. In later years of adult life there can be a period of pre-retirement where preparation for years outside formal work is required. While many countries have been used to having a specific age for retirement this is increasingly fluid and becoming later in some higher income countries. In many countries people are forced to work into old age because of poverty and lack of social provision and the concept of retirement has no great significance. Others may choose to continue to work, especially in agricultural economies, throughout life.

Again not unique to this age group, but of particularly high importance, can be the number and impact of transitions at the individual and the social level. At an individual level increased levels of change in family structures arising from separation and divorce and geographical mobility are impacting on long-standing, extended family structures. In many countries family structures are being affected by the deaths of young adults from HIV/AIDS. Social and political changes can have significant implications, positively and negatively for mental health. In the last decade these have included the ending of apartheid in South Africa and the breakdown of the USSR.

A particular issue is the impact of conflict and violence, whether at the macro- or micro-level. These impact directly on mental health and also indirectly through the impact on other influences on mental health. The effects can result from overt violence or from the threats posed by the fear of possible violence. At the macro-level many parts of the world are affected at the time of writing: Iraq, Sudan, Sri Lanka, parts of the Middle East. Violence at the interpersonal level has long-term effects on the adults involved as well as on other family members as discussed in earlier chapters.

Box 6.1 Summary points: factors that may impact on mental health and well-being in adulthood

1   Increasing responsibility, 25–45 years:
   - having and bringing up children;
   - workplace security/insecurity;
   - relationship issues.
2   Middle-age, 45–65 years:
   - bringing up a family;
   - work and community responsibilities;
   - caring for ageing parents;
   - preparing for retirement.
3   Adulthood, 25–65 years:
   - changing family structures;

- individual and social transitions, life events;
- age/sex/race discrimination;
- conflict and violence.

Determinants of, and influences on mental health

In common with other life stages there are multiple influences on mental health, operating at micro, meso and macro levels. While major influences can be considered on an individual basis the complex interactions between influences need to be recognized. The influences will be discussed broadly according to the model in Chapter 4, Figure 4.1, which categorizes influences into those which are related to the individual's biology and physical health, individual competences and lifestyle behaviours, and environmental factors, divided broadly into socio-economic and cultural factors, and those of the natural and human-made environment. While the categories are not fully distinctive they form a convenient basis for organizing discussion.

Individual biological/physical determinants

The mental health of people with disabilities and with long-term conditions can be affected as a consequence of the stigma and the way their conditions are treated in the wider social environment. Studies have shown that the risk of depression is significantly higher among disabled adults compared with able-bodied adults. This risk is increased even further by external factors such as unemployment (Turner and Turner 2004), and physically disabled adults are more likely to be involuntarily unemployed. Even high achieving women with physical and sensory disabilities have been found at various points in their lives and careers to experience low self-esteem, lack of confidence and stress as a result of prejudice and lack of support (Noonan et al. 2004). These women describe the availability of disabled role models and mentors, social support and education as being pivotal in the way they approached their careers.

It almost goes without saying that HIV/AIDS can have a serious impact on mental health. So far most research has focused on the mental health of HIV patients. Recent studies have shown that the association between depression and HIV/AIDS is linked to gender, an experience of greater impact of negative life events, poverty, drug use and disability (Olley et al. 2004; Braitstein et al. 2005). In other words, it is the synergistic effect of other life events and socio-economic and personal factors which determines the level of risk of depression. The impact of HIV/AIDS on the mental health of carers and other close members of the family and community is also significant (bearing in mind that they may also be HIV infected).

Individual competencies and behaviours

The question about why some people seem to be 'protected' from mental ill health despite being subjected to a range of risk factors has been the focus of research into coping mechanisms and resilience. Resilience, which is described in more detail in

Chapter 5, is said to develop as a result of the individual experiencing adverse life events, such as involuntary change, poverty, trauma, conflict or disasters. Coping strategies seem to evolve and develop throughout life to adjust to physical or cognitive changes as people age. However, this does not mean that these skills improve or decline, but rather perhaps that people, over time, strive towards an equilibrium of mental wellness.

Research investigating resilience among marginalized groups, such as refugees, gay, lesbian and bisexual populations, and geographically isolated populations, has found that social support, education and social engagement are utilized to develop resilience. A review of research into stress and mental health among gay, lesbian and bisexual adults noted that resilience is developed by learning to cope with stigma and stress, and through self-acceptance and family support (Meyer 2003). It can therefore be assumed that the interaction between resilience and stress impacts on individuals' mental health. Group cohesiveness, support and identity may also provide additional resources for coping as a member of a minority group.

To date very little research has considered coping skills and resilience of refugees and asylum seekers. Most research has investigated psychiatric mental health problems, such as post-traumatic stress disorder, rather than looked at refugees' coping strategies in dealing with adversity and stress. A British study noted that Kosovan refugees arriving in the UK had a high prevalence of depression and post-traumatic stress disorder, but that many demonstrated a high level of resilience. Separation from family was associated with the severity of people's distress (Turner et al. 2003).

Individual behavioural and lifestyle factors

There are strong associations between behavioural factors and mental health, both in terms of maintaining well-being and as coping mechanisms. The main behavioural factors that affect mental health and well-being are physical activity and exercise, smoking, diet, alcohol and medication.

There is a growing body of evidence that shows the benefits of exercise and physical activity in promoting mental health and well-being. Exercise has been found to improve self-esteem, psychological and subjective well-being, reduce anxiety and depression, and enhance cognitive functioning (Maltby and Day 2001; Callaghan 2004). Qualitative studies have demonstrated that physical activity promotes work and life satisfaction (satisfaction with self), self-confidence, a sense of belonging and purpose and a sense of physical health (DoH 2004a; Crone et al. 2005).

The use of tobacco as a stimulant or as 'coping device' is well known and there is evidence to suggest an association between mental ill health and smoking. The White Paper, *Smoking Kills* (Secretary of State for Health 1998), goes as far as to suggest that the reason people with serious mental illness die prematurely is because they are heavy smokers. Studies have shown that tobacco dependence is a construct of psychological need, physiological dependence and social reinforcement (Graham and Der 1999). The main factors associated with smoking and also with smoking cessation are socio-economic circumstances (including education and poverty); domestic circumstances (partners smoking); psychiatric problems; and drug and alcohol dependence (Graham and Der 1999; Degenhardt and Hall 2001). Life transitions, particularly pregnancy, can be major triggers to giving up smoking. Degenhardt and Hall (2001) suggest that for smoking cessation programmes to be effective they need to take into account co-existing mental health problems and other drug use.

Alcohol use and mental health are related in several ways. The Institute of Alcohol Studies (Institute of Alcohol Studies 2004) summarizes this relationship by stating that mental health problems can result from excessive drinking, but that problem drinking can lead to mental health problems. In addition, external or genetic factors can contribute to both mental health and alcohol related problems. Studies have found that the effects of alcohol and the acceptability of alcohol consumption are influenced by culture, the social environment, psychological and genetic factors (Tolvanen et al. 1998). The expectancies of the effects of alcohol also influence how people drink. Young and middle-aged adults who have positive expectancies of the effects tend to consume more alcohol, although research findings are less consistent regarding the impact of negative expectancies (Satre and Knight 2001). This suggests that individuals who use alcohol as a coping strategy have a positive expectation that the effects of alcohol will help to reduce the impact of stress inducing factors.

Some research suggests that light to moderate drinking improves mood, increases social contacts and helps people to relax and deal with stress. The debate is still open on this issue, with some researchers claiming that the positive effect is simply a placebo effect, with others maintaining that social drinking can be beneficial for people's mental well-being. Undoubtedly, culture, social expectations and social demands play a role in the way people's expectations of the mental health benefits of alcohol are formed.

Adults can use medication in the same way as alcohol or illegal drugs to cope with stressors in their everyday lives. Although the issue of prescription drugs misuse is beyond the scope of this book, we need to acknowledge that the reasons for prescription drug use may be part of wider strategies to address mental health problems in local communities.

Environmental: Socio-economic and cultural

Social determinants
The different ways that people live together – whether in nuclear or extended families, widely dispersed or closely knit urban or rural communities – can impact on mental health. In recent years this has been explored through 'social capital', which is described in more detail in Chapter 2. There is now increasing evidence that there is a strong association between social capital and subjective well-being, happiness and life satisfaction (Helliwell and Putnam 2004). This may also provide some explanation for the way childhood experiences define how we as adults approach life, cope, see ourselves in relation to others and inter-relate with our social networks.

The influence of childhood experiences on adult health is well researched, and we know that there is a strong association between social and environmental risk factors, such as abuse and family dysfunction, and poor mental health in adulthood. Studies suggest that children experiencing adverse childhoods (ACEs) may develop into dysfunctional adults/parents, who in turn may have a negative influence on their own children (Lesesne and Kennedy 2005). It is, however, not the intention of this chapter to discuss experiences that may require interventions, such as psychotherapy, being outside the scope of mental health promotion. Life events, such as parental death, loss and separation, are predictors of decreased psycho-social functioning and of depression over time (Pagano et al. 2004). In addition, Pagano et al. found that positive life events predicted improvements in functioning in interpersonal relationships, although this association was less clear. Family and neighbourhood stability have also been found to be associated with positive self-perceived mental health in midlife (Bures 2003).

The impact of informal caring

Becoming a parent is commonly recognized as a major life transition which affects both mothers and fathers. It can impact on psychological, economic and social life. Most mothers can experience typical responses to life changes: anxiety, reduction in self-esteem and even depression. In many cases, effects are short-lived but in other cases longer lasting postnatal depression can occur. The capacity to manage this life change, like others, comes from a combination of individual and social factors. Those with lower resilience skills and who experience a range of disadvantages are more likely to have difficulties. Provision of support during the antenatal and postnatal period has been associated with better psycho-social health outcomes (Oakley et al. 1996). In a survey of 11,000 mothers, eight months after birth, material disadvantage was more strongly related to depression and anxiety than it was to physical conditions (Acheson 1998).

It is of course not just childrearing which as a long-term commitment affects our mental well-being. The consequences of caring for ageing parents or other family members are often neglected by support services, and yet caring is a life event which can have a major impact on the well-being of the whole family. About 7.5 percent of the adult population in the UK is involved in caring for an older relative or close friend. Women are, however, one and a half times more likely than men to provide care and 22 percent more likely to be in full-time employment while providing care (Leontaridi and Bell 2001; Social Policy Research Unit 2001). This is discussed in more detail in Chapter 7.

Changing relationships

Societal values and norms have, through the ages, provided people with guidance and structure for what is considered acceptable in our social relations. Such norms vary between cultures but nonetheless give individuals a form of knowledge security regarding attitudes, behaviour and expectations within their culture. Social norms include those relating to family relationships and structures. The rapidly changing nature of relationships occurring in many cultures is therefore understandably having an effect on life satisfaction and mental well-being. Much research has focused on the effects of parental divorce on adult children, both immediate and long-term. Data from a British birth cohort showed that parental divorce during childhood or adolescence continues to have a negative effect on the individual's mental health well into their middle-age. However, some of the negative effect may be due to conflicts that were present before the parents separated (Cherlin et al. 1998; Gahler 1998). There also seems to be a complex interaction between economic deprivation following the divorce and the parents' social class, which has a long-term impact on the individual's mental health.

Population migrations

Social relationships are of course reconfigured in other ways as well. Large scale population migrations may impact on people's concepts of self, sense of control, resilience, and may influence how they utilize their coping strategies. They may need to deal with bereavement with regards to the loss of people and places that have been left behind.

Box 6.2 Special issue in adulthood: forced migration

According to Bhugra (2004) people migrate for different reasons, ranging from voluntary decisions to move, to being forced to leave their place of residence because of wars or natural disasters. Migration occurs through a series of events, each of which in turn require different skills and have different impacts on people's mental health. Someone who is forced to migrate will be less mentally (and practically) prepared for the departure, and this may affect their mental health as well as that of their family members. Factors that influence how individuals respond to the stressors of migration include:

* Age and gender. Young adults may struggle to identify their cultural identity; women may be less in control than men; men may lose their role as bread winner.
* Language and occupation. Individuals of high- and low-level education may be more at risk of stress.
* Family and household. Single men have been shown to be more resourceful at coping.
* Level of resilience and coping mechanisms. Biological, psychological, social vulnerabilities social support (or social pressures).
* Religion or faith. These may play a role in coping strategies.
* Stigma of mental illness.

(Bhugra 2004)

Each migration event will generate a range of different mental health risk factors. For each of these risk factors individuals will utilize a variety of available resources (psychological, mental and community) and adapt accordingly. Bhugra (2004) lists stress of adaptation, discrimination, occupational difficulties and feelings of 'not belonging' as some of the main stressors in the settling down period. This period is considered by many researchers as the critical period when both external and internal factors could trigger psychological distress and mental illness.

The manner in which the host country accepts the migrant population has a major impact on adult migrants' mental health (Samarasinghe and Arvidsson 2002). A small study in Yorkshire found that refugee women identified language classes as their main source of mental health promotion because the classes gave them a chance to get out of the house and meet others in a similar position (Green 2006). These findings are echoed in a study in Australia (Jirojwong and Manderson 2001), where Thai women identified language barriers and inability to gain employment through lack of social support and limited options for information as having major impact on their mental well-being.

Not all involuntary migration has a negative impact on people's health. A study in Sweden of refugees who had arrived in the country as unaccompanied children in the 1980s, for political reasons, found that most of the participants were settled and content with their life in the new country (Wallin and Ahlström 2005). Those who expressed greatest sense of well-being had a well established social network consisting of friends mainly belonging to the same ethnic group.

Homelessness

The expression 'homelessness' has been defined as including 'states of rooflessness, houselessness, living in insecure accommodation, or living in inadequate accommodation' (Wright and Tompkins 2005: 5). It is often thought that homelessness or sleeping rough is a youth problem. In fact several surveys have shown that over half of homeless people are aged 24 years and over. Almost half of homeless people are women (but only 8 percent of those sleeping rough). The length of time and the number of times individuals experience homelessness varies. In Britain those who have been homeless for longer and/or for more than one episode tended to be single, male and over the age of 24 (St Mungo 2005).

It is well known that homelessness is associated with mental health problems, although in many cases the causal direction is less clear. Research has shown that people who sleep rough often have problematic family backgrounds, and many are heavy drinkers, drug users or are mentally ill. The main triggers for sleeping rough are relationship breakdown and domestic violence (Rebecca's Community 2005; St Mungo 2005). Perceived lack of love and affection in childhood, lack of social support and poor family and social networks have been identified as the main contributors to homelessness among mentally ill homeless people in a five city study in Europe. However, although most homeless mentally ill people describe their situation as 'difficult', they also consider their situation as transitory and express hope for the future that 'things will get better' (Leonori et al. 2000). This obviously suggests that there may be a range of public health interventions that could help to improve the well-being of homeless adults.

Being in prison

Adults in prison face a range of mental health risk factors such as boredom, homesickness, bullying (by staff and other inmates), isolation and lack of activity, which result in anger, frustration, depression and anxiety (Nurse et al. 2003). External risk factors such as poor education, deprivation, negative life events, mental illness and substance misuse may also impact on mental health in the prison environment. Figures show that over half of women in prison have experienced domestic violence and about one-third, sexual abuse. Surveys suggest that between 60 and 70 percent suffer from some form of mental health problem (WHO Regional Office for Europe 1999; Condon et al. 2006). Suicide rates in prisons are known to be high. We should, however, also bear in mind that prisons can have a positive impact on mental health through for example, access to education and vocational training, support to deal with destructive feelings, access to health care and to sports and fitness facilities (WHO Regional Office for Europe 1999).

Economic determinants

Work
There has been considerable attention to the negative mental health effects of work but it is generally agreed that the health consequences arising from lack of work – when this situation is involuntary – are higher (DoH 1999b). A significant part of the published literature on work and health is derived from higher income countries. The health impacts can result from loss of status, loss of work related social interaction and the reduction of self-esteem. These effects can be exacerbated by poverty and other factors which follow from job loss. An important study of the effects of a threat of job change or job loss is the Whitehall II Study of civil servants, carried out during a period of civil service privatization. Potential psychiatric illness increased significantly for men both before and after change, in comparison with those in a control group (Ferrie et al. 1995, 1998).

Box 6.3 Special issue in adulthood: work related mental health problems

In higher income countries musculoskeletal disorders followed by stress, anxiety and depression are the leading categories of self-reported work related illness. The Bristol survey of self-reported illness (Smith et al. 2000) estimated that about half a million people believed they were experiencing work related stress which was making them ill and an estimated 12.8 million working days were lost as a result. This survey did not report data for ethnic minorities whose occupational health is under researched (University of Warwick 2004). Although figures for work related stress rose through the late 1990s they appear to have levelled off during the last five years. In Britain certain professional groups are more likely to report work related stress including teachers, nurses and public sector professionals and managers. Work related stress, anxiety or depression have increased significantly in those reporting higher workloads, tighter work deadlines, lack of support at work and physical attacks or threats at work.

(Health and Safety Executive 2005)

Approaching retirement
While many studies have investigated the prevalence of mental health problems in the transition years between employment and retirement (Butterworth et al. 2006), fewer studies have considered the actual adjustment to retirement. In a British study senior managers approaching retirement and their wives identified their hopes, fears and expectations as 'the general emotional quality of the relationship; the opportunity to share time and its antithesis; the need for personal space and independence; implications for change in the management of the household; potential bereavement and loneliness' (Hilbourne 1999: 172). Most concerns were related to the marriage

relationship, both positive and negative, rather than to the practical consequences of retirement. There were, however, some clear gender differences, such as women being concerned about their personal space and independence, while men being worried about bereavement and loneliness. Although this group does not necessarily represent the expectations and worries of all adults approaching retirement, the study highlights that expressed pre-retirement concerns are not just about practical matters, but also about people's personal emotional well-being.

Socio-economic position and poverty

People from the poorest areas in the UK are nearly three times as likely to be admitted to hospital for depression and three times more likely to commit suicide (ESRC 2006). There are some significant mental health differences between gender and social class. In men there is a strong class gradient for alcohol and for drug dependence but the gradient is less marked for women and overall rates are lower. In the case of women there is a strong socio-economic gradient for anxiety and depression (Acheson 1998).

Socio-economic position can impact directly on mental health through lack of material resources, as well as indirectly through the anxieties arising from lack of resources. Low resources impact significantly on opportunities for inclusion in many areas of life and, therefore, on self-esteem and on mental health. Insecure and poor housing as well as homelessness are features of low socio-economic status all over the world. Poor housing is directly associated with poorer mental and physical health (Acheson 1998).

Culture

Culture as a term describes the pattern of life, beliefs and customs of whole populations or subsections of populations including specific ethnic groups. Cultures generate their own sets of beliefs about the meaning of mental health, the factors that influence it, interpretations of ill health and appropriate responses to it. In most cultures there are degrees of stigma associated with mental ill health as a whole or with particular illnesses, and this influences with whom, to what extent, and how such problems are shared.

Ethnicity

There are some clear associations between ethnicity and mental health. International data can be drawn from the WHO and nationally from the main data sources and research studies. A particularly useful large scale source of data in the UK was the *Fourth National Survey of Ethnicity* (Nazroo 1997) where the main ethnic groups were compared in relation to social circumstances and health, including mental health. The difficulties of assessing mental health in ways appropriate to all groups was recognized since most available measures had not been developed cross-culturally. Comparable issues to those identified in the UK are likely to occur in most countries.

Box 6.4   Special issue in adulthood: ethnicity and mental health

Suicide is the main contributor to mental health related mortality in all ethnic groups although the rates vary across groups and the combination of factors leading to suicide may differ (Nazroo 1997). There are some significant differences in morbidity across ethnic groups. In the UK, for example, both women and men from South Asian populations have lower rates of consultations for mental health problems although figures may, in part, reflect a reluctance to report problems (Nazroo 1997). In general there are cultural differences between ethnic groups in the presentation of symptoms of mental ill health (Nazroo 1997).

Differences in mental health can be explained in terms of cultural or socio-economic and environmental factors. There are problems in using either of these as single explanations. In the former the promotion of mental health through changing culturally related beliefs, attitudes and behaviours can be victim blaming while adoption of materialist explanations can lead to relevant cultural factors being overlooked. Many commentators have drawn on both materialist and cultural contributions and McNaught (1994) concluded that ethnic minority health – including their mental health – was a result of a combination of factors:

- socio-economic status;
- strength of observance of certain cultural norms;
- physical access to health services;
- housing tenure and conditions;
- racial discrimination;
- quality of written and spoken English.

Gender

Gender differences in mental health can partly be attributed to biological differences but are largely the product of social experiences. In the UK suicide figures are higher for men than women with the highest rates found for men between 25 and 44 years and over 75 years. Seventy-five percent of those who commit suicide are male. In the UK the age standardized rate for suicide in men from 1975 to 2002 stayed the same but this figure obscured a 20–30 percent rise in men under 44 years and a fall of about the same amount in men over 45 years. In the case of morbidity most countries record higher rates of depression for women than for men. In the UK, 18 percent of women have what is defined as a neurotic disorder (anxiety, depression, phobias and anxiety attacks) compared with 11 percent of men. Men, however, are three times more likely to be dependent on alcohol and drugs and to hide symptoms of mental illness (ESRC 2006).

Data on mental health differences between men and women may reflect real differences in experience as well as different ways of responding to problems, which can impact on recorded data. For example, symptoms of anxiety in men may be dealt with through alcohol use while women may refer these symptoms to the GP. In general men are lower users of health services and more reluctant to present symptoms of mental ill health. Health professionals' responses can also differ, with women more likely to be labelled as anxious or depressed (Morgan et al. 1990). Multi-causal explanations for the mental health differences between men and women are offered. A systematic review of gender differences in depression (Piccinelli and Wilkinson 2000) attributed them to adverse experiences in childhood and adolescence, socio-cultural roles and associated adverse experiences, psychological attributes and individual differences in coping skills. Rogers and Pilgrim (2003) have observed that explanatory factors for gender differences are far from agreed.

Conflict and violence

Violence within the domestic sphere and that associated with armed conflict are two major forms of violence which affect mental health, but are not clearly distinct. For example, the sexual violence against women is frequently enhanced in conflict situations. The WHO *Report on Violence and Health* (2002) divided violence into three categories (self-directed, interpersonal and collective violence) and divided the effects of violence into physical, sexual and psychological. Less than 10 percent of violence related deaths occurred in high income countries. About half of the 1.6 million violence related deaths were suicides, one-third were homicides and about one-fifth were war related. As the WHO stresses deaths are the tip of the iceberg as far as the violence related health burden is concerned. Domestic violence is a prevailing concern worldwide (see Box 6.5).

Box 6.5 Special issue in adulthood: domestic violence and mental health

There is a strong relationship between gender and domestic violence with most violence carried out by men on women. The term 'gender-based violence' recognizes this fact with the United Nations defining it as 'acts or threats of acts intended to hurt or make women suffer physically, sexually, or psychologically and which affect women because they are women or affects women disproportionately' (UN 1993, in Fishbach and Herbert 1997: 1162). Heise et al. (1994) noted the problems in accurately estimating the global health burden associated with violence because of the absence of evidence from many countries and significant under-reporting in others. According to the Council of Europe (2002), one in four women experiences domestic violence in their lives.

Violence in relationships tends to escalate over time and is associated with physical, mental and social problems. The mental health consequences can be both immediate and long-term, and include depression, increased suicide and post-traumatic disorder (Fischbach and Herbert 1997). The factors contributing to gender-based violence are many and complex and include the influence of beliefs and attitudes that legitimize violence and justify male control of females (Donellan 2005).

It can be difficult for men to report domestic violence – they do not expect to be believed; there is the stigma of being seen as a battered partner; and there is a lack of knowledge of where to obtain support. Surveys have revealed that fathers are particularly disadvantaged by the bias and prejudice against male victims, with the police and courts reluctant to take action against violent mothers (Donellan 2005).

Health and social services

Services have responsibilities for promoting positive mental health as well as for prevention at primary, secondary and tertiary levels. Health services are provided through primary care and secondary level hospital services. Social services make a particular contribution at tertiary level of prevention. Mental health promotion can be provided to adults through the activities of health and social care professionals as well as through specialist health promotion services in the countries where these exist. Over time the main emphasis of services has been on secondary and tertiary prevention with limited emphasis on primary prevention and little or no attention to positive mental health promotion. In some countries this situation is beginning to change with greater emphasis on the promotion of mental health and primary prevention.

A particular issue has been the reluctance of people from some ethnic minorities to take up mental health services because of communication problems, dissatisfaction with services received and the concern that services can be discriminatory and racist (Bowes and Domokos 1995; Nazroo 1997). A study of young Asian women and self-harm (Chantler et al. 2001) revealed a number of service related issues:

- many statutory and voluntary sector services were not known to the young women;
- the general practitioner was not part of the pathway to care. Women who self-harmed only accessed services at crisis point and some kept the self-harm hidden;
- barriers to seeking support included lack of knowledge of services, fear of loss of confidentiality and cultural and family stigma from seeking support.

The natural and built environment

Both the natural and the built environment can impact on mental health. In countries which experience long hours of darkness in winter seasons there are well documented negative impacts on mental health (Rosenthal et al. 1984; Lam et al. 1990). The impacts of climate change are also being explored and some mental health effects identified (Kovats et al. 1999). The design of built environments – structures and landscapes – to meet aesthetic requirements has a long history but health and social considerations are also increasingly recognized. There is, for example, a growing literature on the influence of the structure of environments on social capital. Cattell's study (2001) reported on two nearby communities in the East of London, and suggested that differences in social networks may have resulted from styles of housing and urban planning. Generally, poorer people live in poorer environments assessed by design, layout and facilities of housing; accessibility of shops and other resources; and the balance between built structures and green areas. These can impact directly or indirectly on aspects of well-being.

Box 6.6   Summary of the main determinants affecting mental health in adulthood reviewed in this chapter

Individual biological/physical determinants:	• Physical disability and long-term conditions • HIV/AIDS
Individual competencies and behaviours:	• Coping and resilience among marginalized groups such as geographically isolated populations, refugees, gay, lesbian and bisexual populations
Individual behavioural and lifestyle factors:	• Exercise and physical activity • Smoking • Alcohol consumption • Medication

Environmental–socio-economic

Social determinants:	• Influence of childhood experiences • Caring for an older relative • Changing relationships • Population migrations • Homelessness • Being in prison
Economic determinants:	• The community • Work • Unemployment • Approaching retirement • Poverty • Health and social services
Cultural determinants:	• Ethnicity • Gender • Conflict and violence: domestic or armed conflict
The natural and built environment:	• Impact of seasons • Building design • Housing • Social capital

Promoting mental health and well-being among young and middle-aged adults

In this section we turn our attention to how mental health and well-being can be promoted and maintained in adulthood. First we discuss what factors adults consider are important for their mental health and how much in control of these factors they think they are. Next we review the research evidence for effective interventions. Finally we describe examples of good practice, including relevant policy documents and the implementation of community-based activities and how these relate to the evidence.

The meaning of mental health/mental well-being for adults

Most surveys with adults regarding mental health have focused on mental illness rather than mental health, attempting to identify the prevalence of mental health problems (not necessarily clinically assessed) in the community, and people's attitudes to mental illness (see for example Taylor Nelson Sofres 2003). In Scotland two surveys have been conducted about public attitudes to mental health, mental well-being and mental health problems with people aged 16 and over (Braunholtz et al. 2004). The findings show that good relationships with family and friends, having enough money, exercise, hobbies, leisure activities and a social life are considered to have positive effects on mental health, whereas not having enough money and physical ill health are considered to be negative factors. Not surprisingly perhaps, younger and middle-aged people were more likely to say that relationship problems affected mental health negatively, while older people mentioned bereavement. Men, younger people and people who were financially secure were more likely to state that they had control over the factors that affected their mental well-being.

Evidence of effective mental health promotion interventions in this age group

Much of the research evidence in these age groups comes from research on parenting (skills), community programmes, workplace and domestic violence.

Parenting
Parenting presents opportunities for enhancing mental health and also for challenging it. Programmes to support this stage have been widely implemented and as noted in Chapter 4 are also designed with the health of infants and young children in mind. In most countries first time mothers are encouraged to access health services in the antenatal period when opportunities for education can be provided. Where antenatal classes are available attendance levels vary and those who are in the more disadvantaged circumstances are typically less like to attend.

A number of systematic reviews have brought together evidence of effectiveness of antenatal and early parenthood programmes. Gagnon (2004) was only able to identify seven studies which met methodological criteria for a review. The studies were of differing sizes, had differing aims and activities and were of variable quality. Positive outcomes were identified in individual studies, for example in maternal role preparation and maternal attachment behaviours but no firm conclusions were drawn from the review. Antenatal education does not appear to be an area readily amenable to RCT style evaluations and a wider range of studies needs to be examined to get a flavour of programme activities and their effectiveness.

Antenatal and postnatal parenting programmes have used both one to one and group methods. The effectiveness of group-based interventions was reviewed by Barlow and Coren (2004) for their impact on maternal psycho-social health. A wide range of outcomes were recorded across the studies including positive mental health as well as illness: self-esteem; social support; relationship with partner/spouse; depression; and anxiety/stress. Some of the studies were used for a meta-analysis. Statistically significant results were found from those in interventions groups for depression; anxiety/

stress; self-esteem; and relationship with partners but no evidence of effectiveness on social support. A meta-analysis on follow up data showed a continued improvement in self-esteem, depression and partner adjustment but findings were not significant. The reviewers concluded that parenting programmes can make a significant short-term impact on psycho-social health of mothers but there was a lack of evidence on longer term impact.

The Pippin programme (www.pippin.org) designed for both women and men aims to promote positive early family and parent–infant relationships and straddles ante- and postnatal periods. It also offers an externally recognized parent–infant facilitator course for professionals and para-professionals and promotes collaborative and inter-agency research and development. The parent programme consists of 17 weekly two hour sessions beginning in pregnancy and continuing to three to five months after birth, plus a one hour home visit soon after birth. Six months after birth men and women in the intervention group were significantly more positive than those in a control group for emotional well-being, satisfaction with couple relationships; the parent–child relationship and the parenting role; and child centred attitudes towards infant care.

Home visits by community nurses to young parents are common in many countries. Visits provide an opportunity to offer advice and support and identify situations where mental health may be vulnerable and support required. A systematic review of domiciliary health visiting drew on international as well as UK examples and reported positive outcomes (Elkan et al. 2000). Although home visiting can be a population-wide provision the studies included in the review mostly focused on disadvantaged families or on families where children had been identified as at risk or with developmental difficulties. Activities in the programmes included advice on child development and interaction with children; advice on childcare and management of behavioural problems; provision of help in the home; and efforts to improve social support for mothers. Another meta-analysis recorded a highly significant positive outcome of home visiting on parent–child interaction and the quality of the home environment (Elkan et al. 2000).

All over the world experienced mothers in communities give support to new mothers with grandmothers often playing a major role. Drawing on such community experience has been a feature of a number of formal programmes of which the Community Mothers Programme in Ireland is a well publicized example (Johnson et al. 1993). This programme was set up in disadvantaged areas defined according to housing, social class, education, employment and level of births. Community mothers were recruited and trained in their own homes. The community mothers were experienced mothers from the same communities and were expected to share their experiences and raise the self-esteem and confidence in parenting of young first time mothers. During the first year of a child's life visits took place on a monthly basis (at least) and included a long visit to discuss a child's development in relation to individual family circumstances. The programme was evaluated against a control group receiving routine support from a public health nurse. In a seven year follow up positive outcomes were reported and the conclusions drawn that the intervention improved several aspects of childrearing in the first year, the benefits also extended to later children and some benefits were sustained over several years (Johnson et al. 2000).

A similar programme in the US was developed in response to the low uptake of pre-natal care by Latina mothers (McFarlane and Mehir 1994). Barriers to use were cultural, linguistic and access barriers such as lack of transport and childcare. Following needs assessment volunteer mothers were recruited as health promoters. They carried out peer education, counselling and day care services. The theoretical basis for the programme was Freire's concept of empowerment. A range of outcomes were recorded including impact on self-esteem and higher satisfaction with parenting.

Preventing the onset of depression has been an important consideration in the postnatal period. There has been a particular interest in the effectiveness of brief listening visits by health professionals in the early postnatal period. A systematic review examined the effectiveness of psycho-social and psychological interventions incorporating a variety of activities (Dennis 2005; Dennis and Creedy 2005). They concluded that women who received the psycho-social interventions were just as likely to develop depression as those receiving standard care. One promising intervention was the provision of intensive postpartum support by public health nurses or midwives. Activities in the postnatal period alone were more effective than those which also included the antenatal period.

Workplace

Workplace health promotion has a relatively long history. It has been dominated by interventions directed towards specific health behaviours and lifestyles rather than holistic health promotion within a settings-based approach. The workplace has often been used as a context to reach parts of communities not easily reached by other health education, with programmes designed in response to professionally defined rather than worker defined needs. In the mental health field programmes have typically consisted of stress management or physical exercise where mental health gains can result alongside physical health ones. The majority of programmes have consisted of education, skills development and various kinds of support. Some have combined such activities with attention to the organization of the workplace in order to promote mental health and reduce stress.

A systematic review by Peersman et al. (1998) did not include any mental health interventions and they noted the need for programmes to addressing the psycho-social environment at work. Platt et al. (2000) reviewed workplace health promotion and looked particularly at existing reviews of stress reduction as well as at individual studies. Two main reviews were identified – one focusing on organizational level interventions and one on individual stress management (Burke 1993; Murphy 1996). Burke reported on organization level interventions designed to reduce stress. Programmes included various activities including increased job autonomy, reduction in role stress and reduction of work–family conflict. The conclusion was that interventions had a beneficial effect. Murphy (1996) reviewed stress management programmes designed to help employees modify their appraisal of stressful situations or deal more effectively with symptoms. The most common activities included were relaxation, meditation, biofeedback, cognitive–behavioural skills and various combinations of these activities. Effectiveness varied according to the aspect of health being assessed with multi-component programmes more effective than single component ones. Most programmes were ineffective in producing changes in job satisfaction or in absenteeism. The author concluded that to produce changes in these measures the sources of stress in the work environment would need to be addressed. Platt et al. (2000) examined three further studies of controlled stress management programmes. Arnetz (1996, 1997, in Platt et al. 2000) showed that programmes affected levels of a stress sensitive hormone. The review authors reported that the conclusions to be drawn from the individual studies were limited due to methodological weaknesses but taken together with the two reviews suggested that stress management interventions targeted at individuals could be effective in reducing physical and psychological symptoms of stress. Organizational outcomes, they argued, needed to be tackled through interventions which addressed the sources of stress in the total work setting.

Loss of employment

As discussed earlier the impact of loss of employment and unemployment has many negative impacts on mental health. Addressing the underlying determinant of lack of work is essential through policy and other measures. The longer unemployment continues the more difficult it can be for people to rejoin the workforce. Maintaining positive health and developing skills which facilitate return to work are important. A programme which was evaluated over a number of years provided good evidence of the effectiveness of a well designed intervention (Caplan et al. 1989; Price et al. 1992; van Ryn and Vinokur 1992). The aim of the programme was to prevent the negative effects of mental health on unemployment and to enable people to secure high quality re-employment. The programme consisted of group sessions based on coping resources theory including the development and rehearsal of job searching skills; increasing self-efficacy, skills to cope with set-backs and social support. The interventions were evaluated through a randomized controlled trial with short-term and longer term (two and a half years) follow up. Among the participants classified as high risk of mental ill health the programme impacted on incidence and prevalence of the more severe depressive symptoms and the results were maintained over the full period (Vinokur et al. 1991). This study was with people who returned to employment. Its impact on depressive symptoms would not necessarily be achieved with people experiencing long-term employment. A similar programme has also been evaluated with long-term unemployed adults in Finland with positive mental health results: increases in self-esteem; and decrease in psychological distress and symptoms of depression (Vuori et al. 2002).

Domestic violence

A variety of programmes directed towards the reduction of violence have been implemented in both high income and low income countries although many in the latter have not been subjected to systematic evaluation (Patel 2005). In addressing the prevention of violence coordinated actions are needed at societal, community, family and individual basis. A variety of strategies and actions can be implemented: support for women and developing skills to leave a situation of abuse; provision of refuges; general parental support programmes; education on gender issues; education of professionals and police; provision of helplines; and so on.

An excellent example of a programme which seeks to reach several levels and is also theory-based is the South African, *Soul City*, a multi-media health promotion project using mass media for social change. Working in partnership with the *National*

Network on Violence Against Women, domestic violence was the focus for its fourth series. It used prime time radio and TV dramas plus printed materials and integrated social issues into entertainment formats. The use of radio as well as TV meant that marginalized rural communities could also be reached. It drew on Bandura's social-cognitive theory. The intervention aimed to catalyse community dialogue, mediate shifts in social norms, facilitate collective action and create an enabling legal environment. The evaluation combined quantitative and qualitative aspects. Table 6.1 shows the full range of objectives at the differing levels.

Table 6.1   The *Soul City* partnership for social change

Levels of change	Objectives
Societal:	Increase public debate in the national media; and advocate for the speedy implementation of the Domestic Violence Act.
Interpersonal and community:	Promote interpersonal and community dialogue; promote community action; and shift social norms
Individual:	Shift attitudes, awareness, knowledge, intentions and practice; enhance self-efficacy; increase supportive behaviour; and connect people to support services.

Soul City reached 86 percent of its target TV audience, 65 percent of its radio audience and 25 percent of the target audience had seen or read print material. Knowledge shifts were achieved with increases in those knowing about the helpline. A number of attitudinal shifts and changes in subjective norms were also recorded. The qualitative data supported the quantitative outcomes suggesting that the intervention played a role in enhancing self-efficacy, effective decision-making and facilitated community action. The implementation of the Domestic Violence Act was attributed to the intervention.

Community-based programmes
Health Action Zone (HAZ) projects were set up in England in 26 health authority areas with a history of deprivation and poor health, and covered one-third of the population. Within the broad programmes there were explicit mental health promotion activities and action on several determinants of mental health. HAZ was evaluated both nationally and locally using the theory of change/realistic evaluation model.

In making measurable impact on health inequalities, the three year funding period was a short time over which to achieve changes. The resources available to the projects were modest in relation to addressing the root causes of ill health. In reviewing achievements, challenges and opportunities, Bauld and Judge (2002) concluded that progress had been made on the seven HAZ principles: achieving equity; engaging communities; working in partnership; engaging frontline staff; taking an evidence-based approach; developing a person centred approach to delivery; and taking a whole systems approach. Within the individual HAZ projects a wide variety of innovative activities had been undertaken and positively evaluated.

Where mental health was concerned the HAZ projects could make an indirect impact through addressing the root causes of mental health inequalities, and more direct impact through health and social service changes and community located projects. These projects could be specifically labelled as being connected to mental health, or to other health topics such as exercise with mental health consequences or general community development. Most operated on a small scale and evaluations were modest although positive mental health outcomes were reported, especially from some projects working with ethnic minority groups and women with young children (Tilford et al. 2002).

Raeburn (2001) has reported on a number of community-based projects which have included mental health outcomes. Superhealth (Abbott and Raeburn 1989) was designed to meet health promotion goals identified through community needs assessment and focused on coping style, social support and social and health skills. People met in small groups, participated in a range of activities including discussions, practical exercises and group support. Facilitators were community members who had already participated in the programme. The programme was evaluated through a quasi-experimental design study where two forms of the intervention, one informational and the other behavioural, were compared with a control population. Both interventions showed changes but these were greater in the behavioural form. This was a low cost programme which could easily be disseminated widely.

Housing, architecture, space and design
Systematic reviews of mental health promotion have included few, if any studies, reporting on studies evaluating these issues in relation to mental health. Goodchild (1998) makes the point that housing measures have undoubted potential as a health intervention but they must be treated as a single aspect of coordinated programmes and policies that upgrade the quality of life of people living in poverty. A recent systematic review suggests, on the basis of seven studies, that housing interventions may improve mental health, perceptions of safety and social participation (Thomson et al. 2001). The authors suggest that methodological difficulties (poor housing co-existing with other problems of deprivation) and political obstacles may be some of the reasons for the lack of evaluation studies on health and housing. A further controlled trial in the UK showed that housing improvements can reduce anxiety, depression and self-reported mental problems (Thomson et al. 2003).

Homelessness
Although the needs of homeless people have been investigated in great detail, there is very little evidence available as to what mental health promotion interventions actually work. There is some evidence that behavioural interventions for mental health problems and associated drug and alcohol problems may be effective. It has also been suggested that peer involvement would increase the effectiveness of interventions, but there is little actual evidence available to show this (WHO Regional Office for Europe's Health Evidence Network (HEN) 2005). An American review outlines the characteristics of successful outreach programmes with homeless people as applying a non-threatening approach; providing flexible services; having regular contact; responding quickly to personal needs; taking sufficient time to develop motivation among the homeless (Dickey 2000). A comparison of the uptake of outreach services in London and New York found that the variables specified by the theory of planned behaviour

(attitudes, subjective norms, perceived behavioural control, intention) were useful in predicting homeless adults' behaviour. The researchers postulated that certain psychological variables could therefore be used to develop intervention strategies (Christian and Abrams 2004).

Exercise

Although there are studies showing the mental health benefits of exercise, the level of the actual research evidence regarding the effects of exercise on mental well-being is medium (DoH 2004a). A review found that exercise interventions improved some aspects of physical self-esteem (although not for middle-aged adults) or self-concept, such as satisfaction with body image, physical self-worth and physical health (Fox 2000). Walking and endurance exercise were found to be particularly effective with middle-aged adults. A more recent evaluation of an exercise referral intervention confirmed these findings. The ten week exercise programme led to improvements in perceptions of physical condition, physical self-worth and physical health (Taylor and Fox 2005). According to the authors, 'self-perceptions' are useful as outcome measures for exercise because they are directly related to global self-esteem and to mental well-being.

Gardening as a social form of exercise has received increased attention. A three year horticultural and gardening project concluded that the project provided participants with social opportunities, increased their confidence and self-esteem and improved psychological well-being (Sempik et al. 2005). The possibility to consume the resulting produce was an added bonus. The authors concluded that communal gardening which emphasizes everyone's contributions is particularly suitable for vulnerable individuals, such as people with learning difficulties or with mental health problems.

Informal carers

The evidence of effectiveness of interventions intended to maintain and improve the mental well-being of carers is discussed in Chapter 7.

People in prison

Health in prison has received increased interest since the World Health Organization established its Health in Prisons Project in order to support a range of initiatives across Europe to improve prisoners' health, particularly with regards to communicable disease, mental health and drug misuse (WHO 2006). At the time of writing the evaluations of many of these projects are still waiting to be published. However, the WHO suggests that a number of public health initiatives may be effective, including the provision of psycho-social support for prisoners, information and training for staff, prisoners and their families on mental health issues, and at a policy level ensuring that the needs of prisoners are included in national mental health policies (WHO 2005). In the UK an information campaign to promote mental health in young offender institutions was found not to be effective. Possible reasons for the results were: lack of clarity regarding the objectives and focus of the campaign; lack of needs assessment and involvement of the target group in the design of the materials; and lack of guidance for staff on how to best use the materials (Caraher et al. 2000). Other initiatives such as peer education are yet to be evaluated.

Debates about evidence of effect in less researched areas of mental health promotion
Apart from the 'obvious' areas of mental health promotion interventions, there are
several others which are evolving and debated, for example the impact of advocacy or
diet on mental health.

The potential link between diet and mental health has only recently started
receiving attention. The Mental Health Foundation in the UK claims that there is
strong evidence that what we eat affects our mental health (Mental Health Foundation 2006). One of the arguments used is that changes in food consumption and
production in the UK mirror increases in mental health problems. However, we must
not forget that other societal changes have also occurred in that period and the sug-
gestion that food is the only (or main) factor involved may be an over simplified
explanation to a complex issue. Although there is some evidence to suggest that certain foods (vitamins, minerals) may improve mental health, a lot more research is
required before we can state what dietary interventions may be of benefit in mental
health promotion.

Advocacy has been utilized in several ways to further the promotion of mental
health. At a mental health service user level advocacy is used to promote the needs of
people with mental health problems. The purpose of advocacy is to enable service users
to have a voice and empower them to find information, make representation to service
providers and make informed choices about the services they require. It could therefore be argued that advocacy also offers the means to combat stigma of mental illness.
For these reasons advocacy is of great interest to mental health service users. However,
at the time of writing the research evidence is fairly weak regarding the effectiveness of
advocacy and user involvement. In addition, service user involvement and advocacy
falls outside the scope of this book because of its focus on mental illness, and readers
would be better referring to a book which considers the role of the user in mental
health services, such as Rogers and Pilgrim's (2005) *The Sociology of Mental Health and
Mental Illness*. WHO (2004b) adds another dimension to advocacy, that of generating
public demand for mental health and ensuring that mental health is prioritized. The
WHO acknowledges that currently there is little research evidence to demonstrate
the effectiveness of such interventions, but suggests that community advocacy in
low-income countries might be an effective way of promoting mental health in
communities.

At the time of writing there is increased interest in the effectiveness of art, music
and dance in promoting mental health and some research projects have been established. A useful website for anyone interested in developments in these fields is the
National Network for Arts in Health (www.nnah.org.uk).

Box 6.7   Summary of evidence of effective adult mental health promotion interventions

- There is good evidence in support of parenting programmes both home-based and in
  the community using professionals or community workers. Many of these programmes have been with disadvantaged mothers.
- Programmes such as Sure Start have the potential to reach a significant proportion of
  mothers of young children in disadvantaged communities.

- Workplace mental health promotion can impact on mental health outcomes with the recommendation that interventions include organizational as well as individual elements.
- Community wide programmes of the Health Action Zone type have the potential to impact on a number of determinants of mental health, if resourced adequately.
- Well designed programmes for people who are unemployed can facilitate return to work and reduce mental health problems.
- There is some evidence that housing interventions may improve mental health and social participation and reduce anxiety and depression.
- A range of different forms of exercise have been shown to improve self-esteem, confidence, psychological well-being and self-perception.
- There is increasing research which suggests that well designed, clearly defined public health interventions in prisons impact positively on prisoners' mental health.

Significant international and national policy that impacts on mental health promotion of adults

It would be impossible to do full justice to all mental health promoting policies. To begin with it is not just specific mental health promotion policy that impacts on adults' mental health. If we consider the wider determinants of mental health it is obvious that policies on transport, housing, public health, family services, work security, health and safety, disability and so on will have an impact on people's mental health. In this section we will only consider the main current policies, which focus on the promotion of mental health and well-being.

Internationally the World Health Organization and the European Commission have undertaken a number of initiatives to promote the acceptance and implementation of mental health promotion strategies. The World Health Organization published two summary reports which provide a framework for national mental health promotion strategy (WHO 2004a, b). The two documents were followed by a fuller report, which is intended as a resource for developing mental health promoting action (Herrman et al. 2005). These have been paralleled by initiatives in Europe (Berkels et al. 2004; Lehtinen 2004; WHO European Ministerial Conference on Mental Health 2005; Commission of the European Communities 2005) which are summarized in Box 6.8.

Box 6.8   Recommended action in international documents relating to mental health promotion policy relevant to adults

Prevention of Mental Disorders: Effective Interventions and Policy Options (WHO 2004a)

- Programmes should address multiple outcomes of mental health problems and disorders, mental/physical health.
- Cultural adaptation and tailoring of evidence-based programmes need to be ensured.
- Mental health promotion/prevention of mental ill health should be integrated with existing effective health promotion programmes and social policies.

- Integrated national/regional policies should be developed to prevent mental disorders and promote mental health as part of public health policy, treatment and maintenance of mental disorders.

Promoting Mental Health Concepts: Emerging Evidence (WHO 2004b: adapted from page 60)

- Mental health outcomes may be primary or secondary outcomes to other social and economic outcomes.
- Involvement of stakeholders, community ownership and continued resources availability required.

Promoting Mental Health Concepts: Emerging Evidence Based Practice (Herrman et al. 2005)

- Mental health can be enhanced through effective public health and social interventions including non-health policies and practices, such as for improved housing, education, child care.
- Known effective interventions should be implemented and evaluated in culturally appropriate way.

Mental Health Action Plan for Europe (WHO European Ministerial Conference on Mental Health 2005: adapted from pages 11–12)

- Prepare policies and implement activities to counter stigma and discrimination and promote mental well-being.
- Include prevention of mental health problems/suicide in national policies.
- Develop specialist services to address gender-specific issues.
- Prioritize services targeting mental health problems and associated problems of marginalized/vulnerable groups.
- End inhumane, degrading treatment and care; comply with United Nations conventions and international legislation on human rights and mental health.
- Increase level of social inclusion of people with mental health problems.
- Ensure representation of users/carers on committees/groups responsible for planning, delivery, review, inspection of mental health activities.

Mental Health Promotion and Prevention Strategies for Coping with Anxiety, Depression and Stress Related Disorders in Europe (Berkels et al. 2004: adapted from pages 12–13)

- Promotion/prevention activities in mental health are essential to reduce social and economic burdens of common mental health problems and in combating stigma of mental illness.
- Promotion of life skills training for coping with common mental health problems should be developed for different settings.
- Intervention measures need to be focused on transitional life periods as possible stressful life events.
- Civil and human rights of persons suffering from common mental health problems to be fully respected.

Improving the Mental Health of the Population: Towards a Strategy on Mental Health for the European Union (Commission of the European Communities 2005: adapted from page 2, Options for Action)

- Mental health to be promoted and mental ill health addressed through preventive action.
- Social inclusion of mentally ill or disabled people needs to be promoted and their fundamental rights and dignity protected.

In addition the documents set out a range of more general recommendations, such as the importance of sharing good practice, the urgency of developing and disseminating evidence-based policy and practice, the need for effective international, interagency and intersectoral working and the need to support low- and middle-income countries to develop and implement effective mental health promotion programmes. Most of the documents also emphasize the need for research to be able to generate further evidence.

Nationally, countries vary a great deal when it comes to policy relating to mental health promotion. In the UK *Choosing Health: Making Healthier Choices Easier* (DoH 2004b) and the *Mental Health National Service Framework* (DoH 1999a), with its equivalents in Northern Ireland and Scotland (Department of Health, Social Services and Public Safety 2003; Scottish Executive 2003) are the main public health documents that should deal with mental health promotion. Unfortunately *Choosing Health* does little to address mental health. As the Mental Health Foundation (2005: 1) states:

> The document provides little explanation of the fundamental role of mental health or its importance in relation to inequalities in health or risk behaviour. It fails to develop a life span perspective and there is a damaging lack of attention to older people . . . And finally there is an over-reliance on the individual choice agenda, which is not supported by the evidence base that indicates that multifaceted approaches will be most effective.

The *Mental Health National Service Framework* (DoH 1999a: 14) set out, in standard one to: 'promote mental health for all, working with individuals and communities; combat discrimination against individuals and groups with mental health problems, and promote their social inclusion'. It recognized that mental health promotion is most effective when it is applied across sectors and utilizes a range of methods. Based on available evidence three areas were proposed for action: actions across whole populations; programmes for individuals at risk; programmes for vulnerable groups, considered in Table 6.2.

Table 6.2 Mental Health National Service Framework: proposed action and examples of evidence

Action	Evidence – some examples
Action across whole populations:	Exercise promotion – can lead to improvements in life satisfaction, perceptions of physical condition, self-worth and health.
Programmes for individuals at risk due to life events:	Work based interventions – stress • management interventions targeted at individuals can reduce physical and psychological stress. To produce changes in job satisfaction and absenteeism sources of stress in the work environment need to be addressed. • Group-based parenting programmes can make a significant short-term impact on psycho-social health of mothers; longer term impact is less clear.
Programmes for vulnerable groups	
Victims of child abuse:	Little evidence available – some suggestion that training in adaptive coping skills may be effective.
Domestic violence:	Little evidence available. Action needed at societal, community, family and individual level. Activity includes refuges, safe rooms, help-lines, education, the use of mass media.
Race discrimination, refugees, asylum seekers:	Little evidence available. • Specific activities, such as exercise groups (see Chapter 7) for ethnic minority women seem to improve self-esteem. • Refugees and asylum seekers have different needs at different stages. Psycho-social interventions may help initially to reduce depression. Qualitative studies suggest that adult education, including learning the language of the host country may improve confidence and self-esteem.
People who sleep rough:	Behavioural interventions for mental health problems, drug and alcohol dependence, sexual risk behaviour can empower homeless people, achieve long-term health gain and treatment retention.
People in prison:	Little evidence available. Interventions with suggested gain include regular physical activity, participation in education, training, work, art, anti-bullying strategies, cognitive/behavioural interventions, spiritual reflection, regular contact with family and friends.
People with drug and alcohol problems:	Brief primary care interventions; see also above.
Combating discrimination (including stigma) and social exclusion:	Little evidence available. Interventions mostly used: public education, media education, legislation.

Earlier a number of social inequalities, including socio-economic position, ethnicity and gender were seen to be linked with poorer mental health. In order to redress this situation in the UK the *Independent Inquiry into Inequalities in Health* (Acheson 1998) stressed the necessity to have a range of policies designed to achieve general health improvements and greater impacts on the less well off. Two general recommendations were made:

- As part of health impact assessment all policies likely to have a direct or indirect effect on health should be evaluated in terms of their impact on health inequalities and should be formulated in such a way that by favouring the less well off they will, wherever possible, reduce such inequalities.
- We recommend a high priority is given to policies aimed at improving health and reducing inequalities in women of childbearing age, expectant mothers, and young children. (Acheson 1998: 120)

A further 36 recommendations related to specific areas of policy and specific groups experiencing disadvantage. For example, with reference to ethnic minorities to young women and to parents:

- We recommend that the needs of ethnic minority groups are specifically considered in the development and implementation of policies aimed at reducing socioeconomic inequalities;
- We recommend policies which reduce psychosocial ill health in young women in disadvantaged circumstances, particularly those caring for young children;
- We recommend policies which reduce poverty in families with children by promoting the material support of parents; by removing barriers to work for parents who wish to combine work with parenting; and by enabling those who wish to devote full-time to parenting to do so. (Acheson 1998: 126–8)

Elsewhere, for example in New Zealand and Australia, mental health promotion is either included in a wider 'health strategy' or linked to a 'mental health strategy', neither of which is satisfactory from a public health or health promotion perspective. This is bound to change over the next few years as countries sign up to the WHO guidelines and/or the European strategy.

Work and health policy

There are international and national policies addressing work, the times of work, ages and conditions of working. At the European level, there is the Working Times Directive (Department of Trade and Industry 1998). Taking the UK as an illustrative example general public health as well as specific workplace health policies have addressed work related health issues. Following a number of White Papers *Choosing Health* (DoH 2004b) recognized work as a key part of life which offers self-esteem, companionship, structure and status as well as income, with environment at work influences health choices and a force for improving health of individuals and communities. This White Paper focused on actions that employers, employees, governments and others can do to extend healthy choices by:

- reducing barriers to work to improve health and reduce inequalities through employment;
- improving working conditions to reduce causes of ill health related to work;
- promoting the work environment as a source of better health.

The document considered specific aspects of stress at work and recognized that a 'focus on individual stress can be counterproductive, leading to a failure to tackle the underlying cause of problems in the workplace' (DoH 2004b: 161). It also addressed the issue of supporting people experiencing mental health problems in returning to work through Pathways to Work pilot projects.

Examples of good practice

Family support

Home Start
This programme started in the UK and has now extended to a number of countries as Home Start International. The programme increases the confidence and independence of families through home visits over a year by volunteers to offer support, friendship and practical assistance and encouraging parents' strength and emotional well-being. Specific objectives are set in the countries involved relative to community needs. Home Start reaches a large number of families in some countries but small number in those where it is in an early stage of development. It links to families that may be difficult to reach. The websites for the programme in individual countries carry observations which reveal the value of the scheme to families involved and to the volunteers:

> Luckily all these social workers know what is going on with my children but that doesn't always help me. What does help me is my volunteer, as her purpose is only to help me and only if I want help. She also has a family but if she is here she has all the time in the world.
>
> (Mother, the Netherlands)

> I see families prosper
> Once again, going through life with confidence,
> Once again, coming out,
> Of the shadow and
> Into the light.
>
> (Poem by a volunteer, the Netherlands)

> We were thinking about why this programme is especially good and realized that if a volunteer comes to give all his/her attention and energy to a child, then the child would have an adult friend as well as Mum and Dad. We have evidence to show that this fact goes some way to greatly improving the child's self-esteem.
>
> (Group of volunteers in Russia)

Evaluations have reported parental satisfaction, increases in parental self-esteem and coping and reduction in family dysfunction. To date significant long-term differences between families who receive the programme when compared with a comparison group have not been identified (Jané-Lopis et al. 2005).

Mass media

Provision of information

While expectations of what can be achieved through provision of educational materials such as leaflets and booklets have often been too ambitious their role in providing information that people want should not be overlooked. Increasingly such materials are accessed in some countries as much through the Internet as they are through more traditional outlets. They can be valuable on a stand alone basis or complementary to face to face discussions. They can have a particular value at the early stages of coping with a difficult experience such as bullying and harassment at work (ACAS 2004), major life changes and helping people to begin to understand new situations and identify any further help needed and sources of such help. As Simich et al. (2005: 16) suggest, 'popular self help materials are appealing and empowering for consumers because they emphasise well-being and recovery'. The authors provide a good discussion of the development of a multi-lingual resource, *Alone in Canada*, designed to develop awareness of the factors influencing mental health being of immigrants and a direct health promotion resource for immigrants themselves. They emphasize the importance of situating mental well-being within a meaningful social context. A 21 page booklet was produced in 18 languages, and was also available online. The authors conclude that:

> *Alone in Canada* is probably the only tool available to community members that is written in accessible language that speaks of their own experiences of social adaptation and isolation and their mental health effects. It has served to build bridges into immigrant communities, helping individuals along the way.
>
> (Simich et al. 2005: 22)

The use of radio, television, billboards

Mass media is used extensively particularly in developing countries for communicating health education messages. Most of these programmes relate to areas other than mental health.[1] One example of a mental health initiative, the multi-media South African *Soul City* project has already been described. In Singapore the 10-year *Mind Your Mind Programme* has been established to 'promote mental wellness and raise awareness of the importance of early detection and treatment of the major mental illnesses' (Health Promotion Board Online 2005). The programme utilizes a variety of strategies, including mass media to raise public initial awareness. This is followed by workshops and training courses to create a lasting infrastructure for mental health.

The application of health promotion theory and principles to mental health promotion involving adults

As in other chapters there is a mixed picture with regards to the application of health promotion theory and principles to research and practice. There are programmes which have in a number of cases been implemented widely that represent well conceived intentions to reduce psycho-social consequences of disadvantage and to reduce inequalities in mental health. Use of a settings approach is central to health promotion. There is increasing recognition of the need for workplace programmes to address the elements of a health promoting setting approach although there are relatively few evaluations. The health promoting hospital movement has slowly grown but the evaluation activities do not, as yet, parallel those for health promoting schools. The WHO Health in Prisons Project is another example of an international programme based on the principles of a settings approach. However, in the few evaluation studies so far published the theoretical underpinning is less clear. The barriers to securing adoption of the health promotion principles in hospitals have been discussed (Whitehead 2004).

There is now a good evidence base developed from programmes involving parents. Some of the programmes subject to experimental styles of intervention have taken a clear at-risk approach and drawn on psychological theories. Others, such as Sure Start in the UK are strongly rooted in health promotion principles and there is good evidence from local evaluations that the commitment to active participation of parents in decision-making has been achieved. The reporting of the theoretical bases of programmes differs. In some such as *Soul City* which drew on Bandura's social cognitive theory, it was clear and detailed. Likewise the study of an outreach programme for the homeless found that the theory of planned behaviour could be used to predict homeless adults' behaviour and consequently be of value when planning interventions. Studies which have evaluated the effectiveness of exercise have in main utilized a theory base from other disciplines, such as psychology. This is not unusual in health promotion.

Appendix 1 summarizes the theory reported in studies drawn on in the chapter.

Conclusions

In this chapter we have considered the factors that impact on mental health in adulthood, the policy context of mental health promotion and the evidence of effective mental health promoting interventions. One thing that stands out when planning mental health promotion interventions for this age group is the potentially large number of points of transition and life events. Adults in this age group have a large amount of caring, financial and political responsibilities and are faced with life challenges, all of which impact both positively and negatively on mental health and well-being. Some of these life events have been researched extensively, such as parenting and adverse childhood experiences, while others to date have received limited attention, for example pre-retirement, homelessness and forced migration. It would seem that this is also the case with regards to the evidence of effective mental health promoting interventions targeting such life events. The chapter has illustrated that some groups remain more 'hidden' than others and are therefore currently more likely to lose out on mental health promotion support. It suggests that although there is good knowledge, effective activity and good practice in many areas of mental health promotion there are also still major gaps in the delivery of effective needs-based interventions in some settings and with some population groups. Finally, the lack of evaluated cross-cutting mental health promoting interventions, such as housing, transport or benefits advice, in adulthood is notable, despite numerous policy documents suggesting the opposite.

Box 6.9   Questions to reflect on

- How much do culture and cultural norms influence our mental and psychological response in adulthood to changes, such as divorce, that are outside our control?
- In what way might current evidence of effective interventions be utilized to develop acceptable and accessible mental health promoting interventions for marginalized groups?
- What factors impact on adults' resilience and their coping strategies and how can this knowledge benefit mental health promotion?
- What are the greatest mental health promotion challenges globally and how might they be addressed internationally, nationally and locally?

Note

1   For an overview of mass media health education programmes see, for example: www.communicatinghealth.com/Mass.ppt   and   www.communicatinghealth.com/case8.htm

References

Abbott, M. W. and Raeburn, J. M. (1989) Superhealth: a community-based health promotion programme, *Mental Health in Australia*, 2(1): 25–35.

ACAS (2004) *Bullying and Harassment at Work*: advice leaflet. Available at: www.acas.org.uk (accessed 31 July 2005).

Acheson, D. (1998) *Independent Inquiry into Inequalities in Health*. London: The Stationery Office.

Barlow, J. and Coren, E. (2004) *Parent-Training Programmes for Improving Maternal Psychosocial Health*, Cochrane Library, Issue 1, Cochrane Review. Chichester: John Wiley and Sons.

Bauld, L. and Judge, K. (2002) Achievements, challenges and opportunities, in L. Bauld and K. Judge (eds) *Learning from Health Action Zones*. Chichester: Aeneas Press.

Berkels, H., Henderson, J., Henke, J. et al. (2004) *Mental Health Promotion and Prevention Strategies for Coping with Anxiety, Depression and Stress Related Disorders in Europe, Final*

Report 2001–2003. Dortmund/Berlin/Dresden: Federal Institute for Occupational Safety and Health.

Bhugra, D. (2004) Migration and mental health, *Acta Psychiatrica Scandinavica*, 109: 243–58.

Boerner, K.A.R. (2004) Adaption to disability among middle-aged and older adults: the role of assimilative and accommodative coping, *Journals of Gerontology Series B: Psychological Sciences and Social Sciences*, 59B(1): P35–P42.

Bowes, A.M. and Domokos, T.M. (1995) South Asian women and the GPs: some issues of communication, *Social Sciences and Health*, 1(1): 22–33.

Braitstein, P., Montessori, V., Chan, K. et al. (2005) Quality of life, depression and fatigue among persons co-infected with HIV and Hepatitis C: outcomes from a population-based cohort, *AIDS Care*, 17(4): 505–15.

Braunholtz, S., Davidson, S. and King, S. (2004). *Well? What Do You Think? The Second National Scottish Survey of Public Attitudes to Mental Health, Mental Well being and Mental Health Problems*. Edinburgh: Scottish Executive Social Research.

Bures, R. M. (2003) Childhood residential stability and health at midlife, *American Journal of Public Health*, 93(7): 1144–8.

Burke, R.J. (1993) Organisation level interventions to reduce occupational stressors, *Work and Stress*, 7(1): 77–87.

Butterworth, P., Gill, S.C., Rogers, B. et al. (2006) Retirement and mental health: Analysis of the Australian national survey of mental health and well-being, *Social Science and Medicine*, 62: 1179–91.

Callaghan, P. (2004) Exercise: a neglected intervention in mental health care? *Journal of Psychiatric and Mental Health Nursing*, 11: 476–83.

Caplan, R.D., Vinokur, A.D., Price, R.H. and van Ryn, M. (1989) Job seeking, reemployment and mental health: a randomized field experiment in coping with job loss, *Journal of Applied Psychology*, 74(5): 759–69.

Caraher, M., Bird, L. and Hayton, P. (2000) Evaluation of a campaign to promote mental health in young offender institutions: problems and lessons for future practice, *Health Education Journal*, 59: 211–27.

Cattell, V. (2001) Poor people, poor places, and poor health: the mediating role of social networks and social capital, *Social Science and Medicine*, 52: 1501–16.

Chantler, K., Burman, E., Batsleer, J. and Bashir, C. (2001) *Attempted Suicide and Self Harm*. Manchester: Women's Studies Research Centre, Manchester Metropolitan University.

Cherlin, A. J., Chase-Lansdale, P.L. and McRae, C. (1998) Effects of parental divorce on mental health throughout the life course, *American Sociological Review*, 63(2): 239–49.

Christian, J. and Abrams, D. (2004) A tale of two cities: predicting homeless people's uptake of outreach programs in London and New York, *Basic and Applied Social Psychology*, 26(2 and 3): 169–82.

Commission of the European Communities (2005) *Improving the Mental Health of the Population: Towards a Strategy on Mental Health for the European Union*. Brussels: European Union.

Condon, L., Hek, G. and Harris, F. (2006) Public health, health promotion and the health of people in prison, *Community Practitioner*, 79(1): 19–22.

Crone, D., Smith, A. and Gough, B. (2005) 'I feel totally at one, totally alive and totally happy': a psycho-social explanation of the physical activity and mental health relationship, *Health Education Research*, 20(5): 600–11.

Degenhardt, L. and Hall, W. (2001) The relationship between tobacco use, substance-use disorders and mental health: results from the National Survey of Mental Health and Well-being, *Nicotine & Tobacco Research*, 3: 225–34.

Dennis, C.L. (2005) Psychosocial and psychological interventions for prevention of post-natal depression: a systematic review, *BMJ*, 331: 15–22.

Dennis, C.L. and Creedy, D. (2005) *Psychosocial and Psychological Interventions for Preventing Postpartum Depression*, Cochrane Library Issue 2. Chichester: John Wiley and Sons Ltd.

Department of Health, Social Services and Public Safety (2003) *Promoting Mental Health: Strategy and action plan 2003–2008*. Belfast: Department of Health, Social Services and Public Safety Northern Ireland. Available at: www.dhsspsni.gov.uk (accessed 11 November 2005).

Department of Trade and Industry (1998) *Guide to Working Time Regulations*. London: DTI.

Department of Work and Pensions/Department of Health/Health and Safety Executive (2005) *Health, Work and Wellbeing: Caring for our Future*. Available at: www.dwp.gov.uk (accessed 3 March 2006).

Dickey, B. (2000) Review of programs for persons who are homeless and mentally ill, *Harvard Rev Psychiatry*, 8(5): 242–50.

DoH (Department of Health) (1998) *Our Healthier Nation: A Contract for Health*. London: HMSO.

DoH (Department of Health) (1999a) *Mental Health National Service Framework*. London: HMSO.

DoH (Department of Health) (1999b) *Saving Lives: Our Healthier Nation*. London: HMSO.

DoH (Department of Health) (2004a) *At least Five a Week: Evidence of the Impact of Physical Activity and its Relationship to Health*. A Report from the Chief Medical Officer. London: HMSO.

DoH (Department of Health) (2004b) *Choosing Health: Making Healthy Choices Easier*. London: The Stationery Office.

Donellan, C. (2005) *Domestic Violence*. Cambridge: Independence Educational Publishers.

Elkan, R., Kendrick, D., Stewart, M. et al. (2000) The effectiveness of domiciliary health visiting: a systematic review of international studies and a selective review of the British literature, *Health Technology Assessment*, 13: 1–339.

Elton, P.J. and Packer, J.M. (1986) A prospective randomized controlled trial for the value of rehousing on the grounds of mental ill health, *Journal of Chronic Disorders*, 39(3): 221–7.

ESRC (2006) Mental health and illness in the UK, *Society Today*. Available at: http://www.esrcsocietytoday.ac.uk (accessed 3 March 2006).

Ferrie, J.E., Shipley, M.J., Marmot, M.G., Stansfield, S. and Smith, G.D. (1995) Health effects of anticipation of job change and non-employment: longitudinal data from the Whitehall II study, *BMJ*, 311(7015): 1264–9.

Ferrie, J., Shipley, M.J., Marmot, M.G., Stansfield, S. and Smith, G.D. (1998) The health effects of major organizational change and job insecurity, *Social Science and Medicine*, 46(2): 243–54.

Fischbach, R.L. and Herbert, B. (1997) Domestic violence and mental health correlates and conundrums within and across cultures, *Social Science and Medicine*, 45(8): 1161–76.

Fox, K. R. (2000) The effects of exercise on self-perceptions and self-esteem, in S.J.H. Biddle,

K.R. Fox and S.H. Boutcher (eds) *Physical Activity Promotion and Psychological Well-being*. London: Routledge.

Gagnon, A.J. (2004) *Individual or Group Based Ante-natal Education for Improving Maternal Psychosocial Health*, Cochrane Library Issue 1, Cochrane Review. Chichester: John Wiley and Sons.

Gahler, M. (1998) Self-reported psychological well-being among adult children of divorce in Sweden, *Acta Sociologica*, 41: 209–25.

Goodchild, B. (1998) Poor housing – poor health: what is the relationship, *International Journal of Health Promotion and Education*, 36(3): 84–6.

Graham, H. and Der, G. (1999) Patterns and predictors of smoking cessation among British women, *Health Promotion International*, 14(3): 231–9.

Green, D. (2006) How can mental health needs of asylum seekers and refugees be met by public health and health promotion. Unpublished MSc dissertation, Leeds Metropolitan University.

Health and Safety Executive (2005) 2004/5 survey of self reported work related illness (SW104/05). Available at: http://www.HSE.gov.uk/statistics (accessed 1 March 2006).

Health and Safety Commission (2004) *Securing Health Together: A Long Term Occupational Health Strategy for England, Scotland and Wales*. London: HSE Books.

Health Promotion Board Online (2005) *Mind Your Mind Programme*. Singapore: Health Promotion Board. Available at: http://www.hpd.gov.sg/hpb/default.asp?pg_id=978 (accessed 18 March 2006).

Heise, L.L., Pitinguy, J. and Germain, A. (1994) *Violence Against Women: The Hidden Health Burden*, Discussion Paper No 1255. New York: World Bank.

Helliwell, J.F. and Putnam, R.D. (2004) The social context of well-being, *Philosophical transactions of the Royal Society of London Series B-Biological Sciences*, 359(1449): 1435–46.

Herrman, H., Saxena, S. and Moodie, R. (eds) (2005) *Promoting Mental Health Concepts, Emerging Evidence Practice: Report of the World Health Organization*. Geneva: World Health Organization.

Hilbourne, M. (1999) Living together full time? Middle-class couples approaching retirement, *Ageing and Society*, 19(2): 161–84.

Institute of Alcohol Studies (2004) *Alcohol and Mental Health*. Available at: www.ias.org/factsheets/mentalhealth.pdf (accessed 10 February 2006).

Investors in Health (1999) *A Standards Based Accreditation Scheme*. Available at: www.investorsinhealth.org (accessed 10 March 2006).

Jané-Lopis, E., Barry, M., Hosman, C. and Patel, V. (2005) Mental health promotion works: a review, *IUHPE Promotion and Education Supplement* 2: 109–25.

Jirojwong, S. and Manderson, L. (2001) Feelings of sadness: migration and subjective assessment of mental health among Thai women in Brisbane, Australia, *Transcultural Psychiatry*, 38(2): 167–86.

Johnson, Z., Howell, F. and Molly, B. (1993) Community Mothers Programme: randomized controlled trial of non-professional intervention in parenting, *BMJ*, 306P: 1449–52.

Johnson, Z., Molly, B., Scallen, E. et al. (2000) Community Mothers Programme: seven years follow up of a randomized controlled trial of non-professional intervention in parenting, *Journal of Public Health Medicine*, 22(3): 337–42.

Knipscheer, J.W., de Jong, E.E.M., Kleber, R.J. and Lamptey, E. (2000) Ghanaian migrants in the Netherlands: general health, acculturative stress and utilization of mental health care, *Journal of Community Psychology*, 28(4): 459–76.

Kovats, R.S., Haines, A., Stanwell-Smith, R. et al. (1999) Climate change and human health in Europe, *British Medical Journal*, 318: 1682–5.

Lam, R.W., Fleming, J.A.E., Buchanan, A. et al. (1990) Seasonal affective disorder, *Canadian Family Physician*, 36: 1162–6.

Lehtinen, V. (2004) *Action for Mental Health: Activities co-funded from European Community Public Health Programmes 1997–2004*. Luxembourg: European Communities and STAKES.

Leonori, L., Munoz, M., Vazquez, C. et al. (2000) The Mental Health and Social Exclusion European Network: a research activity report on European homeless citizens, *European Psychologist*, 5(3): 245–51.

Leontaridi, R. and Bell, D. (2001) *Informal Care of the Elderly in Scotland and the UK*, Health and Community Care Research Findings No. 8. Edinburgh: Scottish Executive Central Research Unit.

Lesesne, C. and Kennedy, C. (2005) Starting early: promoting the mental health of women and girls throughout the life span, *Journal of Women's Health*, 11(9): 754–63.

Magwaza, A.S. and Bhana, K. (1991) Stress, locus of control, and psychological status in black South African migrants, *The Journal of Social Psychology*, 131(2): 157–64.

Maltby, J. and Day, L. (2001) The relationship between exercise motives and psychological well-being, *The Journal of Psychology*, 135(6): 651–60.

McFarlane, J. and Mehir, J. (1994) *De madres a madres*: a community primary health care program based on community empowerment, *Health Education Quarterly*, 21(3): 381–94.

McNaught, A. (1994) A discriminating service: the socioeconomic and scientific roots of racial discrimination in the National Health Service, *Journal of Interprofessional Care*, 8(2): 141–9.

Mental Health Foundation (2005) *Choosing Mental Health: A Policy Agenda for Mental Health and Public Health*. London: Mental Health Foundation. Available at: http://www.mentalhealth.org.uk/html/content/choosing_mental_health.pdf (accessed 29 December 2005).

Mental Health Foundation (2006) *Feeding Minds: The Impact of Food on Mental Health*. London: Mental Health Foundation. Available at: http://www.mentalhealth.org.uk/html/content/feedingminds_report.pdf (accessed 16 February 2006).

Meyer, I.H. (2003) Prejudice, social stress, and mental health in lesbian, gay, and bisexual populations: conceptual issues and research evidence, *Psychological Bulletins*, 129(5): 674–97.

Morgan, M., Calnan, M. and Manning, N. (1990) *Sociological Approaches to Health and Medicine*. London: Croom Helm.

Murphy, L.R. (1996) Stress management in work settings: a critical review of the health effects, *American Journal of Health Promotion*, 11(2): 112–35.

Nazroo, J.Y (1997) *The Health of Britain's Ethnic Minorities*. London: Policy Studies Institute.

Noonan, B.M., Gallor, S.M., Hensler-McGinnis, N.F. et al. (2004) Challenge and success: a qualitative study of the career development of highly achieving women with physical and sensory disabilities, *Journal of Counseling Psychology*, 51(1): 68–80.

Nurse, J., Woodcock, P. and Ormsby, J. (2003) Influence of environmental factors on mental health within prisons: focus group study, *BMJ*, 327(7413): 480–3.

Oakley, A., Hickey, D., Rajan, L. and Rigby, A. (1996) Social support in pregnancy: does it have long-term effects? *Journal of Reproductive and Infant Psychology*, 14: 7–22.

Olley, B.O., Seedat, S. and Stein, D.J. (2004) Predictors of major depression in recently diagnosed patients with HIV/AIDS in South Africa, *AIDS Patient Care and STDs*, 18(8): 481–7.

Pagano, M.E., Skodol, A.E., Stout, R.L. et al. (2004) Stressful life events as predictors of functioning: findings from the Collaborative Longitudinal Personality Disorders Study, *Acta Psychiatrica Scandinavica*, 110: 421–9.

Patel, V. (2005) Poverty, gender and mental health promotion in a global society, *IUHPE Promotion and Education Supplement*, 2: 26–9.

Peersman, G., Harden, A. and Oliver, S. (1998) *Effectiveness of Health Promotion Interventions in the Workplace*. London: Health Education Authority.

Piccinelli, M. and Wilkinson, G. (2000) Gender differences in depression, *British Journal of Psychiatry*, 177: 486–92.

Platt, S., Pavis, S. and Akram, G. (2000) *Changing Labour Market Conditions and Health: A Systematic Literature Review (1993–98)* EF9915EN. Dublin: European Foundation for the Improvement of Living and Working Conditions. Available at: http://www.Eurofound (accessed 28 January 2000).

Price, R.H., van Ryn, M. and Vinokur, A.D. (1992) Impact of a preventive job search intervention on the likelihood of depression among the unemployed, *Journal of Health and Social Behaviour*, 33: 158–67.

Raeburn, J. (2001) Community approaches to mental health promotion, *International Journal of Mental Health Promotion*, 3: 13–16.

Rebecca's Community (2005) *Houseless Statistics*. Available at: http://www.homeless.org.au/statistics/houselessness.htm. (accessed 31 December 2005).

Rogers, A. and Pilgrim, D. (2003) *Mental Health and Inequality*. Basingstoke: Palgrave Macmillan.

Rogers, A. and Pilgrim, D. (2005) *A Sociology of Mental Health and Mental Illness*. Maidenhead: Open University Press.

Rosenthal, N.E., Sack, D.A., Gillin, J.C. et al. (1984) Seasonal affective disorder: a description of the syndrome and preliminary findings with light therapy, *Arch. Gen. Psychiatry*, 41: 72–80.

Samarasinghe, K. and Arvidsson, B. (2002) 'It is a different war to fight here in Sweden': the impact of involuntary migration on the health of refugee families in transition, *Scandinavian Journal of Caring*, 16: 292–301.

Satre, D.D. and Knight, B.G. (2001) Alcohol expectancies and their relationship to alcohol use: age and sex differences, *Aging & Mental Health*, 5(1): 73–83.

Scottish Executive (2003) *National Programme for Improving Mental Health and Well-Being*. Edinburgh: Scottish Executive.

Secretary of State for Health (1998) *Smoking Kills*. London: The Stationery Office.

Sempik, J., Aldridge, J. and Becker, S. (2005) *Health, Well-being and Social Inclusion*. Loughborough: Loughborough University.

Shah, S. and Priestley, M. (2001) *Better Services, Better Health*. Leeds: Leeds Health Involvement/Leeds Health Action Zone.

Simich, L., Scott. J. and Agic, B. (2005) Alone in Canada: a case study of multilingual mental health promotion, *International Journal of Mental Health Promotion*, 7(2): 15–22.

Smith, A.P., Wadsworth, E., Johal, S.S., Davey-Smith, G. and Peters, S. (2000) *The Scale of Occupational Stress: The Bristol Stress and Health at Work Study*. London: HSE Books.

Social Policy Research Unit (2001) *Informal Care Over Time*. York: University of York.

St Mungo (2005) Facts about homeless people. Available at: http://www.mungos.org.facts/demo.html (accessed 31 December 2005).

Taylor, A.H. and Fox, K.R. (2005) Effectiveness of a primary care exercise referral invention for changing physical self-perceptions over 9 months, *Health Psychology*, 24(1): 11–21.

Taylor Nelson Sofres (2003) *Attitudes to Mental Illness 2003*. London: National Statistics.

Teitelman, J. and Copolillo, A. (2005) Psychosocial issues in older adults' adjustment to vision loss: findings from qualitative interviews and focus groups, *The American Journal of Occupational Therapy*, 59: 409–17.

Thomson, H., Petticrew, M. and Morrison, D. (2001) Health effects of housing improvement: systematic review of intervention studies, *BMJ*, 323: 187–90.

Thomson, H., Petticrew, M. and Douglas, M. (2003) Health impact assessment of housing improvements: incorporating research evidence, *Journal of Epidemiology and Community Health*, 57: 11–16.

Tilford, S., Percy-Smith, J., Moran, G. and Green, J. (2002) Leeds: Leeds Metropolitan University, Centre for Health Promotion Research/Policy Studies Institute.

Tolvanen, E. (1998) I and others: alcohol use among older people as a social and cultural phenomenon, *Ageing and Society*, 18: 563–83.

Turner, J.B. and Turner, R.J. (2004) Physical disability, unemployment and mental health, *Rehabilitation Psychology*, 49(3): 241–9.

Turner, S. W., Bowie, C., Dunn, G., Shapo, L. and Yule, W. (2003) Mental health of Kosovan Albanian refugees in the UK, *British Journal of Psychiatry*, 182(5): 444–8.

University of Warwick (2004) *Review of the Occupational Health and Safety of Britain's Ethnic Minorities*, Research Report 221, HSE. Coventry: University of Warwick.

Usdin, S., Scheepers, E., Goldstein, S. and Japhet, G. (2005) Achieving social change on gender based violence: a report on the impact evaluation of *Soul City*'s fourth series, *Social Science and Medicine*, 61: 2434–45.

van Ryn, M. and Vinokur, A.D. (1992) How did it work? An examination of the mechanisms through which an intervention for the unemployed promoted job-search behaviour, *American Journal of Community Psychology*, 20(5): 577–97.

Vinokur, A.D., van Ryn, M., Gramlich, E.H. and Price, R.H. (1991) Long term follow up and benefit-cost analysis of the jobs programme: a preventive intervention for the unemployed, *Journal of Applied Psychology*, 76(2): 213–19.

Vuori, J., Silvonen, J., Vinokur, A. and Price, R. (2002) The Työhön Job Search Program in Finland: benefits for the unemployed with risk of depression or discouragement, *Journal of Occupational Health Psychology*, 7(1): 5–19.

Wallin, A-M. and Ahlström, G.I. (2005) Unaccompanied young adult refugees in Sweden: experiences of their life situation and well-being. A qualitative follow-up study, *Ethnicity and Health*, 10(2): 129–44.

Whitehead, D. (2004) The European Health Promoting Hospitals (HPH) project: how far on? *Health Promotion International*, 19(4): 247–58.

WHO (World Health Organization) (2001) *The World Health Report 2001. Mental Health: New Understanding, New Hope*. Geneva: World Health Organization.

WHO (World Health Organization) (2002) *WHO Report on Violence and Health*. Geneva: WHO.

WHO (World Health Organization) (2004a) *Prevention of Mental Disorders: Effective Interventions and Policy Options*. A report of the World Health Organisation, Department of Mental Health and Substance Abuse in collaboration with the Prevention Research Centre in the Universities of Nijmegen and Maastricht. Geneva: WHO. Available at: www.who.int/mental_health/evidence/en/Prevention_of_Mental_Disorders.pdf (accessed 8 January 2006).

WHO (World Health Organization) (2004b) *Promoting Mental Health. Concepts: Emerging evidence*. A report of the World Health Organisation, Department of Mental Health and Substance Abuse in collaboration with the Victorian Health Promotion Foundation and the University of Melbourne. Geneva: WHO. Available at: www.who.int/mental-_health/evidence/en/promoting_mhh.pdf (accessed 8 January 2006).

WHO (World Health Organization) (2005) *Mental Health and Prisons*. Geneva: World Health Organization. Available at: http://www.euro.who.int/Document/MNH/WHO_ICRC_InfoSht_MNH_Prisons.pdf (accessed 18 March 2006).

WHO (World Health Organization) (2006) *Health in Prisons Project*. Geneva: World Health Organization. Available at: http://www.euro.who.int/eprise/main/who/progs/hipp/home (accessed 18 March 2006).

WHO European Ministerial Conference on Mental Health (2005) *Mental Health Action Plan for Europe: Facing the Challenges, Building Solutions*. Helsinki: World Health Organization.

WHO Regional Office for Europe's Health Evidence Network (HEN) (2005) *How Can Health Care Systems Effectively Deal with the Major Health Care Needs of Homeless People?* Copenhagen: World Health Organization.

WHO Regional Office for Europe (1999) *Mental Health Promotion in Prisons*. Copenhagen: World Health Organization.

Wright, N.M.J. and Tompkins, C.N.E. (2005) *How Can Health Care Systems Effectively Deal with the Major Health Care Needs of Homeless People?* Copenhagen: World Health Organization, Health Evidence Network.

7 Older people: the retirement years (65–80 years and 80+ years)

Mima Cattan

Editors' foreword

Ageing is an increasingly topical subject because of the perceived social and economical impact of an ageing society. Until recently mental health promotion needs of older people were largely ignored, and this is still, as the author highlights, often the case. This chapter explores the factors that impact on older people's mental health and illustrates the global inequalities that persist with regards to old age. Much of the emphasis is on how older people's own views might help shape mental health promotion strategy in the future. In this book 'older people' has been defined as those aged 65–80 years, the retired active aged, and those aged 80 years and over (the fourth age) the 'survivors'. However, there is rarely such clear distinction and therefore these two functional age groups have only been considered where distinct research and examples are available. The chapter considers how retirement age (if it exists) varies between countries, cultures, men and women. Four special mental health issues for older people are discussed: facing end of life; social isolation and loneliness; retirement; and caring.

Introduction

We are living in an ageing world. Recent figures show that 16 percent of the UK population are aged 65 years and over. One-third of a million are aged 90 years or older (Office for National Statistics 2002). In Australia it is estimated that the proportion of the population aged 65 years and over will rise from 12 percent in 2002 to about 18 percent in 2020 (Australian Bureau of Statistics 2000). This increase is not just limited to more developed countries. In 2030 it is estimated that three-quarters (over a billion) of the world's older people over 60 will be living in developing countries. In more developed countries the equivalent figure will be 362 million (HelpAge International 2002).

Age normally refers to **chronological age** – the number of years a person has been alive. This is not always a particularly useful measure when it comes to measuring a person's **functional or health age**. Whilst it is true that many diseases and disabilities occur more commonly in later life, people of the same age vary a great deal in terms of their health. Some senses, such as hearing and sight, tend to deteriorate with age, but the rate and extent to which they do varies widely.

Chronological age is a particularly misleading measure when it comes to mental health. Although some mental health problems seem to increase with age, this does not mean that they are an inevitable consequence of ageing. Older people have, for example, a higher risk than any other age group worldwide of completed suicide. The main psychological factors associated with suicide in older people are depression and certain personality traits (O'Connell et al. 2004). The prevalence of dementia does increase with age, with figures suggesting prevalence ranging from under 2 percent in people aged 65–9 years to almost a quarter of those aged 85 years and over. A major international review suggests that the occurrence of dementia varies between regions, countries, urban and rural areas, different ethnic groups and so on (Ferri et al. 2005). The issue of dementia in the context of this chapter will in main be dealt with in relation to the older carer.

Although this chapter deals with the chronologically defined population group of 'older people' we need to recognize that mental health issues and mental health promotion are not 'fixed' to older people as a homogenous group. First, old age can span from 60 years upwards and can, therefore, in theory refer to 50 years of a person's life. No one would question the fact that an individual's physical capacity and health status will change over that period. Second, if we accept that chronological age may be misleading for measuring health, we should also accept that the mental health issues explored under 'old age' may not necessarily relate to the same older age group every-where as they will be influenced by environmental, cultural, and social factors. We have chosen to consider mental health and older people from the age of 65 years as this is the retirement age for most (but not all) people in the UK. We have divided 'older people' into two (artificial) age bands; 65–80 years and 80 years and over because studies sug-gest that in developed countries there is a noticeable increase in frailty, dependency and dementia in the 'fourth age' (Coleman and O'Hanlon 2004).

Special mental health issues

Although many mental health issues span all age groups, there are some that are of greater relevance at this stage in people's lives. In the 65–80 year age group retirement is a major factor which impacts on people's mental health. For some people retirement means a positive release from the 'daily slog' and other responsibilities, while for others it may mean the loss of important social networks and their professional role. Other factors include deterioration in physical capability and health, changing environments (for example moving home), and the sense of loss of social, physical or psychological factors.

For people aged 80 years and over the sense of loss may become more chronic through the loss of their partners or close friends, their functional ability and a sense of purpose in life. Linked to this is the fear of losing independence. Loneliness, although not restricted to old age, becomes more prevalent among the 'older old' for a range of reasons (Victor 1989). Caring for someone who is frail or in the early stages of dementia may contribute to an older person's isolation and loneliness. Finally, at this stage in

---

Box 7.1 Summary points: factors that may impact on mental health and well-being for people aged 65–80+ years

For people aged 65–80:

- Retirement; positive active ageing or loss of social networks and a role in life.
- Deterioration in physical capability and physical health.
- Changing environments; moving home.
- Sense of loss; of social networks, 'significant others', physical capability, or perceived belonging.

For people aged 80 years and over:

- Sense of loss more chronic; loss of 'significant others'; sense of purpose; and loss of independence.
- Loneliness and social isolation.
- Caring for someone with dementia or someone who is becoming increasingly frail.
- Facing end of life; dealing with bereavement, death and dying.

---

life people are facing the end of life and develop different strategies for dealing with bereavement, dying and death.

Determinants of and influences on mental health for older people

As with other age groups, older people's mental health is not simply a product of their own behaviour but is influenced by where they live, the state of their environment, their physical health, income, and relationships with friends and family. The determinants of health, as defined by the WHO (2002) provide a useful framework for illustrating the factors that affect older people's mental health.

According to the WHO (2002) the over-arching determinants of 'active ageing' are gender and culture, which in turn influence:

- Social determinants, such as education, literacy, human rights, social support, prevention of violence and abuse.
- Factors in the physical environment, such as urban/rural settings, housing, injury prevention.
- Personal determinants, such as biology and genetics, adaptability.
- Economic determinants, such as income, work, social protection.
- Health and social services, such as health promotion, disease prevention, long-term care, primary care.
- Behavioural determinants, such as physical activity, healthy eating, cessation of tobacco use, control of alcohol problems, inappropriate use of medication.

Although this is a slightly different framework from that used in previous chapters (and not everyone will necessarily agree with the distinction that gender and culture are over-arching determinants), it is used here as an illustration of how the WHO framework can be utilized.

Culture

Cultural values and norms determine how society views older people and how mental health and mental illness are conceptualized. Culture influences how we respond to the world around us, how mental illness symptoms are manifested, and the level of stigma attached to mental illness (Abrahamson et al. 2002). The experience of ageing is an essential element of all cultures and age boundaries are maintained by formal laws and social sanctions. However, concepts of what constitutes 'old age' are culturally variable and may be based on chronological age, social functioning or work capacity (Dein and Huline-Dickens 1997).

Theories relating to ageing

A range of psycho-social theories have evolved to provide explanation and understanding of the complexities of ageing in society. Although it is not possible to provide a complete account of all such theories in this chapter, some of these theories may be useful in exploring the cultural impact on mental health in old age.

The disengagement theory

This suggests that decreased social interaction in later life is a process whereby both society and the ageing person withdraw. Disengagement is therefore a natural process rather than something imposed, and as such is accepted by the older individual. According to the theory a sense of psychological well-being is reached by the very old who have reached an acceptance of decreased social interaction. The assumption that disengagement is an inevitable and irreversible process from the age of 65 years, and that psychological well-being or morale is reached once the process is complete has been disputed by several researchers. Instead it has been suggested that disengagement occurs in response to factors other than age, and that older people choose to withdraw from less satisfying relations and often replace them with new, different social contacts (Dein and Huline-Dickens 1997).

Dein and Huline-Dickens (1997) argue that within Western society alienation, withdrawal from social interaction and segregation only occur as people age because it is imposed. According to the authors Western society does not value older people, but rather views them as a burden. On the other hand in some cultures withdrawing from worldly activities and interests in the last two stages of life are seen as an ideal and does not result in loss of status. In many cultures older people are able to contribute to community life, thus having a purpose in life and enjoying respect (Dein and Huline-Dickens 1997; Abrahamson et al. 2002).

According to Nyangweso (1998) disengagement theory can only explain transformations that have taken place throughout African cultures as a result of Western ideals and values being introduced. In traditional African communities older people were held in high esteem because of the knowledge they had accumulated and consequently as the custodians of community wisdom. As a result of transformations many older people have withdrawn from society because they do not feel they belong, becoming isolated and lonely. It has been suggested that the rising, and disproportionately high incidence of suicide among older women in Japan and in rural China may be due to societal transition, changes in traditional family values and family conflict (Dein and Huline-Dickens 1997; Pritchard and Baldwin 2002).

Activity theory

On the other hand, activity theory suggests that older people have the same activity and social contact needs as middle-aged individuals. A decrease in social interaction and activities are therefore imposed rather than voluntarily sought. Well adjusted older people aim to maintain their accepted lifestyle as long as possible and attempt to replace lost roles and activities. For the ageing experience to be successful substantial levels of social, physical and mental activities need to be maintained or developed. In contrast to disengagement theory the level of engagement or disengagement is not as a result of inevitable and intrinsic processes but influenced by past lifestyles, socio-economic status and imposed social changes. The theory implies that the loss of social function is an undesirable state that older people wish to avoid (Burbank 1986; Havighurst et al. 1998). This perspective seems to be more in tune with observations made in many 'non-Western' cultures. Many types of mental health problems are more prevalent among older Inuits, Africans, Native Americans and some ethnic minority groups in the UK than the equivalent white European (Nyangweso 1998; Abrahamson et al. 2002; Bjerregaard and Curtis 2002; Sproston and Nazroo 2002), although the causal link has been questioned.

Activity theory has been criticized for not acknowledging that personality may play a part in determining relationships between life satisfaction and role activity or recognizing that coping strategies built up over people's lives are utilized to deal with changes in social networks (Bengtson et al. 1997).

Social constructionist theories emphasize that social reality changes over time, and focus on people's social meaning, social relations, attitudes towards age and ageing, and life events and timing. One such theory is Kuyper's and Bengtson's social break-down theory.

Kuyper's and Bengtson's social breakdown theory

This theory suggests that ageist attitudes label older people as incompetent in social mechanisms, ultimately leading to a situation of learned helplessness where the older person relinquishes personal control (Bengtson et al. 1997). This theoretical approach provides different perspectives on mental health promotion interventions and older people than are often implemented in practice. The approach has, however, been criticized for giving limited attention to the impact of the wider social and cultural environment.

Social exchange theories

These aim to explain the impact of emotional, social and financial resources on exchanges of contact and social support, particularly between generations. According to these an explanation for why there is less contact between the young and the old is that older people have fewer resources to offer in the exchange. One of the main criticisms of the approach is that it fails to take into account the quality and the meaning of social contacts, focusing mainly on the number of social exchanges and the prediction of exchange behaviours (Bengtson et al. 1997). Again, we need to recognize that these perspectives have been developed in a Western culture with its particular sets of values and norms. Although we can speculate that social exchange theory might help explain the mental health impact of rapid social transition on older people no studies have been published that might corroborate this.

Gender

It is well-known that women are recorded more frequently as suffering from mental health problems compared to men. A study of 14 European countries reported a clear excess of depression among older women in 13 of the 14 countries. In a survey of psychiatric morbidity among adults in Great Britain older people generally showed a lower prevalence of common mental disorder. However, older women were still more likely than older men to be diagnosed with depression and anxiety (Evans et al. 2003). A survey of ethnic minority psychiatric illness rates found a considerable variation in prevalence among women across ethnic groups (Sproston and Nazroo 2002).

The association between gender, mental health and ageing can easily be over simplified. In many societies women have lower social status than men and consequently less access to services, education, food and employment. Women's traditional role in the family can be a factor in women experiencing increased poverty and deprivation in old age. Women also tend to live longer and are more likely than men to live alone in later life. A consequence of this may be isolation linked to inadequate pension, lack of affordable and accessible transport, loss of property and status and real or perceived threats of violence in the external environment. However, in some cultures older men are more likely to be rejected by their community once they have ceased to be 'productive' due to ageing or poor health (HelpAge International 2002). For an older person the loss of what we perceive as traditional gender roles, whether male or female, with associated loss of status, respect and independence is likely to impact on their mental health.

Bereavement

Bereavement is associated with a range of physical and mental health risk factors. Although the causes are not fully understood, studies have suggested that there are some important links between depression, loss, older age and perceived health, which may be more salient for older men (Tijhuis et al. 1999; Alpass and Neville 2003). The services required (such as therapeutic, spiritual) for older people needing help with dealing with dying and death go beyond the scope of this book. For anyone who is particularly interested in mental health in relation to dying and death in later life there are several books available (see for example Dickenson et al. 2000; Hockey et al. 2001; Owen 2005). However, it should be emphasized that although some older people are not comfortable about talking about dying and death, many are and do (Owen 2005).

Box 7.2   Special issue in later life: facing end of life, bereavement and grief

It has been recognized that there are differences in the grieving process depending on if the death has been sudden and unexpected or anticipated after a long illness, and whether or not the widow(er) was present at the time of their partner's death. Importantly, older widow(er)s can 'rekindle' their grief after many years of acceptance if their personal circumstances deteriorate (Sidell 1996). One of the most serious problems linked to bereavement and grief in later life is loneliness, which in turn is linked to depression. The association between widowhood and loneliness is multi-faceted rather than unidimensional through the interaction of a range of factors such as the ones mentioned above, health, gender or having to move into a care home (Tijhuis et al. 1999; Costello and Kendrick 2000). Lopata (1980) suggested that widow(er)s can be grouped into three main categories depending on the type of loneliness they express: missing the partner; missing the lifestyle; or a sense of inadequacy in relationships with other people. Clearly, if this is the case we could expect that different interventions would be required depending on the type of loneliness identified. This is only partially born out by research with most intervention studies focusing on self-help, education and skills training.

Social determinants

Low levels of education and literacy are associated with increased risk of physical and mental health problems in old age, as well as with higher rates of unemployment and poverty. Basic education in childhood combined with opportunities for lifelong learning may help increase older people's confidence, provide them with the skills to adapt to a changing world and improve their quality of life (HelpAge International 2002; WHO 2002).

Older people are at increasing risk of violence, crime and abuse in many parts of the world. In regions experiencing civil conflict, increased levels of crime and drugs related violence, or high levels of HIV/AIDS older people are particularly vulnerable to violence and abusive behaviour. The impact of these violations is reduced quality of life and increased risk of poor mental health. Elder abuse takes the form of physical abuse, psychological abuse, financial abuse, sexual abuse, or neglect.

The role of family and friends in maintaining mental well-being in later life has been investigated in a large number of studies (see, for example, Bowling 1991; Reinhardt 1996; Phillipson et al. 1998; Seeman 2000). The association between the different dimensions of mental well-being and social contact with family and friends is dependent on several factors. It would seem that there are both cultural and geographical differences in how older people perceive social contacts. Some studies suggest that while adult children are the main source of instrumental support, they are not necessarily the main source of emotional support. However, the availability of a companion or confident is linked to the perceived adequacy of instrumental and emotional support (Matt and Dean 1993). A study in Spain suggests (in contrast to earlier American research) that emotional support from children seems to play an important role in maintaining older parents' mental well-being (Zunzunegui et al. 2001).

In Europe some studies have suggested a north–south divide regarding older people's experiences of loneliness. Two cross-cultural surveys found an inverse macro-level association with more older adults in northern Europe living alone, but a greater proportion of older people in the South feeling lonely (Jylhä and Jokela 1990; van Tilburg et al. 1998). Jylhä and Jokela (1990) hypothesized that this was due to different value systems between the North and the South, while van Tilburg et al. (1998) suggested that the variance was mainly due to differences in individuals' social integration.

Although most research has focused on the benefits of social contacts we must remember that social relations can be both positive and negative. In an overview of the health promoting effects of close social interactions in older people Seeman (2000) notes that negative and/or non-supportive social interactions between close social relations are probably main sources of stress, suggesting that negative relationships may have greater impact on affect and mental health than positive ones. Perhaps this is an area which is not acknowledged sufficiently in mental health promotion.

Box 7.3   Special issue in later life: social isolation and loneliness

In later life social networks change and are reduced in size. With increasing numbers of older people living alone, older women are particularly vulnerable to social isolation as a result of living longer, increasing population mobility and poverty. Interviews with older people suggest that deteriorating general health, loss of mobility, fear of being burgled or mugged could lead to social isolation (Cattan 2002a; Cattan et al. 2003). Loneliness, which is often associated with social isolation, is described by older people as a subjective negative feeling often following bereavement or loss in relation to other life events. A recent study in the UK suggests that there has been a decrease in the number of older people who report never being lonely. There is some debate about whether increased age is a risk factor for loneliness, or whether in fact there is a complex interaction with other factors, such as widowhood, which might provide both vulnerability and protection to loneliness (Victor et al. 2005). Social isolation and loneliness have received public attention because they are thought to reduce older people's quality of life and life satisfaction (Bowling 1993; Wenger et al. 1996). The absence of social isolation and loneliness is therefore seen as a desirable state that one would wish to maintain, while being isolated and lonely could be perceived as having failed in the eyes of 'significant others'. Consequently, a large number of community projects have been established, which aim to prevent or reduce social isolation and loneliness in later life. The effectiveness of some of these interventions has been questioned and the research evidence is discussed later in this chapter.

Factors in the physical environment

It almost goes without saying that a safe and accessible environment is conducive to mental well-being. Older people mention transport, housing and the quality of the external environment as particular barriers to social participation (Cattan et al. 2003) and contributing to the loss of independence. In other words, costly or inaccessible transport, inadequate or unsafe housing, and unsafe external environments may lead to social isolation, increased mobility problems and associated mental health problems. Worldwide, older people living in rural areas are particularly vulnerable because of urbanization and migration of younger people to cities, lack of transport and services. In some developing countries there has been a sharp increase in the number of older people living in slums and shanty towns as they follow younger families seeking employment to the cities. In such circumstances older people are highly vulnerable to violence and crime, and becoming socially isolated. Moving into residential housing of some type can have a positive or a negative impact on an older person's mental health. This transition can occur for a variety of reasons, but usually happens at a point of perceived or real vulnerability. Positive effects can include feeling safe, increased social contact, while negative feelings may be a sense of loss of independence and control and associated depression.

Personal determinants

The process of ageing is determined by, among many factors, biology, genetics and how well the individual adapts to changing circumstances. Some functions, such as reaction time, memory and learning speed, naturally decline with age. Ageist attitudes in society and loss of control over the personal environment are thought to have detrimental effects on older people's cognitive functioning (Coleman 1996; Bengtson et al. 1997). The sense of not being in control in turn is associated with lack of confidence, social isolation and depression, although these relationships are complex and not fully understood.

It is worth noting at this point that there is no known direct association between physical ill health and mental ill health. However, several studies have found that *self-reported health* is associated with depression in later life (Herman et al. 2001; Alpass and Neville 2003).

'Use it or lose it' is a well-known phrase, which refers to the hypothesis that by participating in mentally, socially and physically stimulating activities we protect ourselves against cognitive decline. Although there has been some debate about the nature and reality of this association, for most part it has been accepted. However, the direction of the association is not simple and in one direction but complex and reciprocal (Mackinnon et al. 2003).

One of the myths about old age is that ageing is a long negative experience of having to cope with ill health, loss and loneliness. Many older people despite experiencing major life events such as bereavement and loss, impairment and chronic ill health, in fact adjust to and cope well with the negative effects of these life changes. The Berlin Aging Study provides detailed evidence about the complex inter-relationship between a wide range of indicators linked to well-being, by comparing men and women, and the 'old' (aged 70–84 years) with the 'old old' (aged 85–103 years). Although the findings show that the younger old with more desirable profiles (cognitively fit, extra-verted, not lonely, high social embeddedness) for most part demonstrated higher subjective well-being, this relationship was by no means clear-cut (Smith and Baltes 1997). Some of the 'oldest old' with less desirable profiles (cognitively impaired, high external control, high social loneliness, high levels of anxiety and fearfulness) also expressed moderate levels of well-being.

Another important personal determinant is the desirability to retain control over life events (Andersson 1992). According to Coleman and O'Hanlon (2004: 115) 'Primary control involves the use of proactive strategies directed towards overcoming obstacles and attaining the individual's chosen goals', while 'Secondary control refers to strategies directed towards managing and influencing emotions and perceptions'. For older people having a sense of control is linked to feeling valued and having a purpose in life. Several studies of older people moving into residential care have shown that the perception of control and self-esteem are critical components in adjusting mentally and physically to institutional living (Yoon 1996; Antonelli et al. 2000; Shyam and Yadav 2002).

The link between the impact of falling and depression is well recorded. Research has shown that older people who have experienced a falls-related injury are more at risk of depression if improvement in physical function slows down (Scaf-Klomp et al. 2003). A study in Australia found that older women (aged 75 years and over) considered falls and consequential injury as great risks to their independence and quality of life. The majority declared that they 'would rather be dead than experience the loss of independence and quality of life that results from a bad hip fracture and subsequent admission to a nursing home' (Salkeld et al. 2000: 344).

Community living older people often describe a range of different coping strategies to deal with changes in life, which may be influenced by social and cultural factors. The strategies they use can provide useful clues as to where interventions are needed. In order to develop successful mental health promotion programmes we need to consider what influences individuals' ability to adapt and cope with loss and other changes in later life, and why some older people are better at finding new sources of self-esteem than others.

Economic determinants

Not having enough income or social protection in the form of old age pension can seriously affect older people's vulnerability and consequently their mental health. Older women living alone and those who live in rural areas are particularly at risk of social exclusion, poverty and ill health. The Social Exclusion Unit (2006) highlights that many of the most excluded people are among the very old. According to the report many older people face multiple exclusions because of overlapping problems of poor housing, low income and limiting illness. The mental health risk factors linked to the economic determinants are therefore multi-faceted; loss of job and drop in income may be linked to a change of role, decreased independence and sense of self-worth.

Box 7.4 Special issue in later life: retirement

Retirement affects people's health both positively and negatively. With retirement no longer being determined by old age, research has increasingly started defining retirement as a period of transition, rather than as entry into old age. As Johnson (2004: 40–1) puts it:

> Indeed, when the population of seventy-year-olds includes both the physically fit and active and the bedridden, the very wealthy and the abjectly poor, the socially connected and the socially excluded, the family figurehead and the isolated singleton, then it is no longer evident that age should be regarded as a meaningful social or economic category.

The Whitehall II study of civil service employees found that mental health actually improved after retirement, but only for those in high employment grades (Mein et al. 2003). Although those in lower grades also benefited to some degree from giving up work this may have been outweighed by the relative disadvantage of a lower pension in retirement. For women, who are often in low paid jobs, retirement may mean less security. Retirement may also have an effect on marital relationships. Married women tend to view their retirement less positively and take longer to adjust. It has been suggested that while married men's mental health improves when they retire, married women's experiences may be quite different. Conflict over the amount of time spent together and loss of 'personal space' rather than the economic consequences of retirement are concerns that women raise about retirement (Hilbourne 1999; Rosenkoetter and Garris 2001).

Recent studies in developing countries suggest that older people are at greater risk of poverty than younger age groups because of individual, familial, normative and structural determinants (Ogwumike and Aboderin 2005), and that older widows are among the poorest and most vulnerable groups (HelpAge International 2002). The experiences of older women and their feelings of insecurity and vulnerability could be viewed as predisposing social factors, which impact on their mental health.

Families are often assumed to care for and support older members of the family. In Western society such filial duties are not necessarily expected (or even possible) although the support may still be provided in some form. Contrary to assumptions evidence suggests that familial allocation of scarce resources in poorer countries is linked to a normative hierarchy of generational priorities – young people are seen as 'the future' and are therefore prioritized above the old. In contrast to past filial duties to honour parents and support them in return for the care they provided in childhood, decisions to support parents may be taken on the basis of a judgement of 'past conduct and deservedness'. This type of discrimination seems to affect older men more than older women (Aboderin 2004). In some countries older women are more likely to be living in multi-generational families than older men (Gomes da Conceicao and Montes de Oca Zavala 2004), and thereby receive more support in their old age. Explanations for these gender differences may be that older women are seen as 'more desirable' by adult children because they are more likely to offer their services as cook and child minder in exchange for financial support. Although older men tend to be more financially secure than older women, this type of situation is particularly severe for older men in poor health who lack income or other forms of security.

Health and social services, including health promotion

This area will be covered in more detail in the next section. A European review of mental health indicators suggested that the utilization of mental health services may depend on a range of variables other than the clinical condition of the individual (Korkeila et al. 2003). Therefore, the use of (mental) health services may not be a good indicator of the state of a population's mental health.

Diversity among older people

It is impossible in one chapter to give justice to the mental health factors associated with all different population groups among older people. However, some issues for further consideration in mental health promotion can be noted. The diversity of old age is illustrated below:

- Black and minority ethnic older people
- Older lesbians, gay men and bisexual men and women
- Older prisoners
- Older homeless people
- Grandparents
- Caregivers

Because of the 'invisibility' of some of these groups there is little research available regarding their mental health and any particular mental health promotion needs (see for example D'Augelli et al. 2001; Fazel et al. 2001; Stergiopoulos and Herrman 2003; Social Exclusion Unit 2006). We need to be cautious, however, not to make too many assumptions about the 'special' status of these groups of older people. Studies indicate that it is because they are invisible that their mental health needs are not recognized or addressed, rather than because they are older lesbians, caregivers or prisoners. Being older brings with it certain risk factors with regards to mental health, and being homeless or a caregiver for example, adds another dimension to the individual's vulnerability, but also potentially to their experience and resilience. It follows that for mental health promotion to be responsive to the needs of these groups it would need to take into account the multitude of factors that impact on their mental health and well-being.

There is evidence to show that there is a high risk of mental health problems such as depression and anxiety among people who take on the role of informal caring (Social Policy Research Unit 2001; Doran et al. 2003).

Box 7.5   Special issue in later life: caregivers/informal carers

Worldwide older people have become the primary informal carers of family members, friends or neighbours. In developing countries this tends to be linked to caring for family members with HIV/AIDS and for orphaned grandchildren (HelpAge International 2002). In the little data that is available 'grandparents' are taken as one group without making a distinction between grandmothers and grandfathers. More than a fifth of people in their fifties in England and Wales provide informal, unpaid care. Even among people aged 85 years and over 5 percent provide some form of care in the home. Women tend to be the main carers but among people aged 65 years and over, men are more likely to provide care for a family member. Added to this, a substantial number of these carers are themselves permanently sick or disabled (National Statistics 2004). These figures do not take into account the contribution grandparents make. A similar picture is found in other countries. Research shows that there are differences between women's and men's responses to their caring role (with women twice as likely to report increased distress) the types of care they provide and the kind of support they receive (Social Policy Research Unit 2001). With regards to mental health promotion there are differences which may in part determine the suitability of the intervention. Just as women may require different types of support than men in their caring roles, it has been suggested that the health impact of caring for a family member with dementia may be different from the impact of caring for an older person with terminal illness (Grunfeld et al. 1997), and consequently require distinct interventions. Current demographic trends will undoubtedly change the capacity of families to cope with informal caring roles.

Behavioural determinants

Mental health in old age is also linked with behavioural lifestyle factors. These factors often interact and the association between mental health and lifestyle is probably quite complex (van Gool et al. 2003; Cassidy et al. 2004). There is a clear association between the positive effects of physical activity and mental well-being and a significant association between depression and low levels of physical activity. This suggests that participation in regular physical activity promotes mental well-being, but importantly, psychological well-being also seems to be a predictor for staying physically active in later life (Ruuskanen and Ruoppila 1995; Satariano et al. 2000). The main reasons older people give for remaining physically active are the social aspects of exercise and physical activity (Stathi et al. 2002), self-acceptance and a sense of purpose (Crone et al. 2005). Never-married older men are less likely to be members of informal groups than older men with a partner. However, those who are widowed are more likely than partnered older men to participate in sports and other social clubs (Perren et al. 2003).

Linked to the opportunity to stay active is an increasing dependence, especially in developed countries, on the ability to drive. Many older drivers take a conscious decision to reduce then stop driving. American studies have found that driving cessation, particularly among older men, is linked to an increased risk of depression (Fonda et al. 2001). Driving cessation is also a gender issue. Siren et al. (2004) found an association between increased depression and driving cessation, although the direction of the causal link was not clear from their study. Access to reliable public transport is linked to elevated quality of life, and older people report that improvements in public transport would improve their quality of life (Gilhooly et al. 2005). Consequently, older people's mental health could be assumed to be linked to the level of access to public transport.

The association between alcohol consumption and mental health in later life has been debated a great deal. The main triggers associated with heavy drinking are said to be bereavement and widowhood, mental stress, physical ill health, social isolation and loneliness, loss, racism and social pressures from the family (Francis 1995; Alcohol Concern 2002). It is not clear whether social isolation has an impact on drinking habits or whether heavy drinking might lead to reduced social networks and social isolation. Another aspect to the consumption of alcohol and mental well-being in later life is that of social light or moderate drinking. A Finnish study of older people's accounts of their use of alcohol suggests that alcohol consumption is a reflection of cultural habits and norms attached to drinking (Tolvanen 1998), rather than of old age or ageing. Social drinking within cultural limits was viewed as both acceptable and enjoyable, while drinking outside the norms and conventions was not.

The relationship between nutrition and mental health is complex and not well documented. In a study of psycho-social correlates of nutritional risk in older adults Johnson (2005) found that older people at risk of malnutrition had significantly lower levels of social support and higher depression scores than those not at risk. He suggests that there may be a two-way interaction between nutrition and depression in that older people may be at risk of poor nutrition because they are unable to acquire and eat nutritious food without social support. Therefore the perceived quality of social support may have a direct impact on malnutrition. The European Nutrition for Health Alliance has stated that there is a clear association between malnutrition and loneliness, social isolation, lack of motivation and depression, which should not be ignored (Baeyens 2005).

Box 7.6 Summary of the main determinants affecting mental health among older people reviewed in this chapter

Cultural determinants:
- Social interaction/social function
- Cultural transformation
- Stigma/ageism

Gender:
- Depression
- Social status
- Poverty/deprivation
- Gender roles

Bereavement:
- Dying and death
- Bereavement and grief

Social determinants:
- Education/literacy
- Violence and abuse
- Social contact/social support
- Social isolation/loneliness

Physical environment:
- Transport
- Housing
- Quality of external environment
- Rural isolation

Personal determinants:
- Coping
- Retaining control/perceptions of control
- Resilience
- Impact of injury

Economic determinants:
- Retirement
- Social security/pension
- Poverty
- Contacts with family

Health and social services/health promotion:
- Diversity among older people
- Caring responsibilities

Behavioural determinants:

- Physical activity/'other' activity
- Driving
- Alcohol consumption
- Nutrition
- Health risk behaviour and social control

Promoting mental health and mental well-being among older people

So far we have looked at the risk factors, wider determinants and particular vulnerabilities with regards to mental health and older people. Now we will consider what can be done to promote mental health and well-being in later life. First we will look at how older people themselves view mental health and well-being, then we will review the research evidence for effective interventions. Lastly, we will consider examples of good practice, such as the development of policies and strategies and the implementation of community-based services and activities intended to maintain and improve older people's mental well-being and how these relate to the evidence.

The meaning of mental health: older people's perceptions of mental well-being and mental ill health

It is important to understand how older people perceive and describe mental health because without that understanding it simply is not possible to develop sustainable, responsive and acceptable mental health promotion interventions for older people. Most older people in a Scottish survey found it quite difficult to define 'mental well-being' because they felt that it encapsulated everything that contributed to feeling mentally well, such as family and friends, leading active lives, good health, maintaining independence, having a positive attitude to old age, financial security and a continued role in retirement (Bostock and Millar 2003). This illustrates the wide notions of mental health. However, a contributing reason may be that older people are unaccustomed (and reluctant) to discuss issues around their personal mental health.

A survey conducted in the UK as part of the *Inquiry into Mental Health and Well-being in Later Life* showed that almost half the respondents took the phrase 'mental health and well-being' to be negative and more about mental ill health. Dementia was cited frequently, as was 'being fearful', 'being thankful for their own good mental health and well-being' and 'feeling sorry for people suffering mental ill health' (Third Sector First 2005: 14). However, phrases also used included 'healthy mind', 'healthy body' and 'happiness'. Happiness was described as contentment, having a sense of self-esteem, having a balanced outlook, and being positive and cheerful. Finally, some saw mental health as being able to cope with life and being in control. Although the survey did not identify any significant gender differences, there were significant differences between age groups regarding mentioning 'happiness'. Far more people aged 60–9 years cited happiness than those aged 80–9 years, and no one over the age of 90 said that mental health was about feeling happy.

When older people have been asked about the things that worry them and what upsets their mental well-being the main issues they list are: their own physical health; losing capability and independence; social isolation from family and friends; finances and retirement; not being respected as individuals; not being able to maintain physical or mental activity; and world affairs (Bostock and Millar 2003; Third Sector First 2005).

The main worry for the 'young old' (50–9 age group) is finance, while those aged 90 and over are mostly concerned about the possibility of having to go into residential care, and consequently losing their independence. When asked what makes them feel good and motivated the four most commonly given answers focused on being with others and getting out of the house for reasons such as 'interests', 'friends', 'outings' and 'family'. These findings are similar to issues raised by older people about combating social isolation and loneliness (Cattan 2002a).

Evidence of effective mental health promotion interventions among older people

There are, to date, few studies that have evaluated the effect of mental health promotion interventions (direct or indirect) in older people. Some intervention studies have included older people in their study group as adults/older adults. The few studies that are available can broadly be divided into public health or other interventions that specifically target known risk factors in mental health and wider environmental and political interventions that are intended to improve the quality of life among older people. Those that have evaluated the effectiveness of interventions targeting known risk factors in mental health have considered home-based support and home visiting, social support, the impact of exercise and reminiscence, interventions which improve self-esteem and morale, activities targeting social isolation and loneliness, and support for carers.

Home-based support

There is continued debate about the effectiveness of home-based support such as befriending and home visiting schemes on mental well-being. On the basis of three systematic reviews (van Haastregt et al. 2000; Elkan et al. 2001; Cattan et al. 2005) the effectiveness of home-based support in improving psycho-social function, functional status or social isolation and loneliness remains unclear. Van Haastregt et al. (2000) go as far as suggesting that unless the effectiveness of preventive home visits is improved such support should be discontinued. We should perhaps be a bit cautious before taking such drastic steps. It could be that the measures used in the studies were insensitive to any subtle changes in morale or mental well-being. It may also be that research so far has not incorporated the 'right' elements of home visiting to measure. We know through qualitative studies that older people respond favourably to home visiting, stating that the visitor/befriender 'gives them a reason to get up'; 'is someone to share interests and worries with'; and 'offers both practical help and companionship' (Dean and Goodlad 1998; Cattan 2002b). Older people also emphasize the importance of reciprocity, which may be more likely to occur when the visitor/caller and the 'recipient' are of the same generation, share a common culture and social background, and have common interests (Cattan et al. 2003). A possible explanation for why the reviews were unable to demonstrate effect may be that the interventions included in the reviews were all concerned with direct service provision, rather than with social support and did not include the factors mentioned by older people themselves.

Group activities

Group-based social support interventions for older people with mental health problems, widows, women living alone and caregivers have been found to reduce distress, stress, social isolation and loneliness, and increase self-esteem, morale and social activity (CRD 1997; Tilford et al. 1997; Cattan et al. 2005). Most interventions have included some form of structured activity, such as a negotiated and agreed peer and professionally led educational programme, self-help support, directed group discussion or supported social activation. Participant planned and led activities seem to improve effectiveness. Preconditions for successful social network and social support development have been identified as:

> the existence of people who were interested in socialising and in participating in activities; that the activity was frequent and regular and provided the practical means to participate; that there was a leader, either a professional or an older lay person with the relevant skills and interest who acted as a co-ordinator and a fixed resource for the group
>
> (Hedelin and Svensson 1999: 120)

Exercise and music

The value of exercise and music in improving mental well-being is increasingly recognized (Tilford et al. 1997; Cattan et al. 2005; Young and Dinan 2005). Music has been said to provide people with ways of understanding emotions, their self-identity in relation to others and spirituality. Music is used to express emotions, communicate feelings and ultimately to improve and maintain a sense of well-being (Hays and Minichiello 2005). The researchers argue that music can provide a cultural and normative 'bridge' between individuals and is frequently used to form contacts and social links with others. In interviews with older Australians music was found to enhance older people's self-esteem and lessened their feelings of isolation and loneliness.

Several evaluation studies show the benefits of exercise for older people's mental health. In the UK, low intensity exercise to music has been shown to result in significant improvements in happiness and well-being (Tilford et al. 1997), enjoyment and other social and psychological benefits (Paulson 2005). Both tai chi and moderate intensity exercise can improve self-rated sleep quality (King et al. 1997; Li et al. 2004), which is associated with quality of life, risk of depression and suicide (Rabheru 2004). In addition it has been shown that tai chi reduces the fear of falling and enhances self-esteem in older people (Wolf et al. 1996). Home training combined with twice weekly group training demonstrated greater mental health benefits than home training on its own, suggesting that the social activity effects of the group may improve the overall effects of exercise (Helbostad et al. 2004). A programme which combined health education with exercise sessions demonstrated a significant reduction in loneliness among older people in The Netherlands (Hopman-Rock and Westhoff 2002). Gardening as a form of physical activity has been found to provide mental stimulation, while the social contact aspect of communal gardening has major effects on older individuals' sense of worth and mental well-being (Milligan et al. 2005).

Reminiscence

For the past 30 years reminiscence has become an almost natural part of activities in care work. For anyone particularly interested in reminiscence and life review, Coleman and O'Hanlon (2004) provide a comprehensive overview of the historical background, types, functions and evaluations of reminiscence with older people. Reminiscence enables older people to recall past events and life experiences, while life review focuses on the individual's past life as a whole. Reminiscence is conducted in groups or on a one to one basis. It is used for a variety of reasons, for example to find meaning and purpose in life, to reduce boredom, to teach and inform. It has been used therapeutically, to deal with depression and traumatic memories, with residents in sheltered housing to improve well-being, and with demented older people. Interestingly, it would seem that some ethnic groups utilize reminiscence more than others, although as Coleman and O'Hanlon (2004) point out, it is not clear whether this is because some cultures have a stronger oral tradition or because these groups have a greater need to promote self-understanding, preserve identity and educate ensuing generations.

Carers' support

There is a large body of research which has evaluated ways of improving the mental well-being of those who care for frail older people, older people with Alzheimer's disease and dementia. The main types of interventions that have been evaluated include respite care, psycho-social interventions, group education and support. So far there is little evidence that any of these interventions result in significant long-term improvements in stress, distress, coping skills, depression or anxiety (McNally et al. 1999; Pusey and Richards 2001; Cattan et al. 2005). McNally et al. (1999) suggest that the lack of evidence may be because although respite provides immediate relief from caring duties, it fails to help maintain socially supportive relationships, which are needed once respite has come to an end. A more carer-centred approach, they say would take into account factors such as the carer-patient relationship, the carer's active social networks, the effect of respite on the care recipient, the carer's attitude to respite, any feelings of guilt, and the level of self-efficacy with regards to their ability to make use of the respite time. Their suggestions are in part supported by research, which has shown that the carer–cared-for relationship improves more in one to one support and carer burden is reduced through cognitive-behavioural interventions (including education, stress management and coping skills). However, in one study carers attending supportive group activities guided by peer leaders demonstrated a significant increase in network size (and consequently a reduction in social isolation) one year after the intervention (Toseland et al. 1990). There is some indication that psycho-social interventions that include the use of problem-solving and a behavioural component may be effective with carers of people with dementia (Pusey and Richards 2001). Although these interventions show some promise in providing support for carers Marriott et al. (2000) note that the implementation of the cognitive-behavioural intervention is lengthy and therefore has resource implications and requires specialist training. Such critical observations need to be taken seriously when planning mental health promotion support for carers of frail older people.

Volunteering

Volunteering is often put forward as one of the most effective ways of increasing social-ization and maintaining mental well-being in later life (Seymour and Gale 2004; Social Exclusion Unit 2006). Volunteering undoubtedly has beneficial effects in terms of men-tal health, mainly because of the social aspects of the activity and because it can give a sense of worth. It may also be that the reciprocity of volunteering adds to an indi-vidual's sense of well-being, by giving a sense of social support. This is supported by two reviews (van Willigen 2000, in Seymour and Gale 2004: 56; Wheeler et al. 1998). These reviews are mainly based on American studies, and therefore the findings are not neces-sarily directly transferable to other cultures. It would be wrong to suggest that volun-teering is not beneficial in maintaining and improving mental well-being among older people. The main difficulty regarding effect is that we cannot assume that older people's perceptions and experiences of volunteering are identical in all cultures.

Computer technology

Despite major advances in computer technology hardly any studies so far have evalu-ated the effectiveness of the use of computer technology to improve mental health among older people. Evaluation of computer assisted support for carers of older people indicate that with appropriate support the use of the Internet may meet some of carers' support needs (Brennan et al. 1995; Pusey and Richards 2001). This is obviously an area where the lack of evidence does not necessarily mean that the intervention is not effective. It is more likely that computer/telephone assisted support for carers requires further evaluation before we can make a judgement about its effectiveness. The use of the Internet to reduce social isolation has also been investigated. Despite the interven-tions not leading to significant reductions in perceived social isolation or loneliness there was an indication that education groups set up in congregate housing (White et al. 2002) and an Internet forum for caregivers (Brennan et al. 1995) were used for social contact and social support.

Lifelong learning

Lifelong learning has been hailed as an effective means of maintaining mental well-being and alertness, and even in preventing Alzheimer's disease. These claims relate to the notion that by participating in interesting and stimulating activities people can protect themselves against cognitive decline. Although there is some evidence to sug-gest that mentally stimulating activities can reduce the risk of Alzheimer's disease the reasons for why this might be the case are not clear. There is little research evidence to demonstrate that lifelong learning has a positive impact on older people's mental health. Improvements in self-esteem, social confidence and self-understanding have been cited as outcomes of lifelong learning. Likewise, gaining hope and purpose and a sense of competence have been mentioned (Hammond 2004). For some people lifelong learning can have a negative impact, for example in terms of confidence and sense of competence. We can speculate that this is because people have had a bad experience of a teacher or because they have set themselves unrealistic targets.

Wider environmental and political interventions intended to improve the quality of life among older people

There is little 'non-health specific' evidence of interventions that impact on older people's mental well-being. The main exceptions are housing and transport. The majority of studies on housing have not considered the health impact on older people specifically, but have included them in broader studies on re-housing and housing adaptations (see Chapter 6). A study on Teesside of medical priority re-housing found a reduction in the prevalence of mental health problems and less frequent use of health services (Blackman et al. 2003). Again the study did not focus specifically on older people but included them in the general study population. Consequently, we know very little about the specific mental health benefits of housing for older people.

The effectiveness of transport interventions in improving population health has been evaluated extensively (Morrison et al. 2003). However, most of this research has focused on injury prevention and on children and young people. We mentioned earlier that driving cessation increases depressive symptoms in older drivers. These consequences should obviously be taken into account when older drivers are advised about a possible transition to not driving and alternative driving strategies developed sensitively. The introduction of local traffic calming schemes has been found to be associated with increased pedestrian activity but not with improved mental health (Morrison et al. 2004). Here again the study did not distinguish between age groups, which could have highlighted possible differences in need and response between older people and younger adults.

Box 7.7 Summary of evidence of effective mental health promotion interventions for older people

- There is good evidence that group-based social support activities are effective in reducing social distress, social isolation and loneliness.
- There is increasing evidence that exercise promotes self-esteem, happiness and well-being, and reduces depression.
- There is conflicting evidence regarding the effectiveness of befriending and home visiting schemes for older people. Qualitative research suggests that they are acceptable and helpful.
- Despite a significant body of research there is little evidence that respite care, psychosocial interventions, group education and support impact significantly on depression, stress or coping skills in older carers.
- There is some evidence (based on mainly American research) to suggest that volunteering has a positive effect on older people's mental health.
- To date there is little research and consequently evidence to demonstrate the effectiveness of reminiscence, computer technology and lifelong learning in improving or maintaining mental health in later life.

The policy context

The promotion of mental health in older people has not until recently featured particularly highly in international, national or local policy documents. The European Community consultative Green Paper states:

> An ageing EU-population, with its associated mental health consequences, calls for effective action. Old age brings many stressors that may increase mental ill health, such as decreasing functional capacity and social isolation. Late life-depression and age-related neuro-psychiatric conditions, such as dementia, will increase the burden of mental disorders. Support interventions have shown to improve mental well-being in older populations.
>
> (Commission of the European Communities 2005: 9)

This is illuminative of how seriously the European Commission is taking the mental health of its ageing population. Preceding the Green Paper was a survey of good practice (Berkels et al. 2004). One of the sections focused on older people aged 60 years in various settings. The survey aimed to identify and evaluate strategies and models of best practice to develop a common strategy for coping with these problems. Some of the projects are described in the next section in this chapter. The document made ten recommendations for future policy development:

1 Stop discrimination by age and acknowledge the heterogeneity of older people.
2 Promote personal autonomy and possibilities for independent living to the fullest possible extent.
3 Provide adequate means to endorse social participation in all relevant settings.
4 Improve access of older people to effective psychological therapies.
5 Ensure that vulnerable risk groups are reached by special programmes.
6 Promote an increase in the social participation of older people.
7 Apply available evidence-based methods aimed at preventing and reducing physical morbidity, impairment, and at increasing mobility.
8 Ensure that help and support programmes for those in crisis situations (e.g. bereavement, wish to die) should be available and visible in the community, and encourage older people to make use of them.
9 Include adequate amounts of gerontological education in the training of professionals working with older people.
10 Make interventions targeting major risk factors, such as social isolation and physical ill-health, available for all European citizens.

(Berkels et al. 2004: 144–5)

Two other important points were made. First, the active participation of older people themselves is a key factor for any programme to be successful. Second, that it is still unclear how easily and successfully effective projects are transferable to different settings and different countries. In other words, to what extent are the projects dependent on cultural settings, local circumstances or even individual characteristics of those who implement the activities?

Within the UK, England, Wales, Scotland and Northern Ireland have approached the strategic development of mental health promotion from different perspectives. England does not have a national mental health promotion policy. Instead two national service frameworks (NSF) have been published as long-term strategies for improving health of older people and mental health of the population at large (DoH 1999, 2001). Unfortunately, it seems that the promotion of mental well-being among older people has fallen between two stools and is consequently covered fairly superficially in the two documents. In the *Mental Health NSF* older people are not mentioned specifically, even though there is opportunity to include older people under 'vulnerable or socially excluded groups' or as 'carers'. Where the *Mental Health NSF* has been used as a vehicle for developing local mental health promotion strategies older people have for most part not been one of the priority target groups.

The focus of mental health promotion in the *NSF for Older People*, which sets out 'to promote good mental health in older people and to treat and support those older people with dementia and depression' (DoH 2001: 90) is almost entirely on the management and treatment of mental illness, such as depression, and a large part is devoted to the care of dementia. Tackling social isolation, providing bereavement support and suicide prevention are also raised as ways of improving mental health. The promotion of physical activity is specifically mentioned as a means of promoting social interaction and mental well-being. Other wider initiatives which could impact on mental health are also suggested, such as home improvements, policies to reduce fear of violence and crime, affordable and accessible public transport, road safety, and policies to ameliorate the consequences of disability for those living alone. However, no evidence of the effectiveness of the proposed interventions is provided.

The final report on older people from the Social Exclusion Unit suggests that social relations and participation need to be supported by reducing the prevalence of social isolation, improving access to leisure, learning and volunteering, preventing homelessness and enabling older people to 'remain active and independent for as long as possible' (Social Exclusion Unit 2006: 13).

Initiatives to tackle ageism, such as Better Government for Older People have started to produce a cultural shift in our perceptions of older people. The Better Government for Older People (BGOP) programme was established in 1998 to improve public services for older people by better meeting their needs, listening to their views and encouraging and recognizing their contributions (Hayden and Boaz 2000). The over-arching notion of 'independence and well-being' is taken forward through a focus on: housing and the home; neighbourhoods; social activities, fun and social networks; learning and leisure; getting out and about; income; information; health and healthy living; employment; lifelong learning; mental health services; black and minority ethnic older people; age diversity (Better Government for Older People 2005). Although not initially set up specifically to improve and maintain older people's mental health, the programme seems to have had a major impact on participants' mental well-being simply through its ethos of participation and policy influence and the types of activities that have evolved as a result.

One of the BGOP 'off-shoots' has been Moving Out of the Shadows (MOOTS), an initiative intended to 'harness the voices of older people who experience a range of mental health problems, to inform and influence future policy, practice and experiences'

(Bowers et al. 2005: 1). Although the main emphasis of the initiative is on older people with mental health problems, many of the principles and priorities apply to *all* older people.

MOOTS includes mental health promotion in its priorities and states that promoting mental health is about:

- More advice, information and practical assistance for people aged 50 years and older.
- Education for people of all ages about mental health in later life.
- Making policy makers, commissioners, service providers and practitioners aware of mental health and 'active ageing'.
- A broad approach to achieving and sustaining good mental health in later life which includes learning, housing, leisure, environment and transport.
- A focus on preventative approaches to promote and sustain independence and good health.
- More research into what helps older people living alone to combat isolation and loneliness, such as personal strategies, improved public and community transport.
- Access to independent advocacy and counselling support.
- Ensuring that older people with ongoing mental health problems are treated as individuals.

(Bowers et al. 2005)

The three year Joint Inquiry into Mental Health and Well-being in Later Life project (2004–06) intended to 'make a positive difference to the mental health and well-being of all older people' (Seymour and Gale 2004: 1). It also set out to champion older people, develop a common understanding of mental health in later life, improve the quality and range of mental health services for older people, influence policy and planning to take into account mental health for older people, and to raise the profile of mental health in later life as an important issue (Seymour and Gale 2004).

These two national initiatives illustrate the way older people and their representative organizations are beginning to lobby the Government and raise awareness of mental health issues in later life and the rights of older people to maintain their mental well-being.

Elsewhere national strategies promoting the mental well-being of older people are thin on the ground. The *Welsh Strategy for Older People* (Welsh Assembly Government 2003), for example, is conspicuously void of any reference to the promotion of older people's mental health, although it could be argued that many of the key areas, such as transport, housing, learning and employment, will impact on the mental well-being of older adults. On the other hand the Scottish Programme for Improving Mental Health and Well-Being includes older people as one of the priority areas. The Action Plan which builds on available evidence proposes 'to support older people to make an active contribution for as long as they wish [or are able] and to support their continuing connectedness with their families, friends and communities' (Scottish Executive 2003: 10). In New Zealand the *Health of Older People Strategy* (Associate Minister of Health and Minister for Disability Issues 2002) incorporates mental health as one of the main strands of maintaining health. One of the action points in the strategy is to reduce depression, social isolation and loneliness through a range of collaborative community development approaches.

Despite the lack of national policy and strategies, local strategies which have included mental health promotion and older people have been developed in several countries. With over 1200 cities and towns in more than 30 countries in the European region, the WHO Healthy Cities Programme (WHO 2005) has provided a useful frame-work for the development of local strategies and action plans to promote mental well-being in later life. One of the three core themes in phase IV is 'healthy ageing', which recognizes the rights of people to equity as they age. It emphasizes positive attitudes towards ageing and understanding between generations. Different cities have taken different approaches within this theme, including the provision of housing and pensions, social support and social activity, transport, community and home safety. Principles have included reducing social and health inequalities, encouraging inter-generational work, reducing social isolation and loneliness, encouraging participation and tackling ageism.

Stockholm County Council's public health policy is a good example of a multi-sectoral initiative. The policy recognizes the impact of the social determinants of health on older people's physical and mental health by proposing a range of cross-cutting strategies to enable older people to lead an active and fulfilling life (Stock-holms läns landsting 2005). The mental health promotion strategies range from the development of an environment (including 'meeting places') which is conducive to mental well-being to capacity building and the reduction of social isolation and loneliness.

In the UK the National Service Frameworks have been used as levers to develop local action with mixed results. An example of this is the development of *Leeds Strat-egy to combat Social Isolation and Loneliness in Older People* (Leeds Older People Social Isolation Strategy Group 2004). The strategy evolved from *All of Us*, Leeds Mental Health Promotion Strategy (Leeds National Service Framework Steering Group 2002). The success of the strategy has to a great extent been due to careful thought going into the initial development process. From the start older people were involved as equal partners. Cattan's research (2002a,b) was used as a building block and to guide action but the solutions evolved locally. As the strategy developed there were visible spin-offs at local and neighbourhood level, such as awareness-raising events, liaison with related organizations and small scale surveys conducted by members of the strategy planning group (Cattan and Ingold 2003). The development of the Social Isolation and Loneliness Strategy demonstrated that it was feasible to link research with practice as long as there was local ownership of the strategy and its ensuing action. The process was mapped using the Leeds Model of Mental Health Promotion (Table 7.1).

Many other local policy and strategy documents have been developed. Few specif-ically mention the theoretical underpinning of their proposed plans, although it could be assumed that by utilizing research evidence some theoretical underpinning will exist indirectly. An exception is the Social Exclusion Unit's report on older people, which draws on an adapted version of Beattie's structural analysis of health promotion approaches (see Chapter 3, Figure 3.1) to illustrate the range of participative activities which are potentially most beneficial (Social Exclusion Unit 2006: 63).

Table 7.1 Leeds Model of Mental Health Promotion applied to alleviating social isolation and loneliness of older people

Factors which demote mental health		Level	Factors which promote mental health	
From practice	*From research*		*From practice*	*From research*
• Not being able to get out and about • Fear of 'not managing'	• Retirement • Bereavement • Loneliness • Lack of confidence • Low self-esteem • Poor mental health • Deteriorating physical health • Loss of mobility • Older people patronized • Fear of crime	***Individual***	• Valuing individuality • Recognizing diversity of older people • Reminiscence	• Buddying • Feeling safe • Beliefs in personal ability to carry out tasks • Resourcefulness • Exercise and physical activity
• The complexity of identifying socially isolated older people	• Stigma of old age and loneliness	***Community***	• Raising awareness • Reducing stigma • Share ideas and ways of working • Being valued	• Group activity • Desired social networks • Social support • Practical support e.g. transport • Reciprocity • Carers' support • Volunteering
• Older people not involved in planning or consulted about project development • Lack of wider representation from ethnic minority groups / older people with sensory impairments	• Transport • Housing	***Structural / policy***	• Ethos of older people as active citizens • Strategy based on what older people say • Links with initiatives with supporting goals • Working collectively	• Older people enabled to be involved and consulted at all levels of planning and developing work • Ensure services and activities are delivered equitably and enable those at most need to gain access
Setting • Care homes • Transport	• Housing • Lack of transport		**Target group** • People with sensory impairments • People with mobility problems	• Recently widowed older people • Women living alone • Caregivers and receivers • Men • Women • Ethnic minority communities • Older people with mental health problems

Source: Adapted from Cattan and Ingold 2003: 18

Box 7.8   Common factors of policies and strategies intended to promote mental health and well-being among older people

1   Based on:
    - demographic trends;
    - current research evidence and good practice;
    - population forecasts;
    - political will;
    - social determinants of mental health.
2   Mostly concerned with:
    - prevention of mental ill health/mental illness;
    - support for older people with mental health problems;
    - a wider policy/strategy on mental health or ageing.
3   Major gaps:
    - policies and strategies that focus on mental health promotion for older people rather than singly on the prevention of mental ill health.

Examples of good practice

There are of course many examples of 'good practice' that have been based on 'long-term experience and a well-based gut feeling' (Cattan 2002a: 218), rather than necessarily on theory or research evidence. Several attempts have been made to collect and disseminate such information without making claims about comprehensiveness (see for example Cattan 2002b; Berkels et al. 2004; Seymour and Gale 2004).

Awareness raising:
Pyramid Theatre Company, UK (theatre in health education, see:
www.pyramidtheatrecompany.co.uk/pyramid)
'Who's Helen?' is a one act, one person play which has toured the UK for several years. The aims of the play are to illustrate the problems of loneliness in old age and ensuing concerns, fears and frustrations; to generate empathy and understanding of the problems; to act as a catalyst for subsequent discussion; and to provide information about local services and activities (Liverpool City Council 2004). The story raises issues around depression; loneliness; fear of being taken into care; the value of friends; and the adjustment to a new role in life. Following the play a hot-seating session takes place where the audience is invited to ask questions of Helen. Workshops frequently follow the question–answer session, which enable the issues to be explored further. The play has been used successfully with older people, service providers and with younger audiences. Interestingly, the questions raised by these groups are quite different. For example, older people frequently ask if Helen ever contemplated suicide, while service providers mainly ask about practical matters and service provision.

Centres for older people:
day centre in Oxfordshire, UK
The effectiveness of day centres has been controversial. This day centre has attempted to listen to the actual needs of the older population likely to use its services and has developed an effective outreach model. Local consultation sessions are held regularly and every opportunity is taken to widen the network in the community. The centre provides drop-in services such as chiropody, trips out, home visiting, social activities, transport to health services, etc. Older people's involvement in the development of the activities is seen as critical to the success of the centre (Thewlis 2001).

Community involvement:
Norwegian community mental health profile
Although the community involvement scheme is not specifically aimed at older people, older people are identified as one of the high risk groups. The aims of the project are to reduce psycho-social risk factors, to strengthen protective factors, to decrease levels of depression and anxiety and to increase social integration. The project may be initiated as a result of some societal change (for example, enforced move because of property development). Following a survey the target group is supported and empowered to develop and implement the intervention(s) in collaboration with community services (Dalgard 2005).

Prevention of depression:
the Mood Project, Scotland
The Mood project aims to identify older people who are at risk of depression in order to devise a range of relevant resources to help and support them in the community. Before joining one of the activity groups each individual is interviewed to ascertain the most appropriate activity. The groups include self-help, specific interest groups, carpet bowling, music, photography, local history and carer support. The purpose of the groups is to raise self-esteem and confidence and to support the development of further friendships. In addition the project is attempting to encourage inter-generational work through making contact with schools. Evaluation is said to be encouraging (Cook 2005).

Ethnic minority mental health promotion
1   *Black and Minority Ethnic Elders Group (BMEEG) Scotland.* The Black and Minority Ethnic Elders Group was established in 2000 in partnership with Age Concern. It was set up by older people together with local community activists. The aim is to ensure that ethnic elders are given the same opportunities for consultation and participation as their majority elder counterparts, and to drive forward common agendas and approaches in care development and management of services to ethnic elders and their carers (Age Concern Scotland 2005). BMEEG intends to bring together older people from a wide range of cultural and ethnic backgrounds in one forum. It advocates for social inclusion of all older people, and promotes equality of citizenship and opportunity to develop better access to housing, health, social work and education by providing culturally sensitive services.
2   *Active Sisters! Enhancing the community capacity for physical activity of Islamic women, Brisbane, Australia* (see: www.health.qld.gov.au/pahospital/qtmhc.asp).

The Queensland Transcultural Mental Health Centre in Brisbane piloted the two year Active Sisters! project in partnership with the Islamic Women's Association of Queensland Inc. The project aimed to enhance the capacity of the Islamic women's community to promote regular physical activity, maintain supportive and safe environments for physical activity and increase social contacts between isolated older women. Strategies included mentoring of a project coordinator, developing skills among bilingual community workers in peer education and peer support, supporting Islamic women swimming instructors to become accredited and nego-tiating with a leisure centre to accommodate the special needs of the women. Implementing the culturally appropriate swimming and local walking groups increased the social contacts of women from many cultures. At the end of the programme the women were maintaining regular physical activity and reported feeling more in touch with the community and experiencing a greater sense of well-being and self-confidence.

Supporting independence:
Good Neighbour Scheme, UK
Age Concern's Good Neighbour Scheme, Dudley, is one of a large number of befriend-ing schemes in the UK. The aim of the scheme is to provide regular support for socially isolated older people in their own homes to enable them to retain independence for as long as possible. Activities include escorting people to medical appointments, daytime activities and shops, reading mail for the visually impaired, befriending, dog walking and emotional support. An important facet of the project is that volunteers are trained in listening skills, dementia awareness and support for bereavement and loss. Evaluation suggests that the scheme has improved self-esteem and emotional health and that many participants have received more company and increased time spent outside their home.

Supporting isolated older people:
Otley Action for Older People, UK
The project was initiated by older people in Otley to provide activities and support for older people in the area. The uniqueness of the project is that it is run by older people for older people. A project coordinator was engaged to act as a facilitator for activities that are put forward by project members. After identifying that loneliness and isolation was a major problem in the community, the project successfully bid for a large grant to tackle loneliness and a Community Development and Social Inclusion Project was established. The coordinator stated: 'Clearly there are no simple remedies or any one-size-fits-all solutions'. The project is primarily concerned with providing support and services through meaningful activities for individuals, while at the same time rais-ing awareness of social isolation and loneliness. The aim is to reduce the prevalence of loneliness among older people.

Suicide prevention:
Wisdom and well-being language specific Telephone Support Groups for older people, New South Wales, Australia
The aim of the Telephone Support Group pilot project is to improve protective factors against suicide and reduce suicide risk factors for older people from non-English

---

Box 7.9   Common factors for 'good practice' projects

- They are either based on some form of evidence or on long-term knowledge and experience of an area/population.
- They take into account the cultural and social circumstances that contribute to older people's attitudes, beliefs, values and motivation which influence how they approach activities.
- They enable older people to be involved in the development, implementation and evaluation of the activities.
- They approach evaluation systematically and creatively.
- They retain the purpose of the project while acknowledging that activities can be improved upon.

---

speaking backgrounds. The project utilizes telephone conferencing to bring people together in groups, so that people who are isolated due to living in remote areas, to poor physical mobility or to lack of adequate transport are able to participate. Groups are run in different languages. The project also supports self-help initiatives by having the group facilitator available for one to one telephone discussion with group members during a few hours after each group discussion. Well-being covers topics related to mental well-being as well as physical and social well-being. Although the groups are guided by a group facilitator, members are involved in the choice of topics, which has broadened the discussions to include spiritual, financial and environmental well-being (Diversity Health Institute 2005).

As we have seen there is an abundance of schemes in the community which aim to maintain and improve mental health and mental well-being among older people. Many such schemes are based on 'common know-how' of people's behaviour and some have been evaluated at a local level. Some, but not all, involve older people at all stages of the development, implementation and evaluation of the activity, although research has shown that older people want to have the opportunity to be involved (Cattan et al. 2003). Very few have been established as a result of research evidence.

The application of mental health promotion theory and principles to mental health promotion practice for older people

In Chapter 2 we noted that mental health promotion draws on a range of disciplines for its theoretical basis. However, as with most health promotion interventions, theory is rarely used directly to underpin and develop mental health promoting activities for older people. We reviewed the theoretical basis for all included studies in a systematic review (Cattan et al. 2005). Not unexpectedly the majority of the studies that stated their theoretical basis (a third did not) based their research on some form of behavioural theory, such as cognitive or educational theory, social learning theory, and the theory of reasoned action (for a brief overview of these theories see for example Nutbeam and Harris 2004). In some of the studies behavioural theories were linked to other theories such as Weiss's theory on loneliness (Weiss 1982) or to Burbank's disengagement theory (Burbank 1986). Hopman-Rock and Westhoff (2002) uniquely utilized diffusion of innovation theory (Rogers 1995) to develop their exercise programme intended to improve older people's health and reduce loneliness. If we consider that most interventions are intended to promote mental health of the individual through behaviour change it is hardly surprising that behavioural change theory, rather than community or organizational change theory, underpins most research on mental health promotion.

If we look at the examples of good practice it can be seen that the concepts of community change and community capacity building lie at the heart of many of the activities. Frequently knowledge (or assumption) of health risk is used to instigate behaviour change. This risk awareness is frequently determined by professionals working in the field rather than stated by older people, which goes against the grain of community development approaches. The aim of many of the schemes is either to improve older people's social networks and to raise their self-esteem and confidence or to empower people to take control over their own (mental) health. The Norwegian community mental health profile is a good example of a programme which is based on an empowerment model of promoting health in order to bring about community change. It could also be argued that theatre in health education contains elements of the empowerment model, although the main strand of the activity focuses on health education.

The purpose of most community centre activities is to improve older people's social contacts and to raise their confidence in participating in the variety of activities offered by the centre. However, if we analyse the methods used in such interventions the notion of empowerment rarely informs the intention to raise older people's self-esteem and confidence. This illustrates that theory has not been used to develop the programmes, but could still be utilized to evaluate them. Communal gardening programmes do, however, engage older people in both creative and social activities through empowerment, thereby raising both their self-esteem and sense of personal control. Home visiting schemes on the other hand could be said to be based on theories concerned with resilience and/or coping skills, an approach which was recommended by the European Commission (Berkels et al. 2004). Therefore, the (implicit) theoretical basis for home visiting schemes is social learning (cognitive) theory (Bandura 1977). The intervention does not seek to improve social networks, but rather to increase self-esteem and a sense of control as postulated by social learning theory.

These examples illustrate that older people mostly have things 'done to' them rather than being 'included in' or 'in control of' mental health promotion. Social engagement or active citizenship as measured through, for example, social capital does not feature as a driving force in promoting mental health among older people, despite ecological social capital having the potential for being used to develop community enhancing interventions. In conclusion theory has to date had limited function in the development and application of interventions intended to improve and maintain mental well-being of older people.

Box 7.10 Questions to reflect on when considering mental health promotion for older people

- Consider what the main influences are on older people's mental health
- Why can diversity among older people impact particularly adversely on older people's mental health?
- What particular issues of inequality in later life should be taken into account when planning mental health promotion interventions for older people?
- How might older people's own perceptions of mental health and mental ill health be utilized when interventions are developed?
- What are the main gaps in the evidence base of effective mental health promoting interventions for older people?
- How might policy be drawn on to ensure acceptable, effective mental health promotion interventions for older people?
- What role might theory have in ensuring that mental health promoting activities for older people are meaningful?

Conclusion

In this chapter we have considered the factors that impact on mental health and well-being of older people, their mental health promotion needs and some of the theory that might help explain these factors (in addition to those presented in Chapter 2) and help develop effective interventions. Because the population is ageing there is increased interest nationally and internationally, in developing appropriate services and activities to promote and maintain mental well-being among older people. As we have seen, however, older people are not a homogenous group and therefore their needs and expectations vary across age groups, cultures, ethnic groups and gender. One of the most important aspects of ageing and mental health is that older people are people first and older second. What unfortunately often seems to happen is that older people are discriminated against two-fold: first because they are 'aged' and second because of who or what they are as a person. By considering the wider factors that impact on older people's mental health, the research evidence, examples of 'good practice' and the theoretical framework for mental health promotion we should be able to develop effective, appropriate projects, services and activities that older people actually want to take part in.

References

Aboderin, I. (2004) Intergenerational family support and old age economic security in Ghana, in P. Lloyd-Sherlock (ed.) *Living Longer: Ageing, Development and Social Protection.* London: Zed Books.

Abrahamson, T.A., Trejo, L. and Lai, D.W.L. (2002) Culture and mental health: providing appropriate services for a diverse older population, *Mental Health and Mental Illness in Later Life*, Spring: 21–7.

Age Concern Scotland (2005) *Black and Minority Ethnic Elders Group (BMEEG) Scotland.* Available at: http://www.ageconcernscotland.org.uk (accessed 9 December 2005).

Alcohol Concern (2002) Alcohol misuse among older people, *Acquire*, 34: i–viii. Available at: http://www.alcoholconcern.org.uk/servlets/doc/50 (accessed 10 October 2005).

Alpass, F.M. and Neville, S. (2003) Loneliness, health and depression in older males, *Aging and Mental Health*, 7(3): 212–16.

Andersson, L. (1992) Loneliness and perceived responsibility and control in elderly community residents, *Journal Of Social Behavior and Personality*, 7(3): 431–43.

Antonelli, E., Rubini, V. and Fassone, C. (2000) The self-concept in institutionalized and non-institutionalized elderly people, *Journal of Environmental Psychology*, 20(2): 151–64.

Associate Minister of Health and Minister for Disability Issues (2002) *Health of Older People Strategy. Health Sector Action to 2010 to Support Positive Ageing.* Wellington, New Zealand: Ministry of Health.

Australian Bureau of Statistics (2000) *Australian Social Trends 1998.* Canberra: Australian Bureau of Statistics. Available at: http://www.abs.gov.au/Ausstats/abs@nsf (accessed 1 September 2005).

Baeyens, J-P. (2005) Are your grandparents starving to death? *Guardian*, 7 October.

Bandura, A. (1977) Self-efficacy: toward a unifying theory of behavioral change, *Psychological Review*, 64(2): 191–215.

Bengtson, V.L., Burgess, E.O. and Parrott, T.M. (1997) Theory, explanation, and a third generation of theoretical development in social gerontology, *Journals of Gerontology Series B-Psychological Sciences and Social Sciences*, 52(2): S72–S88.

Berkels, H., Henderson, J., Henke, N. et al. (2004) *Mental Health Promotion and Prevention Strategies for Coping with Anxiety, Depression and Stress related Disorders in Europe* Final Report 2001–2003. Dortmund/Berlin/Dresden: Federal Institute for Occupational Safety and Health.

Better Government for Older People (2003, 2005) *BGOP Fundamentals.* Available at: http://www.bgop.org.uk/index.aspx?primarycat=2&secondarycat=4 (accessed 13 November 2005).

Bjerregaard, P. and Curtis, T. (2002) Cultural change and mental health in Greenland: the association of childhood conditions, language and urbanization with mental health and suicidal thoughts among the Inuit of Greenland, *Social Science & Medicine*, 54(1): 33–48.

Blackman, T., Anderson, J. and Pye, P. (2003) Change in adult health following medical priority rehousing: a longitudinal study, *Journal of Public Health Medicine*, 25(1): 22–8.

Bostock, Y. and Millar, C. (2003) *Older People's Perceptions of the Factors that Affect Mental Well-being in Later Life.* Edinburgh: NHS Health Scotland.

Bowers, H., Eastman, M., Harris, J. and Macadam, A. (2005) *Moving Out of the Shadows. A Report of Mental Health and Wellbeing in Later Life.* Bournemouth: Help and Care Development Ltd.

Bowling, A. (1991) Social support and social networks: their relationship to the successful and unsuccessful survival of elderly people in the community. An analysis of concepts and a review of the evidence, *Family Practice*, 8(1): 68–83.

Bowling, A. (1993) The concepts of successful and positive ageing, *Family Practice*, 10(4): 449–53.

Brennan, P.F., Moore, S.M. and Smyth, K.A. (1995) The effects of a special computer network on caregivers of persons with Alzheimer's disease, *Nursing Research*, 44(3): 166–72.

Burbank, P.M. (1986) Psychosocial theories of aging: a critical evaluation, *Advances in Nursing Science*, 9(1): 73–86.

Cassidy, K., Kotynia-English, R., Acres, J. et al. (2004) Association between lifestyle factors and mental health measures among community-dwelling older women, *Australian and New Zealand Journal of Psychiatry*, 38: 940–7.

Cattan, M. (2002a) Preventing social isolation and loneliness among older people: effectiveness of health promotion interventions. Unpublished PhD thesis, University of Newcastle.

Cattan, M. (2002b) *Supporting Older People to Overcome Social Isolation and Loneliness*. London: Help the Aged.

Cattan, M. and Ingold, K. (2003) Implementing change: the alleviation of social isolation and loneliness among older people, *Journal of Mental Health Promotion*, 2(3): 12–19.

Cattan, M., Newell, C., Bond, J. and White, M. (2003) Alleviating social isolation and loneliness among older people, *International Journal of Mental Health Promotion*, 5(3): 20–30.

Cattan, M., White, M., Bond, J. and Learmonth, A. (2005) Preventing social isolation and loneliness among older people: a systematic review of health promotion interventions, *Ageing and Society*, 25(1): 41–67.

Coleman, P. (1996) Psychological Ageing, in J. Bond, P. Coleman and S. Peace (eds) *Ageing in Society: An Introduction to Social Gerontology*. London: Sage Publications.

Coleman, P. G. and O'Hanlon, A. (2004) *Ageing and Development*. London: Arnold.

Commission of the European Communities (2005) *Improving the Mental Health of the Population: Towards a Strategy on Mental Health for the European Union*. Brussels: European Union.

Cook, R. (2005) MOOD project, personal communication. 5 December.

Costello, J. and Kendrick, K. (2000) Grief and older people: the making or breaking of emotional bonds following partner loss in later life, *Journal of Advanced Nursing*, 32(6): 1374–82.

CRD (NHS Centre for Research and Development) (1997) Mental health promotion in high risk groups, *Effective Health Care*. York: University of York.

Crone, D., Smith, A. and Gough, B. (2005) 'I feel totally at one, totally alive and totally happy': a psycho-social explanation of the physical activity and mental health relationship, *Health Education Research*, 20(5): 600–11.

D'Augelli, A.R., Grossman, A.H., Hershberger, S.L. and O'Connell, T.S. (2001) Aspects of mental health among older lesbian, gay, and bisexual adults, *Aging & Mental Health*, 5(2): 149–58.

Dalgard, O-S. (2005) Centres for elderly, community mental health profile, personal communication, 2 December.

Dean, J. and Goodlad, R. (1998) *Supporting Community Participation? The Role and Impact of Befriending*. Brighton: Rowntree Foundation.

Dein, S. and Huline-Dickens, S. (1997) Cultural aspects of aging and psychopathology, *Aging and Mental Health*, 1(2): 112–20.

Dickenson, D., Johnson, M. and Samson Katz, J. (eds) (2000) *Death, Dying and Bereavement*. London: Sage.

Diversity Health Institute. (2005) *Wisdom and Well-Being Language Specific Telephone Support Groups for Older People*. Available at: http://www.dhi.gov.au/tmhc/projects/older_people.htm (accessed 4 December 2005).

DoH (Department of Health) (1999) *Mental Health National Service Framework*. London: HMSO.

DoH (Department of Health) (2001) *National Service Framework for Older People*. London: HMSO.

Doran, T., Drever, F. and Whitehead, M. (2003) Health of young and elderly informal carers: analysis of UK census data, *British Medical Journal*, 327: 1388.

Elkan, R., Kendrick, D., Dewey, M. et al. (2001) Effectiveness of home based support for older people: systematic review and meta-analysis, *British Medical Journal*, 323: 719–24.

Evans, O., Singleton, N., Meltzer, H., Stewart, R. and Prince, M. (2003) *The Mental Health of Older People*. London: Office for National Statistics.

Fazel, S., Hope, T., O'Donnell, I., Piper, M. and Jacoby, R. (2001) Health of elderly male prisoners: worse than the general population, worse than younger prisoners, *Age and Ageing*, 30: 403–7.

Ferri, C.P., Prince, M., Brayne, C. et al. (2005) Global prevalence of dementia: a Delphi consensus study, *The Lancet*, 366: 2112–17.

Fonda, S.J., Wallace, R.B. and Herzog, A.R. (2001) Changes in driving patterns and worsening depressive symptoms among older adults, *Journals of Gerontology: Social Sciences*, 56B(6): S343–S351.

Francis, J. (1995) Call time, *Community Care*, 23–9 November.

Gilhooly, M., Hamilton, H., O'Neill, M. et al. (2005) Transport and ageing: extending quality of life via public and private transport, *ESRC Society Today*. Available at: http://www.esrcsocietytoday.ac.uk/ESRCInfoCentre/Plain_English_Summaries/envionment/mobility/index150.aspx (accessed 7 November 2005).

Gomes da Conceicao, C. and Montes de Oca Zavala, V. (2004) Ageing in Mexico: families, informal care and reciprocity, in P. Lloyd-Sherlock (ed.) *Living Longer. Ageing, Development and Social Protection*. London: Zed Books.

Grunfeld, E., Glossop, R., McDowell, I. and Danbrook, C. (1997) Caring for elderly people at home: the consequences to caregivers, *Canadian Medical Association Journal*, 157(8): 1101–5.

Hammond, C. (2004) Impacts of lifelong learning upon emotional resilience, psychological and mental health: fieldwork evidence, *Oxford Review of Education*, 30(4): 551–68.

Havighurst, R.J., Neugarten, B.L. and Tobin, S.S. (1998) Disengagement and patterns of aging, in M.P. Lawton and T.A. Salthouse (eds) *Essential Papers on the Psychology of Aging*. New York: New York University Press.

Hayden, C. and Boaz, A. (2000) *Making a Difference Better Government for Older People: Evaluation Report*. Available at: http://www.bettergovernmentforolderpeople.gov.uk/reference (accessed 2002).

Hays, T. and Minichiello, V. (2005) The contribution of music to quality of life in older people: an Australian qualitative study, *Ageing and Society*, 25: 261–78.

Hedelin, B. and Svensson, P-G. (1999) Psychiatric nursing for promotion of mental health and prevention of depression in the elderly: a case study, *Journal of Psychiatric and Mental Health Nursing*, 6: 115–24.

Helbostad, J.L., Sletvold, O. and Moe-Nilssen, R. (2004) Home training with and without additional group training in physically frail older people living at home: effect on health-related quality of life and ambulation, *Clinical rehabilitation*, 18: 498–508.

HelpAge International (2002) *State of the World's Older People 2002*. London: HelpAge International.

Herman, D.R., Solomons, N.W., Mendoza, I. and Qureshi, A.K. (2001) Self-rated health and its relationship to functional status and well-being in a group of elderly Guatemalan subjects, *Asia Pacific Journal of Clinical Nutrition*, 10(3): 176–82.

Hilbourne, M. (1999) Living together full time? Middle-class couples approaching retirement, *Ageing and Society*, 19(2): 161–84.

Hockey, J., Katz, J. and Small, N. (eds) (2001) *Grief, Morning and Death Ritual*. Buckingham: Open University Press.

Hopman-Rock, M. and Westhoff, M.H. (2002) Development and evaluation of 'Aging Well and Healthily': a health education and exercise program for community living older adults, *Journal of Aging and Physical Activity*, 10: 363–80.

Johnson, P. (2004) Long-term historical changes in the status of elders: the United Kingdom as an exemplar of advanced industrial economies, in P. Lloyd-Sherlock (ed.) *Living Longer: Ageing, Development and Social Protection*. London: Zed books.

Johnson, C.S.J. (2005) Psychosocial correlates of nutritional risk in older adults, *Canadian Journal of Dietetic Practice and Research*, 66: 95–7.

Jylhä, M. and Jokela, J. (1990) Individual experiences as cultural – a cross-cultural study on loneliness among the elderly, *Ageing and Society*, 10: 295–315.

King, A.C., Oman, R.F., Brassington, G.S., Bliwise, D.L. and Haskell, W.L. (1997) Moderate-Intensity Exercise and Self-rated Quality of Sleep in Older Adults, *JAMA*, 277(1): 32–7.

Korkeila, J., Lehtinen, V., Bijl, R. et al. (2003) Establishing a set of mental health indicators for Europe, *Scandinavian Journal of Public Health*, 31: 451–9.

Leeds National Service Framework Steering Group (2002) *All of Us: A Mental Health Promotion Strategy for Leeds*. Leeds: Leeds North West PCT.

Leeds Older People Social Isolation Strategy Group (2004) Leeds' strategy to reduce social isolation and loneliness of older people (unpublished). Leeds: Leeds North West PCT.

Li, F., Fisher, K.J., Harmer, P. et al. (2004) Tai Chi and self-rated quality of sleep and daytime sleepiness in older adults: a randomized controlled trial, *Journal of the American Geriatrics Society*, 52: 892–900.

Liverpool City Council (2004) Impact evaluation report: Who's Helen? (unpublished).

Lopata, H.Z. (1980) Loneliness: forms and components, in R.S. Weiss (ed.) *The Experience of Emotional and Social Isolation*. Cambridge: MIT Press.

Mackinnon, A., Christensen, H., Hofer, S.M., Korten, A.E. and Jorm, A.F. (2003) Use it and still lose it? The association between activity and cognitive performance established using latent growth techniques in a community sample, *Aging, Neuropsychology, & Cognition*, 10(3): 215–29.

McNally, S., Ben-Shlomo, Y. and Newman, S. (1999) The effects of respite care on informal carers' well-being: a systematic review, *Disability and Rehabilitation*, 21(1): 1–14.

Marriott, A., Donaldson, C., Tarrier, N. and Burns, A. (2000) The effectiveness of a cognitive-behavioural intervention for reducing the burden of care in carers of patients with Alzheimer's Disease, *British Journal of Psychiatry*, 176(6): 557–62.

Matt, G.E. and Dean, A. (1993) Social support from friends and psychological distress among elderly persons: moderator effects of age, *Journal of Health and Social Behavior*, 34(3): 187–200.

Mein, G., Martikainen, P., Hemingway, H., Stansfield, S. and Marmot, M. (2003) Is retirement good or bad for mental and physical health functioning? Whitehall II longitudinal study of civil servants, *Journal of Epidemiology & Community Health*, 57: 46–9.

Milligan, C., Bingley, A. and Gatrell, A. (2005) *Cultivating Health: A Study of Health and Mental Well-being Amongst Older People in Northern England*. Lancaster: Lancaster University.

Morrison, D.S., Petticrew, M. and Thomson, H. (2003) What are the most effective ways of improving population health through transport interventions? Evidence from systematic reviews, *Journal of Epidemiology & Community Health*, 57(5): 327–33.

Morrison, D.S., Thompson, H. and Petticrew, M. (2004) Evaluation of the health effects of a neighbourhood traffic calming scheme, *Journal of Epidemiology & Community Health*, 58(10): 837–40.

National Statistics (2004) *Informal care: National Statistics*. Available at: http://www.statistics.gov.uk/cci/nugget_print.asp?ID=925 (accessed 31 August 2005).

Nutbeam, D. and Harris, E. (2004) *Theory in a Nutshell*. Sydney: McGraw-Hill Australia.

Nyangweso, M.A. (1998) Transformations of care of the aged among Africans study of the Kenyan situation, *Aging and Mental Health*, 2(3): 181–5.

O'Connell, H., Chin, A-V., Cunningham, C. and Lawlor, B. (2004) Recent developments: suicide in older people, *British Medical Journal*, 329: 895–9.

Office for National Statistics (2002) *Census 2001: National report for England and Wales*. London: The Stationery Office.

Ogwumike, F.O. and Aboderin, I. (2005) Exploring the links between old age and poverty in Anglophone West Africa: evidence from Nigeria and Ghana, *Generations Review*, 14(2): 7–15.

Owen, T. (ed.) (2005) *Dying in Older Age: Reflections and Experiences from an Older Person's Perspective*. London: Help the Aged.

Paulson, S. (2005) The social benefits of belonging to a 'dance exercise' group for older people, *Generations Review*, 15(4): 37–41.

Perren, K., Arber, S. and Davidson, K. (2003) Men's organisational affiliations in later life: the influence of social class and marital status on informal group membership, *Ageing and Society*, 23: 69–82.

Phillipson, C. and Scharf, T. (2004) The impact of government policy on social exclusion among older people: a review of the literature for the Social Exclusion Unit, *Breaking the Cycle*. London: Office of the Deputy Prime Minister.

Phillipson, C., Bernard, M., Phillips, J. and Ogg, J. (1998) The family and community life of older people: household composition and social networks in three urban areas, *Ageing and Society*, 18: 259–89.

Pritchard, C. and Baldwin, D.S. (2002) Elderly suicide rates in Asian and English speaking countries, *Acta Psychiatrica Scandinavica*, 105: 271–5.

Pusey, H. and Richards, D. (2001) A systematic review of the effectiveness of psychosocial interventions for carers of people with dementia, *Aging and Mental Health*, 5(2): 107–19.

Rabheru, K. (2004) Special issues in the management of depression in older patients, *Canadian Journal of Psychiatry*, 49(suppl.1): 41s–50s.

Reinhardt, J.P. (1996) The importance of friendship and family support in adaptation to chronic vision impairment, *Journals Of Gerontology Series B-Psychological Sciences and Social Sciences*, 51(5): 268–P278.

Rogers, E.M. (1995) *Diffusion of Innovations*. New York: Free Press.

Rosenkoetter, M.M. and Garris, J.M. (2001) Retirement planning, use of time, and psychosocial adjustment, *Issues in Mental Health Nursing*, 22: 703–22.

Ruuskanen, J.M. and Ruoppila, I. (1995) Physical activity and psychological well being among people aged 65 to 84 years, *Age and Ageing*, 24(4): 292–6.

Salkeld, G., Cameron, I.D., Cumming, R.G. et al. (2000) Quality of life related to fear of falling and hip fracture in older women: a time trade off study, *BMJ*, 320: 341–6.

Satariano, W.A., Haight, T.J. and Tager, I.B. (2000) Reasons given by older people for limitation or avoidance of leisure time physical activity, *Journal of the American Geriatrics Society*, 48: 505–12.

Scaf-Klomp, W., Sanderman, R., Ormel, J. and Kempen, G.I.J.H. (2003) Depression in older people after fall-related injuries: a prospective study, *Age and Ageing*, 32: 88–94.

Scottish Executive (2003) *National Programme for Improving Mental Health and Well-Being*. Edinburgh: Scottish Executive.

Seeman, T.E. (2000) Health promoting effects of friends and family on health outcomes in older adults, *American Journal of Health Promotion*, 14(6): 362–70.

Seymour, L. and Gale, E. (2004) *Literature & Policy Review for the Joint Inquiry into Mental Health & Well-being in Later Life*. London: Mentality.

Shyam, R. and Yadav, S. (2002) A study of depression, self-esteem and social support amongst institutionalized and non-institutionalized aged, *Journal of Personality & Clinical Studies*, 18(1–2): 79–86.

Sidell, M. (1996) Death, Dying and Bereavement, in J. Bond, P. Coleman and S. Peace (eds) *Ageing in Society: An Introduction to Social Gerontology*. London: Sage Publications.

Siren, A., Hakamies-Blomqvist, L. and Lindeman, M. (2004) Driving cessation and health in older women, *The Journal of Applied Gerontology*, 23(1): 58–69.

Smith, J. and Baltes, P.B. (1997) Profiles of psychological functioning in the old and oldest old, *Psychology and Aging*, 12(3): 458–72.

Social Exclusion Unit (2006) *A Sure Start to Later Life: Ending Inequalities for Older People*. London: Office of the Deputy Prime Minister.

Social Policy Research Unit (2001) *Informal Care Over Time*. York: University of York.

Sproston, K. and Nazroo, J. (eds) (2002) *Ethnic Minority Psychiatric Illness Rates in the Community (EMPIRIC)*. London: TSO.

Stathi, A., Fox, K. and McKenna, J. (2002) Physical activity and dimensions of subjective well-being in older adults, *Journal of Aging & Physical Activity*, 10(1): 76–92.

Stergiopoulos, V. and Herrman, N. (2003) Old and homeless: a review and survey of older adults who use shelters in an urban setting, *Canadian Journal of Psychiatry*, 48(6): 374–80.

Stockholms läns landsting (2005) *Folkhälsopolicy for Stockholms läns landsting* (Public health policy for Stockholm County Council). Stockholm: Stockholms läns landsting.

Thewlis, P. (2001) *Lilac from the Garden: Day Services for Older People in Rural Oxfordshire. A Study of Needs and Innovations*. Oxford: Age Concern Oxfordshire.

Third Sector First (2005) *'Thing to do, places to go' Promoting Mental Health and Well-being in Later Life*. Leeds: Third Sector First.

Tijhuis, M.A.R., de Jong-Gierveld, J., Feskens, E.J.M. and Kromhout, D. (1999) Changes in and factors related to loneliness in older men: the Zutphen Elderly Study, *Age and Ageing*, 28: 491–5.

Tilford, S., Delaney, F. and Vogels, M. (1997) *Effectiveness of Mental Health Promotion Interventions: A Review*. London: Health Education Authority.

Tolvanen, E. (1998) I and others: alcohol use among older people as a social and cultural phenomenon, *Ageing and Society*, 18: 563–83.

Toseland, R.W., Rossiter, C.M., Peak, T. and Smith, G.C. (1990) Comparative effectiveness of individual and group interventions to support family caregivers, *Social Work*, 35(3): 209–17.

van Gool, C.H., Kempen, G.I.J., Pennix, B.W.J.H. et al. (2003) Relationship between changes in depressive symptoms and unhealthy lifestyles in late middle aged and older persons: results from the Longitudinal Aging Study Amsterdam, *Age & Ageing*, 32: 81–7.

van Haastregt, J.C.M., Diederiks, J.P.M., Van Rossum, E., de Witte, P. and Crebolder, M. (2000) Effects of preventive home visits to elderly people living in the community: systematic review, *British Medical Journal*, 320: 754–8.

van Tilburg, T., Gierveld, J.D., Lecchini, L. and Marsiglia, D. (1998) Social integration and loneliness: a comparative study among older adults in the Netherlands and Tuscany, Italy, *Journal of Social and Personal Relationships*, 15(6): 740–54.

Victor, C.R. (1989) Inequalities in health in later life, *Age and Ageing* 18(6): 387–91.

Victor, C., Scambler, S.J., Bowling, A. and Bond, J. (2005) The prevalence and risk factors for loneliness in later life: a survey of older people in Great Britain, *Ageing and Society*, 25(3): 357–75.

Weiss, R.S. (1982) Issues in the study of loneliness, in L. Peplau and D. Perlman (eds) *Loneliness: A Source Book of Current Theory, Research and Therapy*. New York: John Wiley and Sons.

Welsh Assembly Government (2003) *The Strategy for Older People in Wales*. Cardiff: Welsh Assembly Government.

Wenger, G.C., Davies, R., Shahtahmasebi, S. and Scott, A. (1996) Social-isolation and loneliness in old-age: review and model refinement, *Ageing and Society*, 16(Pt3): 333–58.

Wheeler, F.A., Gore, K.M. and Greenblatt, B. (1998) The beneficial effects of volunteering for older volunteers and the people they serve: a meta analysis, *International Journal of Ageing and Human Development*, 47(1): 69–79.

White, H., McConnell, E., Clipp, E. et al. (2002) A randomized controlled trial of the psychosocial impact of providing internet training and access to older adults, *Aging and Mental Health*, 6(3): 213–21.

WHO (World Health Organization) (2002) *Active Ageing A Policy Framework*. Geneva: WHO.

WHO (World Health Organization) (2005) *Healthy Cities and Urban Governance*. Available at: http://www.who.dk/healthy-cities (accessed 24 November 2005).

Wolf, S.L., Barnhart, H.X., Kutner, N.G. et al. (1996) Reducing frailty and falls in older persons: an investigation of Tai Chi and computerized balance training. Atlanta FICSIT Group. Frailty and Injuries: Cooperative Studies of Intervention Techniques, *Journal of the American Geriatrics Society*, 44(5): 489–97.

Yoon, G. (1996) Psychosocial factors for successful aging, *Australian Journal On Ageing*, 15(2): 69–72.

Young, A. and Dinan, S. (2005) Activity in later life, *British Medical Journal*, 330: 189–90.

Zunzunegui, M.V., Beland, F. and Otero, A. (2001) Support from children, living arrangements, self-rated health and depressive symptoms of older people in Spain, *International Journal of Epidemiology*, 30: 1090–9.

8 Concluding comments and the future of mental health promotion

Sylvia Tilford

Introduction

In the past the promotion of mental health often had lower priority than the promotion of aspects of physical health. This has changed over the last ten years and mental health promotion is achieving a much higher profile. Evidence of this has been seen in the number of effectiveness reviews, national policy statements, a European Ministerial Conference in 2000, of statements from the WHO and its publication of two major reports (WHO 2004a, b) and a special issue of the *International Union of Health and Promotion Education* (*IUHPE*) journal in 2005. According to Williams et al. (2005: 7) international attention is now being devoted to actively creating social and physical environments that contribute to, and promote positive mental health, while in the IUHPE special issue Mittelmark (2005) concluded that there is a considerable momentum for mental health promotion. As explained in the Preface, this book was written in response to expressed needs for a text which integrated material to inform mental health promotion practice. In this final chapter we will bring together some concluding points from the earlier chapters, reflect further on selected themes which have run through the chapters, and comment on the future needs for mental health promotion.

The book was organized in accordance with a lifespan approach for the reasons given in the Preface. The specific divisions of the lifespan which have been used might be questioned. Phases labelled in some parts of the world, such as 'adolescence' and 'middle years', may not be recognized in other parts of the world. The meanings associated with specific phases may also vary. Chapter 4, for example, noted the differing conceptions of what it is to be a child and the nature of childhood, and Chapter 7 examined the meanings surrounding the last phase of life. To a great extent the categories used to divide and describe different points in the lifespan are provisional, contested and socially created. In most cultures childhood and adulthood are acknowledged, as is older age, but adulthood may not be subdivided. Adolescence, also, which is seen as important in some cultures may receive only token, if any, recognition in others, and a significant transition is from childhood directly to adulthood. Common sense suggests that there are likely to be some similarities across cultures in the mental health promotion issues relating to major life events such as birth and death although there may also be significant differences in the meanings attributed to them. The selection of the specific phases has been made on the grounds that there are some broadly similar experiences at the designated periods in the lifespan which it can be useful to examine together. It was not our intention to adopt a simple ages and stages model or to make any assumptions that what may be relevant to some countries with broadly similar intellectual traditions and histories applies universally.

Chapter 2 analysed the concept of mental health and brought out some of the dilemmas and debates surrounding its definition. While leaving readers to consider their preferred definition of mental health Glenn Macdonald argued against a fully eclectic position. He made a strong case for mental health to be viewed as a positive attribute rather than as a simple absence of ill health. Concern was expressed about the individualistic emphasis of many definitions of mental health. The importance of identifying and understanding concepts of mental health across cultures and developing valid measures was introduced, issues that are now becoming more fully acknowledged as key foundations for the development of mental health promotion programmes. Early chapters commented in general on the determinants of mental health and these were discussed in greater detail in the lifespan chapters. In accordance with dominant thinking in health promotion and public health particular emphasis has been placed on the underlying social determinants of mental health and the argument made that these must be addressed if significant impacts are to be made on the mental health of individuals and populations.

Prior to considering the nature of mental health promotion Chapter 3 outlined the growth of the general discipline of health promotion and described its fundamental principles and values. It has been argued that, ideally, mental health promotion should be conceived and implemented in accordance with these principles. That is, it should seek to promote the mental health of all, foster individual and community empowerment and be committed to equity and the reduction of mental health inequalities. Active participation of individuals and communities in the identification of needs and the planning and implementation of programmes should also be encouraged. In the earlier chapters efforts have been made to describe mental health promotion programmes which adopted these principles and values although many reported studies have had a more restricted focus and commitment to a preventive rather than an empowerment approach.

While each of the lifespan chapters addressed similar issues there were also some differences over and above the content specific to each life phase. There were the special issues selected within each chapter, the extent of detail in discussion of some mental health promotion concerns, the breadth of evidence included, and the individual writers' views on specific matters. Contributors have given differing levels of emphasis to certain concepts discussed across chapters. Resilience is a particular example. This has become a major concept in mental health promotion, arguably rather more so than in other areas of health promotion. It fits in well with the group of individualistic concepts widely associated with mental health. It is important that activities at the individual level are in the context of community and societal actions that address the causes of challenging circumstances. There is a risk that the balance between the individually focused activities and those at meso and macro level may otherwise tip too heavily towards the individual.

Theory

Throughout the book there have been efforts to consider the theoretical foundations of mental health promotion practice and to comment on the theories being used in the programmes discussed. The various contributors have supported the view that general health promotion theory is applicable to mental health promotion (Secker 1998) and it is expected that theory guides the analysis of mental health promotion problems and the design and implementation of solutions. In the reporting of interventions there is differing attention to theory in mental health promotion, in common with health promotion as a whole. Some papers included in the lifespan chapters have provided a careful explication of theory used while others have made little reference. If compared with physical health the particular subject matter of 'mental' health might influence the particular theories drawn on. In published mental health promotion studies psychological theory has frequently been used but this comment could also be made about other areas of health promotion. The use of developmental psychological theory appears to be greater in mental health promotion, in part a reflection of what were identified as differences in the traditions of mental and general health promotion. We have also noted the particular popularity of resilience theory in mental health promotion. What now seems apparent is that there is some broadening of the theory drawn on in mental health promotion in order to support the analysis of the social as well as the individual determinants of mental health, the influencing of policy development, and the planning and implementation of complex interventions. The theories used in designing and implementing programmes will differ according to the type of programme and its objectives.

An important point concerns the relevance of theory to contexts outside the origins of its development, a point frequently made in relation to psychological theory. For example the cross-cultural relevance of the concept of resilience has been questioned but its use has been supported by Johnson (2005) working with different cultures in South Africa. Cross-cultural psychology which has attempted to address the issue of assuming the global relevance of Western concepts has itself been subject to the critique that it has merely helped to legitimize psychology in the international arena (Moghaddam and Studer 1997). It is not only a questioning of the relevance of psychological theories that is needed but a critical stance, in general, to application of Western thinking. This includes scrutiny of what are often highly individualistic definitions of mental health and its associated attributes and the emphasis on individual autonomy, the framing of mental health issues and specification of appropriate solutions. Assumptions cannot be made that Western explanations have universal applicability. This has been discussed by Summerfield (1999) with specific reference to Western responses to dealing with disasters where post-traumatic stress disorder is assumed and Western counselling responses put in place. He suggests that what may be more important is the rebuilding of external social worlds rather than dealing with internal mental states. Although some may challenge his views on this particular issue his general concerns are valid.

Debates

We will return briefly to the debates about mental health promotion which were raised in the early chapters, namely about its purposes, processes and appropriate levels of action. At the beginning of the book tensions between promotion and prevention, population versus individual, and individual versus community approaches were identified. While indicating a preference for emphasis on the promotion of positive health, population level interventions and greater focus on communities rather than individuals, the realities of practice were acknowledged and qualified support was given to the combination of promotion and prevention within mental health promotion as a totality. The importance of securing wider adoption of health promotion principles of empowerment, participation and collaboration was emphasized and interventions which applied these were to be sought in discussing evidence. There is a growing number of reported studies which conform to this account of mental health promotion work but these continue to be outnumbered by those informed by a preventive approach and undertaken with at-risk groups. To have included only those studies with a positive mental health focus and to have ignored that literature which relates to a preventive approach would have meant that the needs of some mental health promoters were unmet. Evidence from studies which have been undertaken in accordance with such a preventive approach is disseminated widely, nationally and internationally. For example, in the UK, dissemination occurs through National Service Frameworks, organizations such as the Mental Health Foundation, NICE, professional networks, and a variety of other publications. In the shorter term the implementation of preventive actions which have been shown to be effective can make a significant contribution to prevention of mental health and some impact on positive health. As noted in the Introduction some mental health promoters will be uncomfortable with this position but, on the other hand, others are pragmatic and appear to accept some combination of promotion and prevention (Barry 2001; Weare 2004). Where the balance between promotion and prevention is located will depend on any individual's ideas about what mental health promotion should be, the contexts of practice, constraints within contexts and people's expressed needs. Where the level of mental health promotion action is concerned many influential commentators are agreed that any significant impact on mental health will require population level actions. While such actions, if measured at the level of the individual, typically make smaller differences but make a greater overall impact on mental health because of the total numbers that are reached through population wide actions. Context of practice will, to a considerable degree, determine the level of activity. What can be advocated is that activities at the individual level are undertaken within contexts which seek to be health promoting settings.

Determinants of mental health

Many determinants of mental health have been discussed in previous chapters and it is important to consider if there are priorities for action. Given the complex interactions between determinants integrated action on major ones is most likely to achieve sustained effect. In earlier discussion, however, emphasis has been placed on some determinants which suggests that priorities can be identified. Addressing poverty has been highlighted because of its relationships with so many other determinants of mental health. A key relationship is with education and this was given particular emphasis in the two chapters on children and young people. Addressing work and mental health issues might also be prioritized. We are of the view that there is a considerable burden of mental ill health which, potentially, could be reduced by a fuller commitment to the promotion of positive mental health and action on major social determinants such as education, level of material resources, social power and exposure to violence and, like poverty is relevant to all phases of the lifespan and also a priority for consideration. With particular reference to low income countries Patel (2005: 28) focused on poverty and gender as major determinants and drew up a number of recommendations which have wider relevance:

- Raise awareness about the association of poverty and gender with mental health amongst public health policy makers, donors and mental health workers.
- Advocate for sustainable economic development to ensure that economic policies do not inadvertently lead to greater inequalities and marginalization of people.
- Advocate for eliminating gender discrimination and violence in society.
- Improve access for health care and social welfare of persons living in poverty.
- Enable community programmes which aim to empower women and the poor.
- Evaluate the impact of globalization on mental health, in particular where globalization influences the livelihood or lifestyles of people.

Although policy actions are needed to make significant impact on international socio-economic and gender inequities Patel et al. (2004) have argued that there are also community-based activities, not necessarily designated as mental health, that can make a measurable impact on the mental health of people concerned including economic empowerment initiatives; the empowerment of women; and violence prevention in the community.

Policy and mental health

Building healthy public policy was identified in the Ottawa Charter (WHO 1986) and in succeeding health promotion documents as a key element of health promotion although the need for a greater investment in mental health policies has been called for recently (Williams et al. 2005). In previous chapters policy has been referred to in differing ways. Some projects have combined policy elements with environmental actions and educational activities to form comprehensive programmes. Health promoting schools, prisons and hospitals projects provide good examples and these can set within national and international policies on the development of such settings. In other cases programmes with individuals and communities can be an integral part of public policy on an issue. For example, Sure Start, the UK programme for children between 0 and 4 years in disadvantaged areas (discussed in Chapter 4) is an integral part of Government policies on child poverty reduction. The *Soul City* programme described in Chapter 6 (Usdin et al. 2005) was designed to integrate with national policy on domestic violence. Each of the lifespan chapters also considered the wider policy context and indicated the range of public policies acting on the determinants of mental health for the phase in question.

If policy to enhance mental health is to be developed and implemented policy makers need to be convinced of the links between any proposed policy and specified outcomes. While the impact of social and economic conditions on mental health is evident in a broad sense it has been emphasized that the understanding of the mediating pathways and causal links and the extent to which the impact can be altered, requires more study (Herrman and Jané-Llopis 2005). A number of questions can be asked: How strong does the evidence have to be? Do we currently have such evidence for the determinants of mental health where we are most concerned to see action? And, even if the evidence does exist will policy makers take action? In the last few years there has been increasing attention to these issues. A recent study (Petticrew et al. 2004; Whitehead et al. 2004) involving policy makers and researchers reported their respective views on influencing the policy making process. Policy makers were of the view that researchers needed a better understanding of the climate within which policy makers worked, needed to think through the policy implications of their work and needed to sell their findings in the right way, recognizing windows of opportunity. In general the policy makers were less concerned about '**gold standard**' studies and more interested to see methods used which were appropriate to the problem in hand, the resources available, and the public health context. They also noted a lack of theoretical underpinnings in much quantitative research and a need for work on the effectiveness and cost effectiveness of interventions.

On the general questions, researchers' views were highly congruent with those of the policy makers. In order to enhance the evidence for policy makers the researchers recommended building a jigsaw of evidence – a synthesis of quantitative and qualitative evidence drawn from diverse sources that, taken together, would contribute towards establishing the knowledge needed on causal links. The points raised in these papers can usefully be reflected on by mental health promotion researchers wishing to advocate for policy developments.

Many of the points made in this study overlap a summary of points concerning evidence into policy drawn up by Davies et al. (2000) (Box 8.1).

Box 8.1   Evidence into policy

Attention is more likely to be paid to research findings when:

- the research is timely, the evidence is clear and relevant, and the methodology is relatively uncontested;
- the results support existing ideologies, are convenient and uncontentious to the powerful;
- policy makers believe in evidence as an important counterbalance to expert opinion and act accordingly;
- the research findings have strong advocates;

- research users are partners in the generation of evidence;
- the results are robust in implementation;
- implementation is reversible if need be.

The future of mental health promotion

The current evidence base for mental health promotion

Throughout the book attention has been given to the evidence base on effectiveness of mental health promotion activities. What conclusions can be drawn at the present time about the state of this evidence? Systematic reviews have brought together evidence derived largely from studies higher on the hierarchy of evidence, designated as least susceptible to bias (Chapter 3). Other reviewers have brought together a broader range of evaluations building up the 'jigsaw' of evidence described earlier. Firm adherents of RCT type evaluations may not be particularly pleased with the current state of evidence. While relatively good evidence has been noted from some areas of mental health promotion there is less in others. It is probably fair to say that those who argue for a broader approach to evidence and are committed to building the 'jigsaw' share a growing sense of some optimism about the amount of evidence that can now be drawn on in planning for practice while, at the same time recognizing the shortcomings. A recent review (Jané-Llopis et al. 2005) has summarized effective programmes for specific contexts, groups and periods in the lifespan. There is, for example, some good evidence from competence enhancement programmes, particularly in school settings. Programmes with parents based on home visit and community activities have shown successes and can be scaled up from small scale to wider implementation. Many interventions such as arts, drama, music and gardening that are popular with participants are being evaluated but the evidence base needs some strengthening. The smaller number of interventions of the population based public health type that address mental health comprehensively has also been noted (Williams et al. 2005) but the number and type of these is increasing. There are evaluations of health promoting school type programmes which are implemented widely and are providing evidence of successes in relation to mental health although most of the stronger evaluations come from a limited number of countries. Other population-based programmes which have been, or are currently being subject to extensive evaluation are the Health Action Zone programmes designed to address health inequalities and the Sure Start (UK) and Headstart (US) programmes. Williams et al. (2005) have picked up the point noted earlier (Whitehead et al. 2004) that there is need for effectiveness and cost-effectiveness evaluations for practitioners and policy makers which provide information on the feasibility and cost of programmes in the diversity of global situations, but especially in low and middle income countries. Even in the studies that originate from the US relatively few have incorporated detailed cost-effectiveness data. The call to broaden the evidence base drawing on mental health promotion activities from across the world is a very positive development and the WHO is making an important contribution to this. An issue that was raised in Chapter 3 continues to be relevant, namely the tendency to publicize more widely studies that have been evaluated in accordance with particular methodologies leading to reinforcement of those same activities (Secker 1998). These tend to be individualized programmes in controlled situations very often with groups designated as at-risk and using psychological models and theories. Often evidence of success is modest and it cannot be readily concluded that success would necessarily be achieved in real life settings. There are areas of evaluation which, to date, have been insufficiently developed. A key one is a detailed examination of environmental actions which have mental health as secondary effects. These include transport, housing, design of the built environment and noise pollution.

Ensuring evidence impacts on practice

Although the task of building the evidence base is ongoing practice can be enhanced through application of the existing evidence. This requires dissemination to those who need to use the evidence, the readiness of practitioners to act on the evidence and the skills to be able to do so. Nutbeam (1996) said that progress in health promotion required that knowledge from research should be applied more systematically to practice. In his view there was a longstanding dilemma on how to improve the research–practice fit.

One of the good things to report from the last ten years or so has been the efforts to improve the process of dissemination, the first stage in developing this research–practice fit. In mental health promotion Internet and paper based summaries of evidence produced by Mentality (mentality.org.uk) and other organizations and documents of the NSF type have made valuable contributions to dissemination. In summarizing evidence for dissemination in user friendly ways there can be a danger that its quality may be exaggerated and it may be presented with insufficient critical assessment. It is rather easy to disseminate an interesting and possible innovative activity which, in accordance with communication of innovations theory, is readily picked up and applied even though the supporting evidence for it may be relatively weak. Practitioners need, therefore, to be able to access the available evidence and also possess the skills to appraise it critically. Passive forms of dissemination are probably not sufficient in themselves. Focused activities appropriate to professional groups combined with some face to face activity have been proposed (Blackburn et al. 1997), a strategy adopted by some UK health authorities in implementing the National Service Frameworks. Once disseminated ensuring that evidence is applied in practice requires an understanding of the processes needed to ensure fidelity of implementation of a successful programme and, in some cases of achieving changes in practice within complex organizations. Barry et al. (2005) have identified a need for 'practice and policy based guidelines based on best available evidence concerning the critical factors needed to ensure the implementation of successful programmes across a range of cultural and economic settings' (2005: 35).

There are a few additional points about evidence, or the lack of it, and the significance of this for practice. The evidence that is widely disseminated is derived very largely from a limited number of predominantly higher income countries. It has been said that 'the evidence for the effectiveness of mental health promotion is least available in areas that have the maximum need, such as low and middle income countries and conflict areas where mental health is especially compromised' (Herrman et al. 2004: 11).

Although the resources for evaluation are often very difficult indeed to access in lower income countries evaluations are taking place. Evidence from them may not meet the stringent criteria imposed by some so the studies are not included in systematic reviews. More typically, the evidence is simply unknown outside its immediate context. McQueen (2001) reported the widely held belief at the WHO Mexico Conference (WHO 2000) that there was a strong evidence base in developing countries particularly concerning the evaluation of community programmes. Current efforts to support the identification and dissemination of these are welcomed (Jané-Llopis et al. 2005).

On many occasions programme activities are carried out when there is, to date, little or no reported evidence and no detailed evaluation is planned. This is sometimes the case when new ideas are being tried out. If subsequently evidence of lack of success is available from other studies should the programme be discontinued? Where a group has been consulted and has identified the need for specific activities designed to improve mental health, and has reported feeling mentally healthier as a result of participation should that not be sufficient reason to sustain those activities? It could be argued that as long as resources given to the activity are not depriving others whose needs may be greater a programme should be able to continue. This response could be seen to fit with health promotion principles. Funders, however, often require evidence of impact which goes beyond what is acceptable at the level of a project in order to justify continuation of funding. Where this is the case projects may need to come up with the necessary evidence, or seek alternative funding. In reality demands to discontinue specific practice are not typically made on the basis of the first evidence to appear. Degrees of scepticism about new evidence are typical and existing practice is 'protected'. Evidence typically needs to be consolidated before changes begin to take place.

Unmet needs

There are many unmet needs for actions on specific aspects of mental health promotion and with specific populations. While emphasis has been placed on population-wide promotion of positive mental health we also acknowledge that progress in addressing the acute needs of some groups will require focused activities. There are less powerful groups and relatively hidden groups in societies whose mental health needs can be overlooked. These include stigmatized groups such as travellers, refugees and asylum seekers who can be reluctant to make themselves visible, and any groups that lack the power to draw attention to the issues that affect them and advocate for change. There is growing evidence that such groups are now being better recognized and local actions developed to promote mental health. Examples have been provided in the good practice sections in Chapters 4 to 7 but more actions are needed.

Those who are experiencing mental ill health continue to be stigmatized in most societies. Recent comments from the UK (Appleby 2006) bear this out. Appleby, the national director for mental health in the NHS, reported that many people find stigma worse than the actual illnesses. The anti-stigma campaign in the UK has held a recent conference to share international experience on this issue. Those involved in mental health promotion continue to have an important role in changing attitudes to mental ill health. There is evidence that this can be achieved but more action is needed.

Priorities for future actions

Priorities can be drawn from issues raised above, in the conclusions of earlier chapters and contributions of others. They are subject to discussion and debate.

- In the light of the widening inequalities in mental health within and between countries it can be argued that activity with disadvantaged and vulnerable populations and groups should be prioritized in combination with population-wide promotion of positive mental health for all.
- Determinants of mental ill health common to all life phases as well as some which mainly affect one or more specific age phases have been identified. Selecting the most important determinants for immediate action is a matter for debate since the knowledge of aetiological pathways is often incomplete and further research is required. Some priorities for consideration are proposed: poverty, education, gender and work.
- Mental and physical health are intimately related and improvements of mental health are associated with improvements in physical aspects. A web of consequences for current and future mental arise from major physical health problems. Globally at the present time much attention focuses on HIV/AIDS because of its direct or indirect impact on all age groups within populations. There are other physical health problems which attract less attention but can also impact significantly. Children and adults experiencing physical disabilities have reduced opportunities to engage fully in social life in most countries and can experience poorer mental health as a result. More action to improve physical health has the potential, therefore, to impact also on mental health.
- The development of evidence must continue based on a broad approach to methodologies, attention to health promotion principles, and in consideration of what is appropriate for specific programmes and the nature of evidence required for specific purposes and specific people such as policy makers. In evaluating programmes consideration needs to be given to their theoretical foundations as well as to issues of effectiveness. Support for evaluation and disseminating evidence from low income countries is especially important.
- Improvements in mental health could be achieved from a more thorough dissemination and implementation of existing evidence. Improvements in the dissemination of evidence have been noted but there is still much to be achieved especially in low income countries. This is needed 'so that the evidence base can be used effectively to inform practice and policy that reduces inequalities and brings about improved mental health, especially where it is needed most' (Barry and McQueen 2004: 117). The suitability of evidence for wider dissemination from contexts in which it has been generated has, at the same time, to be taken into account. Implementing programmes which have been shown to work will require education and training for those involved to ensure that modifications necessary for the context of use are made without undermining the potential of programmes to achieve desired outcomes.
- Mental health promotion is theory-based, evidence-based, and values-based. The

greater use of theory other than that derived from psychology needs to continue. The further scrutiny of theory for its relevance across cultures is necessary. Of particular importance is the need to gain wider acceptance and use of the general principles and values of health promotion throughout mental health promotion.

- Issues for mental health promotion at various points in the lifespan have been identified in Chapters 4 to 7, some general to all phases, others specific to one or more phases. The development of health promoting settings is one general issue especially in health care and workplaces where less progress has been made than in schools. Facilitating the active participation of participants in defining and implementing mental health promotion actions crosses the lifespan but with the particular to ensure these are not given lesser attention with young children and older people. Continued reflection on the ways that societies think about children, young people, adults and older people and their mental health is necessary if mental health promotion programmes are to fit needs.

- The promotion of positive mental health is not an activity simply for those who are well but is equally relevant to those who may be described as experiencing mental ill health. This needs to be actively communicated to all contexts where mental health promotion takes place.

- Finally, the momentum which has developed for the promotion of health needs to be sustained taking all opportunities for advocating for the importance of mental health. While accepting the realities of diversity in thinking and practice the balance should be towards the promotion of positive health, population based approaches, use of non-discriminatory, participative and empowering processes and a firm determination to redress inequalities in mental health nationally and globally.

References

Appleby, L. (2006) It is time we finally removed the stigma of mental illness. *Guardian* 22 March.

Barry, M. (2001) Promoting positive mental health: theoretical frameworks for practice, *International Journal of Mental Health Promotion*, 3(1): 4–12.

Barry, M.M. and McQueen, D.V. (2004) The nature of evidence and its use in mental health promotion, *Mental Health Promotion: Concepts, Emerging Evidence and Practice*. Geneva: World Health Organization.

Barry, M.M., Domitrovich, C. and Lara, M.A. (2005) The implementation of mental health promotion programmes, *IUHPE Promotion and Education Supplement*, 2: 30–9.

Blackburn, C., Graham, H. and Scullion, P. (1997) Disseminating research findings on women's smoking to health practitioners: findings from an evaluative study, *Health Education Journal*, 56: 1113–24.

Davies, H., Nutley, S. and Smith, P. (eds) (2000) *What Works: Evidence Based Policy in Practice in Public Services*. Bristol: Policy Press.

Herrman, H. and Jané-Llopis, E. (2005) Mental health promotion in public health, *IUHPE Promotion and Education Supplement*, 2: 42–7.

Herrman, H., Saxena, S., Moodie, R. and Walker, L. (2004) Promoting health as a public health priority, *Promoting Mental Health: Concepts, Emerging Evidence, Practice*. Geneva: WHO.

Jané-Llopis, E., Barry, M., Hosman, C. and Patel, V. (2005) Mental health promotion works: a review, *IUHPE Promotion and Education Supplement*, 2: 9–25.

Johnson, B. (2005) Mental health promotion in schools: an exploration of factors relating to risk resilience and health promoting schools in order to enhance the well-being of our youth. Unpublished PhD thesis, University of the Western Cape, South Africa.

McQueen, D. (2001) Strengthening the evidence base for health promotion, *Health Promotion International*, 16(3): 261–8.

Mittelmark, M. (2005) Why 'mental' health promotion, *IUHPE-Promotion and Education Supplement*, 2: 55–7.

Moghaddam, F.M. and Studer, C. (1997) Cross cultural psychology: the frustrated gadfly's promise, potentialities and failures, in D. Fox and I. Prillentensky (eds) *Critical Psychology: An Introduction*. London: Sage Publications.

Nutbeam, D. (1996) Achieving 'best practice' in health promotion: improving the fit between research and practice, *Health Education Research*, 11(1): 317–26.

Patel, V. (2005) Poverty, gender and mental health promotion in a globalised society, *IUHPE Promotion and Education Supplement*, 2: 26–9.

Patel, V., Swartz, L. and Cohen, A. (2004) The evidence of mental health in developing countries, *Promoting Mental Health: Concepts, Emerging Evidence and Practice*. Geneva: WHO.

Petticrew, M., Whitehead, M., MacIntyre, S.J., Graham, H. and Egan, M. (2004) Evidence for public health policy on inequalities: the reality according to policymakers, *Journal of Epidemiology and Community Health*, 58: 811–16.

Secker, J. (1998) Current conceptualizations of mental health and mental health promotion, *Health Education Research*, 13(1): 57–66.

Summerfield, D. (1999) A critique of seven assumptions behind psychological trauma programmes in war affected areas, *Social Science and Medicine*, 48: 1449–62.

Usdin, S., Scheepers, E., Goldstein, S. and Japhet, G. (2005) Achieving social change on gender-based violence: a report on the impact evaluation of *Soul City*'s fourth series, *Social Science and Medicine*, 61: 2434–45.

Weare, K. (2004) The International Alliance for Child and Adolescent Health in Schools (INTERCAMHS), *Health Education*, 104(2): 65–7.

Whitehead, M., Petticrew, M., Graham, H., MacIntyre, S.J., Bambra, C. and Egan, M. (2004) Evidence for public health policy on inequalities: assembling the evidence jigsaw, *Journal of Epidemiology and Community Health*, 58: 817–21.

Williams, S.M., Saxena, S. and McQueen, D. (2005) The momentum for mental health promotion, *IUHPE Promotion and Education Supplement*, 2: 6–9.

WHO (1986) *Ottawa Charter for Health Promotion*. Geneva: WHO.

WHO (2000) *Fifth Global Conference on Health Promotion: Bridging the Equity Gap. Mexico, 5–9 June*. Geneva: WHO.

WHO (2004a) *Prevention of Mental Disorders: Effective Interventions and Policy Options*. Geneva: WHO.

WHO (2004b) *Promoting Mental Health: Concepts, Emerging Evidence and Practice*. Geneva: WHO.

Appendix 1

Table A1.1 Theories used in a selection of studies referred to in the book

Study	Theory/theoretical concepts
Children	
Bale and Mishara (2004) Developing an international mental health promotion programme for young children.	Coping skills.
Dubow et al. (1993) Teaching children to cope with stressful experiences.	Coping skills; competence enhancement.
Olweus (1993) Bullying among schoolchildren: intervention and prevention.	Behaviour modification; developmental models of aggressive behaviour; social system theory.
Pedro-Carroll et al. (1992) Evaluation of efficacy of a preventive intervention for 4th–6th grade urban children of divorce.	Competence enhancement; coping skills.
Stewart et al. (2004) Promoting and building resilience in primary school communities: evidence from a comprehensive 'health promoting school' approach.	Resilience theory; health promoting schools; ecological models; social capital.
Adults	
Usdin et al. (2005) Achieving social change on gender based violence.	Ecological models; social mobilization community theory; social learning theory.
Price et al. (1992) Impact of preventive job search intervention on the likelihood of depression among the unemployed.	Coping resources theory: explains variation in the strength of the relationship between stressors and psychological disorder.
Toseland et al. (1990) Comparative effectiveness of individual and group interventions to support family caregivers.	Ecological systems framework.
Johnson et al. (2000) Community Mothers Programme.	Developmental psychology; self esteem empowerment, peer support.
Hopman-Rock and Westhoff (2002) 'Aging Well and Healthily': a health education and exercise program for community living older adults.	Diffusion of innovation theory.

References

Bale, C. and Mishara, B. (2004) Developing an international mental health promotion pro-gramme for young children, *International Journal of Mental Health Promotion*, 6(2): 12–16.

Dubow, E.F., Schmidt, D., McBride, J. et al. (1993) Teaching children to cope with stressful experiences: initial implementation and evaluation of a primary prevention program, *Journal of Clinical Psychology*, 22(4): 428–40.

Hopman-Rock, M. and Westhoff, M.H. (2002) Development and evaluation of 'Aging Well and Healthily': a health education and exercise program for community living older adults, *Journal of Aging and Physical Activity*, 10: 363–80.

Johnson, Z., Molly, B., Scallen, E. et al. (2000) Community Mothers Programme: seven years follow up of a randomized controlled trial of non-professional intervention in parenting, *Journal of Public Health Medicine*, 22(3): 337–42.

Olweus, D. (1993) *Bullying at School*. Oxford: Blackwell Publishers.

Pedro-Carroll, J.L., Gillis, L.J. and Cowen, E.L. (1992) An evaluation of the efficacy of a preventive intervention for 4th–6th grade urban children of divorce, *Journal of Primary Prevention*, 13(2): 115–30.

Price, R.H., van Ryn, M. and Vinokur, A.D. (1992) Impact of a preventive job search interven-tion on the likelihood of depression among the unemployed, *Journal of Health and Social Behaviour*, 33: 158–67.

Stewart, D., Sun, J., Patterson, C., Lemerle, K. and Hardie, M. (2004) Promoting and building resilience in primary school communities: evidence from a comprehensive 'health promoting school' approach, *International Journal of Mental Health Promotion*, 6(3): 26–33.

Toseland, R.W., Rossiter, C.M., Peak, T. and Smith, G.C. (1990) Comparative effectiveness of individual and group interventions to support family caregivers, *Social Work*, 35(3): 209–17.

Usclin, S., Scheepers, E., Goldstein, S. and Japhet, G. (2005) Achieving social change on gender-based violence: a report on the impact evaluation of *Soul City*'s fourth series, *Social Science and Medicine*, 61: 2434–45.

Appendix 2

Definitions of mental health and mental health promotion in international documents on mental health promotion

Mental health is:

- *Prevention of Mental Disorders* (WHO 2004a: 16): Health is 'a state of complete physical, mental and social well-being, and not merely the absence of disease or infirmity'.
- *Promoting Mental Health: Concepts, Emerging Evidence* (WHO 2004b: 12): 'a state of well-being in which the individual realizes his or her abilities, can cope with the normal stresses of life, can work productively and fruitfully and is able to make a contribution to his or her community'.
- *Promoting Mental Health Concepts: Emerging Evidence Practice* (Herrman et al. 2005): As WHO (2004b).
- *Mental Health Action Plan for Europe* (WHO European Ministerial Conference on Mental Health 2005: 1): 'Mental health and well-being are fundamental to quality of life, enabling people to experience life as meaningful and to be creative and active citizens. Mental health is an essential component of social cohesion, productivity and peace and stability in the living environment, contributing to social capital and economic development in societies'.
- *Mental Health Promotion and Prevention Strategies for Coping with Anxiety, Depression and Stress Related Disorders in Europe* (Berkels et al. 2004): Mental health is affected by biological, psychological, sociological, economic, political and cultural forces.
- *Improving the Mental Health of the Population: Towards a Strategy on Mental Health for the European Union* (Commission of the European Communities 2005): As WHO (2004b).
- *Principles of Mental Health Promotion: Prevention of Mental Disorders* (WHO 2004a: 16): 'Mental health promotion aims to impact on the determinants of mental health so as to increase positive mental health, to reduce inequalities, to build social capital, to create health gain and to narrow the gap in health expectancies between countries and groups' (from the *Jakarta Declaration for Health Promotion*, WHO 1997). Preventive interventions focus on reducing risk factors and enhancing protective factors associated with mental ill health.
- *Promoting Mental Health: Concepts, Emerging Evidence* (WHO 2004b): Mental health promotion is an integral part of public health and not just the absence of disease; associated with behaviour at all stages of life; linked to social and economic determinants of health dependent on partnerships across all sectors and the utilization of the full spectrum of health promotion methods.
- *Promoting Mental Health Concepts: Emerging Evidence Practice* (Herrman et al. 2005):

Mental health promotion requires a public health approach. It includes promotion of health, prevention of illness and disability, treatment and rehabilitation of those affected.

* *Mental Health Action Plan for Europe* (WHO European Ministerial Conference on Mental Health 2005: 1): 'Mental health promotion increases the quality of life and mental well-being of the whole population, including people with mental health problems and their carers'.
* *Mental Health Promotion and Prevention Strategies for Coping with Anxiety, Depression and Stress Related Disorders in Europe* (Berkels et al. 2004): Mental health promotion aims to: enhance the well being of individuals, groups and communities; create individual, social, societal and environmental conditions that enable optimal development through a reduction in mental health problems.
* *Improving the Mental Health of the Population: Towards a Strategy on Mental Health for the European Union* (Commission of the European Communities 2005: 8): 'Promotion of mental health and prevention of mental ill health address individual, family, community and social determinants of mental health, by strengthening protective factors (e.g. resilience) and reducing risk factors'.

References

Berkels, H., Henderson, J., Henke, N. et al. (2004) *Mental Health Promotion and Prevention Strategies for Coping with Anxiety, Depression and Stress Related Disorders in Europe: Final Report 2001–2003.* Dortmund/Berlin/Dresden: Federal Institute for Occupational Safety and Health.

Commission of the European Communities (2005) *Improving the Mental Health of the Population: Towards a Strategy on Mental Health for the European Union.* Brussels: European Union.

Herrman, H., Saxena, S. and Moodie, R. (eds) (2005) *Promoting Mental Health Concepts, Emerging Evidence Practice: Report of the World Health Organization, in Collaboration with Victoria Health Promotion Foundation and the University of Melbourne.* Geneva: WHO.

WHO (World Health Organization) (1997) *The Jakarta Declaration for Health Promotion.* Available at: http://www.who.int/hpr/NPH/docs/jakarta_declaration_en.pdf (accessed 8 January 2006).

WHO (World Health Organization) (2004a) *Prevention of Mental Disorders: Effective Interventions and Policy Options.* A report of the World Health Organisation, Department of Mental Health and Substance Abuse in collaboration with the Prevention Research Centre in the Universities of Nijmegen and Maastricht. Geneva: WHO. Available at: www.who.int/mental_health/evidence/en/Prevention_of_Mental_Disorders.pdf (accessed 8 January 2006).

WHO (World Health Organisation) (2004b) *Promoting Mental Health: Concepts, Emerging Evidence.* A report of the World Health Organisation, Department of Mental Health and Substance Abuse in collaboration with the Victorian Health Promotion Foundation and the University of Melbourne. Geneva: WHO. Available at: www.who.int/mental-_health/evidence/en/promoting_mhh.pdf (accessed 8 January 2006).

WHO European Ministerial Conference on Mental Health (2005) *Mental Health Action Plan for Europe: Facing the Challenges, Building Solutions.* Helsinki: WHO.

Appendix 3

Organizations which are involved in mental health promotion policy, campaigning, research or funding of research – national and international: some examples

Alzheimer's Society – leading care and research charity for people with dementia, their families and carers (see http://www.alzheimers.org.uk/).

Bullying Online – provides help and advice on bullying online (http://www.bullying.co.uk/).

Centre for Suicide Research – investigates the causes, treatment and prevention of suicidal behaviour (http://www.psychiatry.ox.ac.uk/csr).

Joseph Rowntree Foundation – one of the largest social policy research and development charities in the UK, and seeks to better understand the causes of social difficulties and explore ways of overcoming them (http://www.jrf.org.uk).

Mental Health Foundation – aim to help people of all ages manage their own mental health; promote innovative action across the UK; do their own research which informs policy, practice development and campaigns (http://www.mentalhealth.org.uk).

Mental Health Foundation for New Zealand – their website is designed to deliver knowledge in the area of mental health, by providing access to quality information and resources (http://www.mentalhealth.org.nz/).

Mental Health Foundation of Australia – an organization of professionals, sufferers and families, related organizations and members of the public. It makes recommendations on mental health policy, encourages and initiates mental health research and works to remove stigma associated with mental ill health (http://www.mentalhealthvic.org.au/).

Mental Health Specialist library – aims to meet the information needs of health care professionals who work in the field of mental health (http://rms.nelh.nhs.uk/mentalHealth/).

Mentality – dedicated solely to the promotion of mental health in the UK. It is part of the Sainsbury Centre for Mental Health and has a wealth of experience in planning, delivering and evaluating public mental health promotion programmes (http://www.mentality.org.uk/).

MIND – the leading mental health charity in England and Wales. They do this by challenging discrimination, influencing policy, campaigning and education (http://www.mind.org.uk/).

National Institute for Mental Health (NIMHE) – responsible for supporting the implementation of positive change in mental health and mental health services. They are part of the Care Services Improvement Partnership, and their main sponsor is the Department of Health (http://nimhe.csip.org.uk/home).

Public Health Observatories – North East – one of nine regional Public Health

Observatories in England and is part of the Government's strategy for improving health and reducing health inequalities. North East Public Health Observatory (NEPHO) is responsible for mental health (http://www.nepho.org.uk).

Samaritans – a 24 hours a day telephone and email service providing emotional support for people experiencing feelings of distress which could lead to suicide (http://www.samaritans.org.uk/).

The Suicide Prevention Resource Center (SPRC) – USA – provides prevention support, training, resources to assist organizations and individuals to develop suicide prevention programmes and policies to advance the National Strategy for Suicide Prevention (http://www.sprc.org).

Young Minds – the national charity committed to improving the mental health of all children and young people (http://www.youngminds.org.uk/).

Glossary

Absolute and relative poverty: absolute poverty refers to a state in which the individual lacks the resources necessary for subsistence. Relative poverty refers to an individual or group's lack of resources when compared with those of other members of society, i.e. their relative standard of living.

Age: *Chronological age*: refers to the years a person has been living.
Functional or health age: refers to the non-linear functional decline over time that occurs during the process of ageing.

Allopathic system: the healing system of Western biomedicine. A set of ideas and assumptions about the causes of ill health and treatment. The term literally means treating by opposites in contrast to homeopathy, treatment by similarities.

Community development: a process of social action in which the people of a community organize themselves for planning and action; define their common needs and problems; make group and individual plans to meet their needs and solve their problems; and execute these plans with a maximum of reliance on community resources.

Coping skills: capacity to apply cognitions and competencies to control, lessen or endure internal or external conditions that are viewed as stressful. Often categorized into different types: e.g.:
problem focused: managing the situation causing the stress; and
emotional *focused*: regulating the emotional response associated with the stress

Critical literacy: The third level of a three-part hierarchy of health literacy proposed by Nutbeam (2000):

- *Basic/functional health literacy*. Sufficient basic skills in reading and writing to be able to function effectively in everyday situations.
- *Interactive health literacy*. More advanced cognitive and literacy skills which, together with social skills can be used to participate in everyday activities to extract information and derive meaning from different forms of communication and to apply new information in changing circumstances.
- *Critical health literacy*. More advanced cognitive skills which, together with social skills, can be applied to critically analyse information, and to use this information to extert greater control over life events and situations; the cognitive and skill development outcomes oriented towards supporting effective social and political action, as well as individual action.

Critical periods: a term used in developmental psychology to describe key points for aspects of development, e.g. in building early emotional relationships through the process of bonding. Also called sensitive periods.

Discrimination: to set up or act on the basis of difference. Can be positive or negative. It is negative where there is a sense of injustice to the distinction and its consequences. Discrimination can be based on one or more differences from a supposed majority or norm: e.g. ethnicity, age, gender, appearance, aspect of health. It is associated with a number of outcomes e.g. labelling, stigma, exclusion, inequality of opportunity and even violence.

DSM IV: *Diagnostic and Statistical Manual of Mental Disorders*, 4th edn (APA 1994).

Empowerment: a process by which individuals gain mastery or control over their own lives and democratic participation in the life of the community. Used as a term in relation to individuals and communities.

- *Psychological empowerment* can be defined as a feeling of greater control over their own lives which individuals experience following active membership in groups or organizations and may occur without participation in collective political action (Rissel 1994).

- *Community empowerment* includes a raised level of psychological empowerment among its members, a political activity component in which members have actively participated. The achievement of some redistribution of resources or decision-making is favourable to the community or group in question (Rissel 1994).

Epidemiological transition: the sequence linked with socio-economic development in which the burden of disease shifts from infectious diseases to broadly degenerative ones.

Equity: access to services or resources in relation to need; equal provision for equal needs. Refers to the idea of fair opportunity. A concern with equity in mental health is evidenced in the creation of equal opportunities for health and reduction of unfair differentials.

Gold standard: a term applied to studies which meet the criteria of randomized controlled trials.

Health literacy: represents the cognitive and social skills which determine the motivation and ability of individuals to gain access to, understand and use information in ways which promote and maintain good health. Health literacy means more than being able to read pamphlets and successfully make appointments. By improving people's access to health information and their capacity to use it effectively, health literacy is critical to empowerment (Nutbeam 1998).

Hidden curriculum: this involves the learning of attitudes, norms, beliefs, values and assumptions in schools which are often expressed as rules, regulations and rituals. They are taken for granted and rarely questioned (Seddon 1983, in Marsh 1992).

Inequity: differences which are unnecessary and avoidable but, in addition, are also considered unfair or unjust. So in order to describe a situation as inequitable the cause has to be examined and judged to be unfair in the context of what is occurring in the rest of society (Whitehead 1990).

Macro: social, national or global level

Meso: organizational and institutional level

Meta-analysis: where several randomized controlled trials (RCTs) on a specific topic have used precisely the same methodology the results can be statistically combined using the technique of meta-analysis to give an overall summary result of significance and effect size. Particularly useful where several studies have been done that are individually too small to give convincing results.

Micro: individual level

Modelling: a concept within social learning theory. The process by which a behaviour is observed and imitated. Many health behaviours are learned through modelling on others.

Paradigm: an agreed way of looking at and interpreting the world or an area of study. A paradigm is drawn on in defining the nature and process of investigation. Frequently used to describe approaches to research e.g. positivist v interpretivist paradigm. See Kuhn* for discussion of paradigms.

Positivism: a philosophical position which states that objective accounts of the world can be produced and causal patterns and theories tested through scientific method.

Positivist belief: that there is one single 'truth' about mental health.

Randomized controlled trial: this is a controlled experimental research design used to test an hypothesis. Seen to be superior to other methods for testing cause-effect relationships. Those taking part are divided through a process of randomization into experimental and control conditions. There is an assumption that randomization ensures that confounding factors are equally distributed between the two conditions. Results can be generalized if conditions of internal and external validity are met (Gomm and Davies 2000).

Reductionist: refers to a theory that any complex system can be fully understood in terms of its simple, component parts

Self-efficacy: the extent to which individuals believe themselves to be capable of a specified action or behaviour.

Self-esteem: the value which an individual places on the set of beliefs held about him/herself. The set of beliefs are the self-concept and the attitude towards them is the self-esteem. It is a subjective experience which an individual conveys to others by verbal reports and other expressive actions.

Social constructionist: the belief that there are many 'truths' about mental health.

Social constructivism: a general term applied to theories that emphasize the socially created nature of social life. These approaches emphasize the idea that society is actively and creatively produced by human beings rather than being given or taken for granted and governed by universal laws. Social worlds are interpretive nets woven by individuals and groups. Constructivism is informed by the work of the Chicago sociologists – phenomenologists such as Shutz, Mead, Berger and Luckman, and Lincoln and Guba (see Marshall 1998).

Social exclusion: the result of living in a society but not being able to take part in the normal activities undertaken by citizens in that society. Normal activities are defined as: a reasonable standard of living; a certain degree of security; involvement in activities valued by others; decision-making powers; and the possibility of support from family, friends and community (Burchardt et al. 1999).

Social inclusion: being able to take part in the normal activities of society as defined above under social exclusion.

Victim blaming: to attribute health problems chiefly to individuals and to neglect the influence of social, economic and environmental factors.

* For example: Kuhn, T.S. (1970) The Structure of Scientific Revolution. Chicago: Chicago University Press.

References

APA (American Psychiatric Association) (1994) Diagnostic and Statistical Manual of Mental Disorders, 4th edn. Washington, DC: APA.

Burchardt, T., LeGrand, J. and Piachaud, D. (1999) Social exclusion in Britain 1991–95, *Social Policy and Administration*, 33(3): 227–44.

Gomm, R. and Davies, C. (eds) (2000) *Using Evidence in Health and Social Care*. London: Sage in association with the Open University.

Marsh, C. (1992) *Key Concepts for Understanding Curriculum*. London: The Falmer Press.

Marshall, G. (1998) *Oxford Dictionary of Sociology*. Oxford: Oxford University Press.

Nutbeam, D. (1998) Health promotion glossary, *Health Promotion International*, 13: 349–64. (This provides useful definitions of most common terms used in health promotion).

Nutbeam, D. (2000) Health literacy as a public goal: a challenge for contemporary health education and communication strategies into the twenty-first century, *Health Promotion International*, 15(3): 259–67.

Rissel, C. (1994) Empowerment: the holy grail of health promotion, *Health Promotion International*, 9(1): 37–47.

Whitehead, M. (1990) *The Concepts and Principles of Equity and Health*. Geneva: WHO.

Index

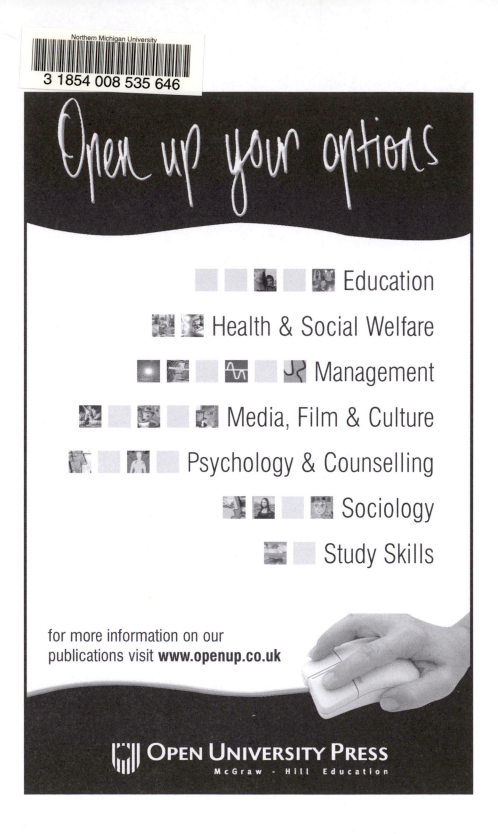